Horse Stable and Riding Arena Design

Horse Stable and Riding Arena Design

Eileen Fabian Wheeler

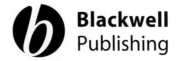

Blackwell Publishing

Eileen Fabian Wheeler is Associate Professor in Agricultural and Biological Engineering at The Pennsylvania State University.

Blackwell Publishing Professional
2121 State Avenue, Ames, Iowa 50014, USA

Orders: 1-800-862-6657
Office: 1-515-292-0140
Fax: 1-515-292-3348
Web site: www.blackwellprofessional.com

Blackwell Publishing Ltd
9600 Garsington Road, Oxford OX4 2DQ, UK
Tel.: +44 (0)1865 776868

Blackwell Publishing Asia
550 Swanston Street, Carlton, Victoria 3053, Australia
Tel.: +61 (0)3 8359 1011

First edition, 2006

Library of Congress Cataloging-in-Publication Data

Wheeler, Eileen.
    Horse stable and riding arena design /
Eileen Wheeler.
        p.   cm.
    Includes index.
    ISBN 13: 978-0-8138-2859-6 (alk. paper)
    ISBN 10: 0-8138-2859-7 (alk. paper)
    1. Stables.   2. Arenas.   3. Corrals.
4. Horses—Housing.   I. Title.

TH4930.W54 2006
636.1'0831—dc22
                              2005013345

The last digit is the print number: 9 8 7 6 5 4 3 2 1

Contents

Preface

This book has been more than a few years in the making. Picture a child drawing horse stable layouts on the back of a restaurant's paper placemat while waiting for the family meal to be delivered. More recently, this book has been a multiyear project to get some solid engineering-based design information to those advising stable managers and builders of horse facilities. In between placemat drawings and my current faculty position, this "child" was educated in animal science and agricultural engineering to better understand the depth and breadth of topics that influence horse stable design. My lifelong interest in horses sparked the desire to become educated, and now to help others to understand the underlying principals influencing function and design of horse stabling.

Pleasant are my memories of entering horse stables containing the mingling smells of hay, horse, and leather. What peace from the satisfied sound of forage being chewed by the horses! Stable spaces that were light and airy felt welcoming. We all seem to know when we have entered a nicely designed and managed stable whether it is plush or spare in its design. I hope this book can aid in the design of such facilities.

One of my motivations in creating this book is to reemphasize the need to provide adequate ventilation for good air quality in stables, because a developing trend is to copy residential construction practices that severely compromise the air quality in horse stable and riding arena environments. I have spent many years working in ventilation of various livestock buildings, and as those systems have made tremendous improvements in providing comfortable conditions and improved air quality, many newly constructed horse facilities have worse environments than the old traditional stables.

My interest is in providing readers with enough background information to make good decisions in horse facility design. Most "nuts and bolts" of construction are available elsewhere. Detailed design and plans can be obtained from builders and professional engineers working in horse stable construction. Through the use of this book, detailed building plans can be checked for features that you have learned are important for horse well-being and human convenience.

Eileen Fabian Wheeler

Acknowledgments

It is hard for me to know how to organize the recognition of people who have contributed so much to the successful completion of this book. Being the sole author of this book implies that this is the work of an individual. True, this book's content comes from my knowledge gained through dedicated education and years of experience that honed that knowledge. Yet, I can't even begin to express my thanks that I owe to myriad individuals who have contributed in concrete ways to this book and the knowledge behind it. In random order, perhaps in the amount of recent time they dedicated directly to the project, let me begin.

As you enjoy this book and the amount of information that it conveys (remember that a "picture" is worth a thousand words), I want you to realize the yeoman's job that William Moyer has done in his capacity as the technical illustrator of this text. Bill has detailed hundreds and hundreds of drawings for me throughout the 10 years that I have been at Penn State University. More than 150 of those drawings are included in this book. Thanks to Bill for such friendly, quick, and dedicated turnaround of the various projects that have meant so much to me. You have built a career on making others look good.

Jennifer Zajaczkowski is another individual deserving extra special attention in the development of this book. Several of the chapters in this book were cowritten with Jennifer Smith, now Zajaczkowski, originally as Extension bulletins on horse housing topics. These were topics not well covered within other available information on horse housing, and Jenn did a great job of fleshing out my draft manuscripts with her own capable horsewoman experiences and information gathered from other animal scientists. Jenn has been an invaluable addition to the applied research in horse housing and riding arena environment that we have conducted over the past several years. Some findings from these studies are incorporated into this book. Jenn is the primary author of the chapter on fire safety, which extends her expertise and interests as an emergency medical technician.

Within my department of Agricultural and Biological Engineering at Penn State, there are three other colleagues who have made this book project a successful effort. Staff assistants Marsha Hull and Amy Maney have contributed in so many big and detailed ways to getting this book done in a professional manner. Marsha is the patient and creative publication artist for the original set of department fact sheets that turned into college bulletins, and now into several chapters of this book. Without her good work the original set of information would not have been so widely noticed, thus setting the stage for development of the information into a book-scale project. Marsha's organization has helped at numerous times in assembling this book from many years' worth of accumulated information. Amy has been so helpful in many detailed aspects of the current tasks of completing this book-writing project while I also maintained other professorial duties. I much appreciate Amy's dedicated professional efforts in timely turnaround of assignments and particularly her attention to detail. Having small and large tasks completed with high quality makes pulling this book together so much easier.

The third department colleague who deserves special thanks is Roy Young, department head of Agricultural and Biological Engineering at Penn State. I appreciate his approval to my spending more time working "out of the office" this past year for concentrated writing effort. I have the type of brain that needs full concentration on technical writing activity. Without that release, this book could not have been completed. Nor could two other books have been completed over the past year, with one being in print and the other going into final layout with its publisher. (By the way, I don't recommend working on three books at once.)

And yes, the family. Who needs a dining room? Work on this (and the other two) book has overtaken the available surface area in my home office, so expansion into what my older son, Ben, now calls my "second office" has crippled the normally clutter-free dining room aura. What a good group of guys I have with husband, Tim, son Ben, and younger son Tucker, putting up with a normally active "mom" stuck at the writing table and computer. My family members, near and far, have been real troopers. The troop brings real joy and laughter to my life and I love them dearly for being them, individually, and appreciate the support they have lent to this book project.

I got into the habit of having my technical writing reviewed long ago because of a career within the research and Extension communities. Having other knowledgeable people look over materials before they go to print is invaluable. It takes additional time; my time and theirs. I welcomed and incorporated their input for the wisdom they have beyond mine in so many nuances of the topics covered in this book. For their efforts this book is greatly strengthened.

The book chapters have benefited from technical review by both agricultural engineers and horse specialists. To make sure that explanations made sense to those without an engineering background, I enlisted the advice of equine scientists or practicing businesspeople with extensive equine experience. This book is not meant to be an engineering text, but the engineer reviewers validated the conceptual framework of the technical discussions.

I've been lucky to have some wonderful reviewers. My heartfelt thanks are extended to each chapter reviewer for taking the time to educate me with even more good information. These reviewers' comments and advice have contributed many thoughtful changes and clarifications. It seemed very important that each chapter provided sensible content that satisfied equine enthusiasts while containing enough engineering technical content to be of use in decision making.

Book Chapter Reviewers in Alphabetical Order:

Dr. Michael Brugger
Associate Professor
Food, Agricultural and Biological Engineering
The Ohio State University
Columbus, OH
Chapters 10 and 11

Dr. John Chastian
Associate Professor
Agricultural and Biological Engineering
Clemson University
Clemson, SC
Chapter 11

Patricia Comerford
Instructor of Equine Programs
Dairy and Animal Science
The Pennsylvania State University
University Park, PA
Chapters 4, 5, 8, 16, and 17

Bonnie Darlington
Safety Chair
Pennsylvania Equine Council
Chapter 9

Dr. Nancy Diehl, DVM
Assistant Professor of Equine Science
Dairy and Animal Science
The Pennsylvania State University
University Park, PA
Chapters 1, 6, 9, and 13

Michael M. Donovan
Principal
Equestrian Services, LLC
Annapolis, MD
Chapter 18

Brian A. Egan
Extension Associate, Equine Programs
Dairy and Animal Science
The Pennsylvania State University
University Park, PA
Chapter 7

James Garthe
Instructor
Agricultural and Biological Engineering
The Pennsylvania State University
University Park, PA
Chapter 14

Dr. Robert Graves
Professor, Agricultural Engineering
Agricultural and Biological Engineering
The Pennsylvania State University
University Park, PA
Chapters 6, 7, 8, and 12

Daniel Greig
District Manager
Chester County (PA) Conservation District.
Chapter 8

Kenneth Guffey
Todd Palmer
Kory Leppo
Agricultural Engineers
RigidPly Rafters
Richland, PA
Chapter 16

Dr. Albert Jarrett
Professor of Soil and Water Engineering
Agricultural and Biological Engineering
The Pennsylvania State University
University Park, PA
Chapters 17 and 18

Nancy Kadwill
Senior Extension Educator
Penn State Cooperative Extension of Montgomery
    County
Collegeville, PA
Chapter 13

Dr. Malcolm "Mac" L. Legault
Assistant Professor
Health, Safety, and Environmental Health
    Sciences
Indiana State University
Terre Haute, IN
Chapter 9

Dr. Harvey Manbeck
Distinguished Professor
Agricultural and Biological Engineering
The Pennsylvania State University
University Park, PA
Chapter 4

Timothy Murphy
Conservation Engineer
Natural Resources Conservation Service
Pennsylvania
Chapter 8

Dr. Ann Swinker
Associate Professor of Equine Science
Dairy and Animal Science

The Pennsylvania State University
University Park, PA
Chapter 14

Emlyn Whitin
Vice President
Stancills, Inc.
Perryville, MD
Chapter 17

Dr. Stacy Worley
Engineering Instructor
Agricultural and Biological Engineering
The Pennsylvania State University
University Park, PA
Chapter 12

Dr. Roy Young
Professor and Department Head
Agricultural and Biological Engineering
The Pennsylvania State University
University Park, PA
Chapter 5

Last, alphabetically, but certainly not least:

Jennifer L. Zajaczkowski
Senior Research Technologist
Agricultural and Biological Engineering
The Pennsylvania State University
University Park, PA

Jennifer was reviewer of chapters 4, 6, and 15 and coauthor on previous versions of five chapters that were first published as Extension bulletins through Penn State's College of Agricultural Sciences: "Stall Design," "Flooring Materials and Drainage," "Manure Management," "Fence Planning," and "Riding Arena Surface Materials." She was also primary author of bulletin, now Chapter 9, titled "Fire Safety."

The photographic figures in this book are from my collection taken over a couple decades of visits to horse stabling facilities. Many horse people have kindly made their farms available for photographs and offered their experiences about horses in relation to housing. A few companies and individuals have shared their photos when I had no suitable photos of my own to use. The following list contains facilities that have photos included in this book. It is in no ways a comprehensive list (see next paragraph). Some farms are more recently visited sites whose owners will likely remember my visit. Other site photographs are from my files and were taken in the 1980s and 1990s.

Some photographed farms are not listed by name. A few photos in this book are curbside "drive-by" photos taken during my other travels and an official farm visit was not involved, so I can offer no farm name. In other cases, farms have changed ownership and name since my visit, so names may no longer match. I have included names of builders and construction companies with whom I traveled for troubleshooting or research project reasons. I don't necessarily list the names of those farms visited during our sometimes whirlwind tour of sites. My apologies if you recognize your facility and do not find your name on the credit list (send me a note to fix this situation!).

Tudane Farm, NY
Cornell University Horse Farms, NY
PenMor Thoroughbreds, NY
Stoned Acres, NY
University of Connecticut Horse Farm, CT
BOCES Horse Program, NY
Saratoga Organic, NY
Champaign Run, KY

Brookdale Farm, KY
Gainesway Farm, KY
Lakeside Arena, KY
McComsey Builders, PA
Red Bridge Farm, PA
Smucker Construction, PA
Greystone Stable, PA
Jodon's Stable, PA
Slab Cabin Stable, PA
Maryland State Fairgrounds, MD
Green Mountain Farm, VT
Tresslor and Fedor Excavating, PA
RigidPly Rafters, PA
Waterloo Farm, PA
Ryerrs Farm, PA
Rigbie Farm, MD
Sinking Creek Stable, PA
Turner Stable, PA
Restless Winds Farm, PA
R&R Fencing, PA
Ev-R-Green, PA
Greystone Farm, PA
Three Queens Farm, PA
Carousel Farm, PA
Detroit Radiant Products Co., MI
Coverall Building Systems, Ontario, Canada
Kalglo Electronics

Introduction

When one thinks of keeping horses, a vision centers on the stable. Horses are housed in stables for many reasons, but they seem to fall into three general categories that include human convenience, providing a less severe environment than that experienced outdoors, and tradition. The first two reasons are related to providing an environment where the handler is comfortable working and the horses are efficiently cared for. The environment and management of the stable is designed to be an improvement over outdoor conditions, or the horse will be disadvantaged by being in a stable. The third reason, tradition, has received little discussion.

Horses have traditionally been kept in stables. Horses as the precursors to "cars" or "trucks," or more appropriately "sport-utility vehicles," were kept in a stable behind the home or business like our cars. In this tradition, horses were used all day, virtually every day, and stored for the night in a stable until they were needed the next day. Compare this with the current Amish expectation where horses are consistently expected to drive dozens of miles each day and auction horses change hands with the ability to drive 20 miles each way to a work site. Now we use our cars every day to move dozens of miles and use most of our horses for recreation with movement restricted to a few miles per day. It may be all right to close our cars in a garage and to let them be idle most of the day, but a living, breathing horse is better suited to being outdoors or in an open airy environment if confined.

The "traditional" use of the horse has dramatically changed, but not our horse housing. Most horses are kept in suburban settings for recreation use rather than for any type of "work." This is fine, but perhaps our thinking about horse stabling needs to change to match the change in how we use horses. Modern horses are often inactive most of the day and confined to a stall where they originally were only expected to rest and sleep for work the next day.

Throughout this book there are several references made to horse housing design in relation to livestock housing design. This upsets some horsemen and horsewomen because they don't think of horses as livestock. Indeed, within our American culture we do not eat or derive food products from horses as we do from hogs, cattle, and poultry. Horses are our companions and treated as family, in many cases, but horses are livestock when it comes to housing. Horses are large, strong animals with instincts and habits that require they be housed in facilities that recognize their needs. As livestock, horses will drop feces and urine on the floor -- large amounts of feces and urine. Companion pets, such as dogs and cats, are trained not to do this throughout our human living environment. As livestock, horses are fed and bedded with relatively dusty materials compared with the food and flooring we find in our own homes. Horses respire large amounts of water into the stable air compared with the moisture we find in our own homes. Horse stables have more moisture, dust, and odor than found in human-occupied environments and, hence, require ventilation rates typical of livestock facilities. In fact, horse stables should have very good air quality to maintain horse health and athletic ability.

The daily activities on horse farms vary according to a farm's primary function, be it breeding, training, or public use. Though each farm requires specialized facilities, the basic goals of facility design and construction are similar. There are many breeds and types of horses and several riding and driving styles. The fundamentals of horse housing remain essentially the same, though. This book is written to house a typical 1000-pound horse. Clearly, scale up proportionally for larger animals. We don't often scale down for smaller equine but in the case of significantly smaller ponies and horses, accommodate their needs with fencing and stall panels that allow them similar safety and ability to see neighbors, respectively, as provided for the typical 1000-pound horse.

One of the biggest challenges in conveying the information contained in this book is that there is such a wide range of suitable horse-housing designs. Designs vary from the simple, low-cost backyard facilities that can be thoughtfully planned and constructed for fully functional horse care to facilities that incorporate expensive and beautifully detailed construction. Stables large and small can be successful with informal features or may incorporate every available convenience. Within large horse enterprises, there is wide variation from "high-end" facilities to average construction. Some readers will be picturing their stable with chandeliers and impressive architectural features, while others want advice on how to most economically achieve horse housing goals. This book has been written to provide recommended practices for an average, well-built stable that will be attractive and with features that others will recognize as thoughtful, functional design. There is an emphasis on labor-saving functional planning. Surely, special features and finishes may be added to enhance visual appeal of the facility once fundamentals of housing the horse in a suitable environment are provided.

This book includes important information on topics that are often not carefully considered in initial stable planning. These topics include environmental control (ventilation), manure management, and fire protection systems. Additional chapters cover recommendations for stall design, flooring, drainage, fencing, utilities, and riding arena features. Individuals using the technical information from this book will be able to more effectively plan and design a facility that best meets operational goals.

Horse Stable and Riding Arena Design

1
Horse Behavior Influence on Design

A designer must understand basic horse behavior for proper design and construction of horse facilities. For designers familiar with farm construction practices, horses have traits that differ from other livestock species. People who have little previous experience with horses or the planned activities of the farm should become familiar with basic horse behavior and functional activities that are expected at the site. Safe and sound designs respect horses' uniqueness and provide convenience and safety for both horse and handler. This short chapter serves to provide an overview of basic horse behavior traits that relate to horse facility construction.

FLIGHT OR FIGHT

Horses have highly developed senses of sight, smell, and hearing. They have a 340° range of vision that makes them very sensitive to motion from almost any direction.

A horse's natural defense mechanism is the *fight-or-flight* instinct. Horses are generally nonaggressive, but when threatened, excited, impatient, scared, or in pain they will typically first try "flight" to escape by running away. Facilities that contain horses need to be sturdy and free of projections that would impale a panicked horse. If escape is not possible, then horses might "fight" by kicking, striking, or biting. A horse's reaction to a threat, real or perceived, is rapid and imparts high force on contact, so construction materials need to be sturdy and handler safety becomes important. Horses are well known for their apparently frantic behavior when entangled in fencing materials or caught with a foot between bars of the stall. Some horses patiently wait to be freed, but unfortunately most seem to struggle in an attempt at flight from the confining situation.

This flight-or-fight defense explains the excitable nature of the horse. The degree of excitability and nervousness varies among individuals and breeding lines. Properly designed handling facilities allow for horse and handler safety while diminishing the horses' instinct or desire to escape by running through or jumping over barriers. Some classes of horses, such as breeding stallions, can be naturally aggressive and require specialized facility design to guard against horse or handler injury.

SOCIAL NEEDS

Horses are social creatures so most will try to join other horses if they can (Fig. 1.1). Isolated horses lack the security of a group and often develop undesirable and possibly health-endangering behaviors not found when a number of horses live together. Horses in stalls quickly become bored, which leads to stable stereotypies (often called "vices," but this implies that these behaviors can be affected by training, which they cannot).

Stereotypies include the following:

- Wood chewing
- Pawing or striking the ground or stall walls with a front foot or repeated kicking out with a back foot
- Weaving nervously by repeatedly shifting weight from one front leg to the other
- Pacing and circling the stall, headshaking
- Placing the upper incisors on a solid object and expanding the larynx, which results in the gulping of air behavior known as *cribbing* (Fig. 1.2)

Horses housed individually are calmer if they can maintain visual contact with other horses. If possible, horses should be allowed to see other horses and outside activities to decrease these stereotypies and to reduce anxiety from being isolated (Fig. 1.3).

DOMINANCE ORDER

Horses kept in groups develop a dominance order. Each horse uses a combination of aggressive and submissive behaviors to place itself in the dominance order within the herd. Pastures and paddocks with corners and other small-enclosed areas that

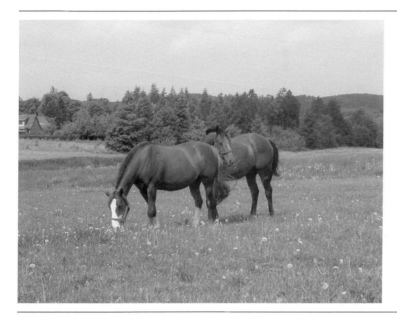

Figure 1.1. Horses on pasture setting exhibit more natural behavior of social contact and time spent eating forages.

allow a dominant horse to trap a submissive one increase the frequency of injury.

In addition, feed, water, and shelter represent limiting resources and access to these are affected by the dominance order.

A good horseman is observant of horse behavior and temperament and can use these to advantage in training and even housing. Grouping horses according to observed relationships at pasture can make turnout, stabling, and trailering safer. Both people and horses can affect another horse's movement by use of the flight zone, much like a person's "personal space." Once a person enters the flight zone, the horse will move away. With training, the flight zone normally decreases. The flight zone is used every day when a person attempts to catch a horse in the field or work the horse in a round pen. A dominant horse may need only enter another horse's flight

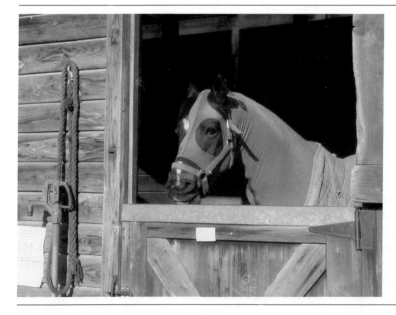

Figure 1.2. Stereotypic behaviors (cribbing shown here) can develop in horses that are kept in situations that deny normal horse behavior.

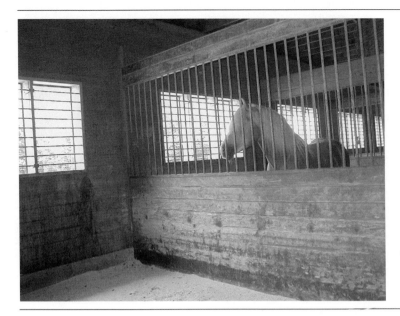

Figure 1.3. Horses kept in stable for prolonged periods seem to benefit from being able to see other horses and activities around them.

zone, without making apparent threats, to make the more submissive individual move away from food, water, or even a grazing spot.

STABLES AS A PLACE FOR FOOD, SECURITY, AND REST

Horses have a major preoccupation with food and security. In a natural setting horses spend a considerable portion of their day grazing than when in confinement where feeding may be a short, regularly scheduled event leaving considerable time to fill with other activities. A stable area typically represents an area for food and security. An excited horse may reenter a burning barn because of this connection between food and security.

Horses often rest or doze standing but will lie down for prolonged sleep. Sleeping patterns mean that horses need a comfortable area to stand and lie down. Horses prefer bedding versus hard, bare flooring. Horses need to get into lateral recumbency in order to get their required daily REM sleep, or at least be able to lie in sternal recumbency and lean against something to mimic lateral recumbency. This is pertinent to horses kept in tie stalls.

Designing facilities to account for horse behavior does not have to be complicated or expensive. Horses have flourished for ages on open grassy plains. Excellent horse husbandry can be achieved with a paddock and simple shelter (the simple "shelter" may include natural things like dense bush or tree stands). Facilities should promote safety as well as the efficient care and handling of horses. Well-planned facilities allow for lower operational costs. Poorly planned or improperly constructed facilities interfere with daily operations, increase costs such as labor and maintenance, and compromise the safety and health of both horses and people.

2
Horse Stable Layout and Planning

A well-designed stable protects horses from weather extremes and keeps them dry while providing fresh air and light and protection from injury. Stables need ample space for the well-being of the horses, chore efficiency, material storage, convenience and safety of handlers, and the enjoyment of riders (Fig. 2.1). Many horses are successfully kept on pasture with a simple shelter (Fig. 2.2). Stables are a popular feature for horse housing irrespective of whether the horse is confined most of the day or only during certain periods.

ADVANTAGES AND DISADVANTAGES OF STABLES VERSUS PASTURE SHELTER

The advantages of a stable are that it

- provides shelter for horse care and handling;
- allows closer observation and individual care of confined horses;
- provides a better opportunity to regulate feed intake with training or exercising programs;
- provides shelter for a horse to maintain condition while clipped for winter working and showing;
- confines horses off pastures during wet, muddy conditions, so that
- they can be kept cleaner; and
- improves security.

The disadvantages of stables are as follows:

- More manual labor and attention to horses is required for such things as cleaning stalls, bedding, feeding at least twice a day, watering, and exercising.
- Improper care and exercise lead to poor health and/or stereotypies.
- Stables are much more expensive to build and maintain than pasture shelters.
- A poorly designed or managed stable can be an unhealthy environment—excess moisture, high ammonia level, stressed horses, hazardous construction, and so forth.

STALL LAYOUT OPTIONS

On the basis of stall and work aisle locations, horse stable floor plans are usually identified as single row, center aisle, or island design (Fig. 2.3). The single-row option is more common in mild climates where the exterior work aisle is comfortable for the human caretakers (Fig. 2.4). The single row is also used where horses are outdoors most of the time with free access to the stall area. The center aisle design is common in the United States for private boarding and showing facilities where the enclosed work aisle is central to horse care functions (Fig. 2.5). The island design is more common with horses that are in intensive training, such as racehorses, where the covered "ring" of aisles is used to cool down or exercise horses (Fig. 2.6).

Single-Row Configuration

- A single-row stable is a one-story structure with side-by-side stalls.
- Horses have access to outside air and sight of activities from the front or rear of stall.
- Stall door(s) opens into the stable yard, individual runs, or communal paddock.
- The work aisle is under a roof overhang or, less typically, is enclosed.

The single-row configuration is attractive and minimizes enclosed space compared with the other two options. Horses are closer to their natural environment, so each horse can have a desirable position within the stable. The handler has less protection from weather unless the aisle is partially enclosed.

Central Aisle Configuration

- The stalls are side by side along opposite stable walls and are separated by a wide alley.
- The alley can be used for tying, grooming, saddling up, and cooling out animals and for cleaning stalls.

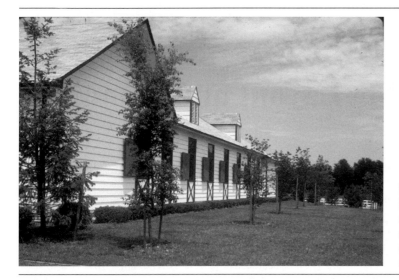

Figure 2.1. Housing the horse in a stable offers many conveniences as long as management of interior environment and horse exercise is sufficient.

This floor plan makes efficient use of interior space, with one work aisle serving two rows of stalls. It provides occupants protection from the outside elements. The central aisle configuration can also be designed to provide each stall with a door to the outside.

Island Design

- An "island" is two rows of side-by-side and back-to-back stalls. An aisle encircles the entire island of stalls.
- Stall doors open into the aisle that encircles all the stalls.

- Another option encloses a central aisle stable as the island with stall doors open to the central work aisle.

In the island floor plan, the aisle can be used to cool horses or, if the ceilings are high enough, to exercise animals. If alleys are used to exercise animals, then dust suppression is important. Sunlight usually cannot reach stalls. This design has the most covered area per horse housed; so unless the extra alleys are frequently used, it is an inefficient design.

Clearly, other stall and work aisle arrangements are successfully used as stables. Particularly with buildings remodeled from other uses, stall and aisle

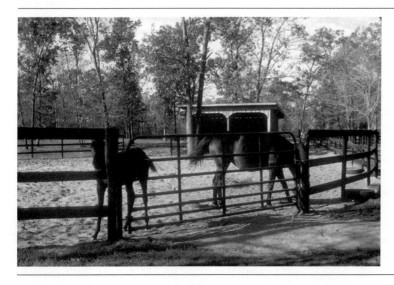

Figure 2.2. A simple pasture shelter with contiguous exercise area is sufficient for most horses, but handlers often desire more amenities in commercial facilities.

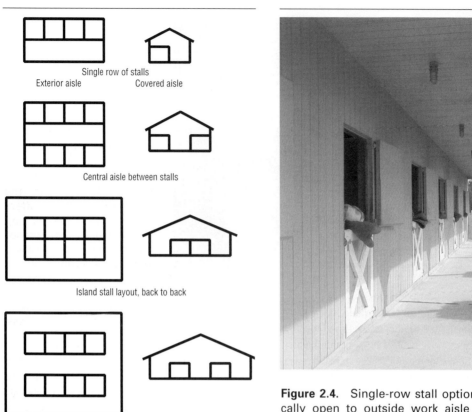

Single row of stalls
Exterior aisle   Covered aisle

Central aisle between stalls

Island stall layout, back to back

Island stall layout with center aisle

Figure 2.3. Common stable floor plan and cross-section configurations.

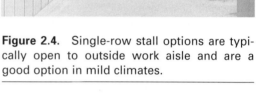

Figure 2.4. Single-row stall options are typically open to outside work aisle and are a good option in mild climates.

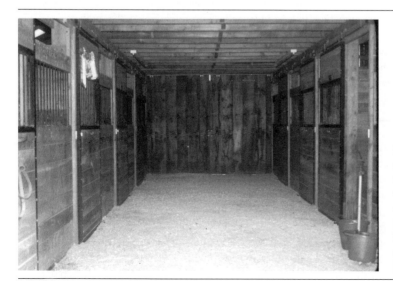

Figure 2.5. Center aisle design, with its enclosed, weather-protected work aisle with stalls on either side, is very common in the United States. This stable features hay storage over the center aisle with no ceiling over the horse stalls.

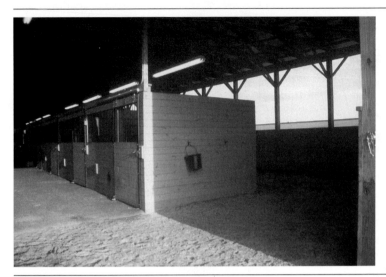

Figure 2.6. Island design puts stalls in the center of the structure with an exercise walkway around the entire perimeter. Shown is a portion of a racehorse stable with a center aisle stable surrounded by an exercise hallway with enough height so that horses can be ridden.

arrangements can be quite variable. Generally, straight, wide aisles are used in stable layout to allow safe and efficient movement of horses with handler, bulky bedding and forage materials, and stall waste removal. Stalls are positioned with direct access to fresh-air openings and to allow a confined horse to see activities within the stable and/or outdoors to decrease boredom. Developing a comfortable area to house horses is the main objective of a good stable design. In addition to comfortable stalls, it is important to design the building to be functional.

PLANNING HORSE STABLES

A stable, large or small, private or commercial, should be well planned, durable, and attractive. Its basic purpose is to provide an environment that protects horses from weather extremes, maintains fresh and dry air during all seasons, and protects horses from injury. A stable is a convenience for handlers and serves a social and recreational function for both private and commercial facilities. Consider safety in features that minimize sharp projections, eliminate fire hazards, and are sturdy enough for horse abuse. Provide enough space for safe passage of horses and handlers through doors, gates, and alleyways. Provide enough dedicated storage space for the tools, tack, and equipment needed for horsekeeping. Additional large storages will be needed for bedding, hay, and manure. Stall barns typically allow animal access to paddocks or riding areas but house individual horses, or mares with foals, in individual stalls.

The type of structure selected depends on size of the operation, climate, amount of capital available, and the owner's preference. Consider general attractiveness and keep facilities well maintained. Locate buildings to take advantage of existing conditions and provide economical use of labor in feeding, cleaning, and maintenance. For all stables and other horse buildings, evaluate the following features. For additional information on a topic, please refer to the suggested chapters.

Flexibility: Assume that remodeling will take place in the future to meet changing needs. The ability to cheaply and easily remodel a stable into another useful function (cabin, garage, storage building) will typically increase the property's resale value (see Chapters 3 and 4).

Attractiveness: Aesthetic value is achieved by a structure with good proportions in harmony with its surroundings and fulfilling its function. Good design enhances value. Landscaping enhances attractiveness (Fig. 2.7).

Space: Both horses and handlers need enough space, but too much of it unnecessarily increases expenses. Provide roofed space for stalls, indoor alleys, tack, and equipment and for storage of hay, bedding, and feed (Fig. 2.8). Some of this roofed space may be in separate buildings (see Chapters 5 and 13).

Safety: Protect both humans and horses from unnecessary risk with good design and construction. Eliminate sharp projections. Provide enough space to allow safe passage of horse and handler through

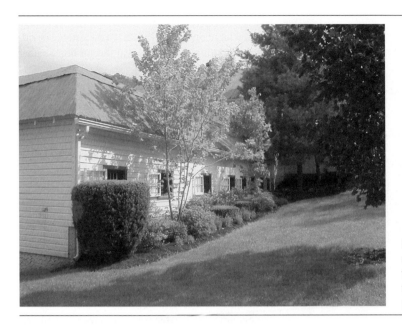

Figure 2.7. Landscaping and buildings in scale with their surroundings contribute to attractiveness and property value.

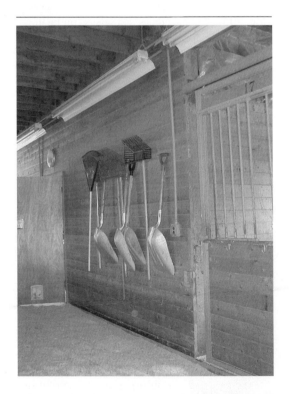

Figure 2.8. Space is needed for storage of tools (shown here) and plenty of equipment, tack, feed, and bedding in addition to the space needed for horse stalls and work aisles.

doors, gates, and alleys. Understand horse behavior in relation to building design features (see Chapter 1).

Floor-to-ceiling height: Low ceilings interfere with ventilation, make the barn dark, and are a safety hazard for people and horses. Common ceiling heights are 10 to 12 feet for stall barns and 16 to 18 feet for riding areas.

Minimized fire risk: Prohibit smoking. Follow a fire prevention program, and prepare to contain and extinguish a fire (Fig. 2.9). Precautions can prevent losses and may reduce insurance premiums. Use fire-resistant materials and fire-retarding paints and sprays where practical. (see Chapter 9).

Interior environment: Barns minimize stress on horses and humans by protecting against rain, snow, sun, and wind. Summer wind cools, but winter wind chills and can drive snow and rain into the building. Get data on prevailing wind direction and velocity to help properly orient buildings. Sunlight entry into a building can provide natural winter heat (Fig. 2.10). Trees are practical windbreaks, summer wind "funnels," screens to obstruct undesirable views, and shades. Some stables will benefit from having critical areas heated for human comfort, moisture control in tack storage, and horse drying in wash stall area. (see Chapters 4 and 12).

Good ventilation: Poor moisture, temperature, and odor control can be major problems in horse stables. Ventilation minimizes moisture buildup during cold

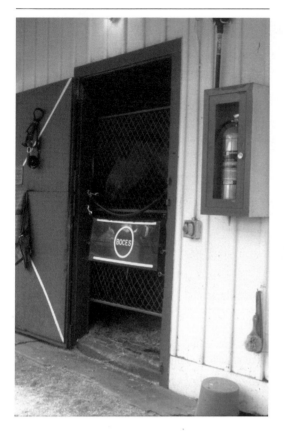

Figure 2.9. Horse facilities are built so as to ensure safety and minimize fire risk. Horse-proof hardware and construction is essential. Provide fire suppression tools as a backup to efforts to prevent fire ignition.

weather and aids in odor removal. The option to provide large openings (Fig. 2.10) on a stable or riding arena will aid heat removal during hot weather (see Chapter 6).

Suitable exercise area: Corrals and paddocks need safe, durable, and attractive fence material on sturdy posts (Fig. 2.11). Provide adequate space in paddocks and access lanes. An efficient traffic plan reduces labor for turning out and bringing in horses. Consider fencing the entire farmstead so loose horses cannot leave the property in conditions where loose horses are particularly undesirable (see Chapters 14 and 15).

Water and feed: Sufficient quantity of good-quality water must be available all year round in stable and turnout areas. Provide feed storage in a rodent-proof and horse-inaccessible location. A storage area for large quantities of hay is best located in a separate building, with a several-day supply (Fig. 2.12) convenient within the stable (see Chapters 10 and 13).

Special features: Special features may include grooming area or wash rack, trailer storage, breeding area, exercise area, office, lounge, and living quarters (Fig. 2.13). These facilities and others can be in one or several buildings. Indoor riding arenas are a popular feature on horse farms (see Chapters 13 and 16).

Labor saving: Three quarters of horse chores are manual, so labor saving is desirable for any sized operation. Labor-saving mechanization is available for large operations (Fig. 2.14). Design to minimize drudgery with a bright and airy interior, compact

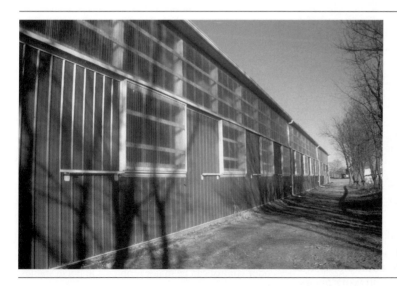

Figure 2.10. Maintaining a good interior environment of stables and arenas is very important. The interior environment should have adequate light level, which may be provided with translucent panels shown here. Admitting fresh air to arenas and stables is essential for horses and human handlers. Having panels like those shown here, which open for warm weather air exchange, is beneficial.

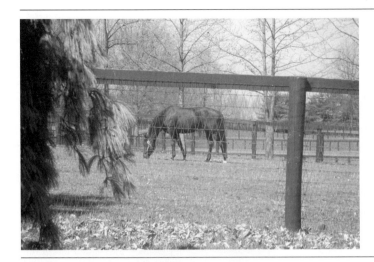

Figure 2.11. A suitable area is needed for daily turnout or exercise of horses.

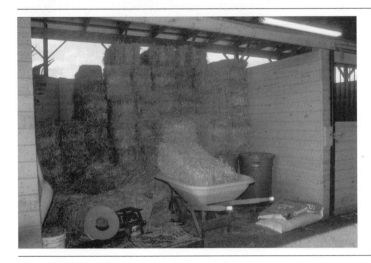

Figure 2.12. Each stable will need at least short-term storage of hay, bedding, various tools, and cleaning equipment.

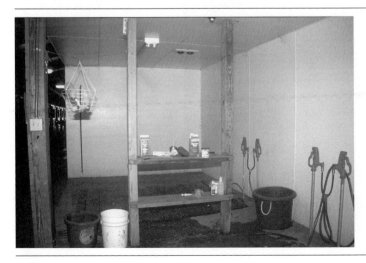

Figure 2.13. Many special features are often included in stables, such as this grooming station. Other features are specific to the main function of the horse facility, such as breeding area or lounge for lesson spectators.

facilities, and efficient chore routines. Put highest priorities on daily chores that consume most time: feeding, watering, cleaning and bedding stalls, grooming, exercising, and turning out and bringing in. Teasing, breeding, worming, veterinary procedures, foot care, halter breaking, and so forth are secondary chores (see Chapters 4, 8, and 11).

Manure management: Plan ahead for storage and disposal of the tons of manure and stall waste that each horse generates (Fig. 2.15). Prioritize convenience in chores associated with stall waste handling. Assure that manure storage locations protect the environment from pollution, such as pile leachate flow into nearby waterways, and from odor and insect nuisances (see Chapter 8).

Drainage: Build on high ground for adequate drainage year round. Proper drainage considers both surface flow and groundwater influences. Poor drainage causes serious problems in the ability to successfully use an otherwise well-planned facility. Fix small drainage problems with grading or subsurface drains (see Chapters 4 and 7).

Construction and maintenance cost: Select materials and construction type for durability, ease of maintenance, cost, advertising value, and intangible values such as pride and satisfaction: Top quality may be most economical in the long run. The primary types of structure construction for horse facilities include post and beam or clear span. Each type has advantages and disadvantages (see Chapter 3).

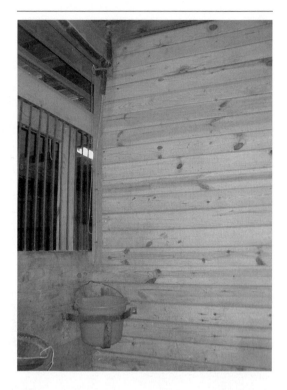

Figure 2.14. Labor-saving features and efficient routines are important because of the high labor demands of horse housing. This stall features a labor-saving overhead water line that supplies the bucket with water after a valve is manually activated.

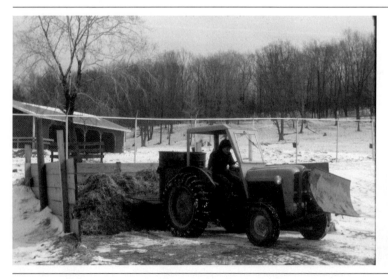

Figure 2.15. Plan for efficiently handling the large quantities of manure and stall waste generated from horse housing.

3
Construction Style and Materials

This chapter provides an overview of common construction styles used in horse stables and indoor riding arenas. Basic construction materials useful in horse facilities are briefly reviewed. Stables and indoor riding arenas are built to provide protection from weather, so there will be regional variation in desirable construction attributes. For example, in a hot, arid climate a more open structure is desirable for cooling breezes while providing protection from sunlight. In climates with cold, snowy winters a more enclosed facility is desirable. Regardless of the type of weather protection sought, the interior climate conditions should be an improvement over outside conditions, with provision of plenty of ventilation to maintain good air quality. Poor interior air quality will compromise building materials with increased absorption of moisture, mold formation, and eventual deterioration of materials. Choose materials that will withstand the higher humidity and dust levels found in horse stabling and riding arena environments.

BUILDING FRAMING STYLES

Building framing styles relate to the structural means of supporting the building shell and influence interior features. The two primary framing styles used in horse stables are "post-and-beam" and "clear-span" construction. Only the latter is used for indoor arena construction. Hoop structures are a variation of clear-span construction, using lighter framing and covering materials than more traditional construction. Post-and-beam and clear-span construction can be designed for natural light entry and ventilation via eave and ridge ventilation openings (see Chapters 6 and 11 for additional detail).

Post and Beam

Post-and-beam construction is common in horse stables because posts support both the structure and the stall partitions (Fig. 3.1). It is an economical construction in many cases, but the drawback of this construction is sacrifice of flexibility as compared with a clear-span barn if remodeling becomes necessary. Post-and-beam construction is the traditional barn construction technique and offers an aesthetically pleasing structure suitable for horse housing.

Clear Span

A clear-span barn is a popular type of structure for stall barns and arenas because there are no interior posts to inhibit movement. Without posts, remodeling is easier than when interior posts and walls need to be moved. Stall walls will need posts for support, but these will not be expected to also support the overall structure. The interior clear span is provided by either truss (Fig. 3.2) or rigid frame (Fig. 3.3) structural support of the roof. Trusses and rigid frames are purchased as engineered products and may be constructed from wood or steel. Trusses are often used in pole buildings. Post or pole construction, with poles embedded in the ground, replaces concrete foundations. Rigid frames and arches are economical when spanning wide distances. The rigid frame or arch is securely attached to concrete foundation supports. Wooden arches are often considered an attractive architectural feature of the building (Fig. 3.4). Rigid frames of either wood or metal material offer a more open appearance to the interior than trusses. Rigid frames offer unobstructed space to the roofline. Trusses offer support for a ceiling, if used.

Hoop Structures

Hoop structures are a newer introduction to horse stabling and riding arena construction. Because of lighter and low-cost construction materials, they offer a lower cost per area enclosed than the more traditional construction approaches discussed earlier. Hoop structures for horse stables and riding arenas provide clear-span attributes that developed from livestock housing and greenhouse construction

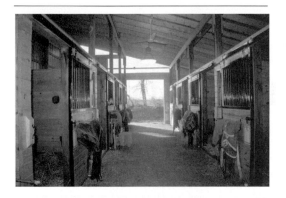

Figure 3.1. Post-and-beam construction that uses stall posts to support roof rafters.

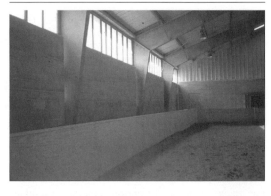

Figure 3.3. Rigid frame clear-span construction is more common in wide indoor arenas than in stables.

practices. The hoop frame construction is of tubular metal design covered with a flexible material similar to a high-quality reinforced plastic tarp (Fig. 3.5). Many hoop structures have translucent coverings over a simple arched metal frame. Any material that admits sunlight will warm the building interior with trapped radiation, which is a benefit in cold weather but a liability in hot weather. Consider the seasonal use of the building if translucent materials are used. Hoop structures can be covered with an opaque material to decrease sunlight penetration. Provide sidewall protection against horse contact, both interior and exterior, because the flexible

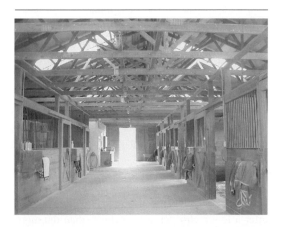

Figure 3.2. Clear-span construction uses trusses that provide an open interior. Stall corner posts attach to the lower chord of some trusses but are not supporting the roof weight.

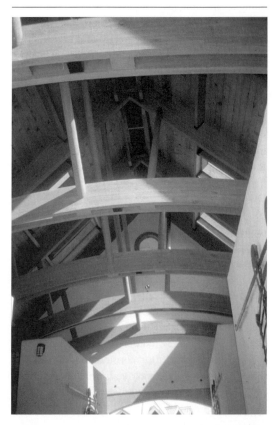

Figure 3.4. Wooden arches of glu-lam construction offer an attractive framing in simple rigid frame style or the more complex formation shown here.

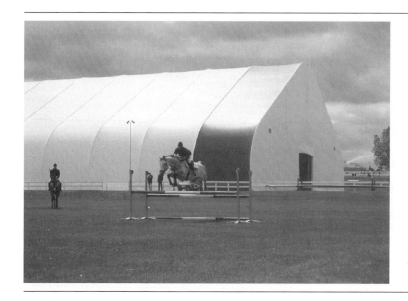

Figure 3.5. Hoop structures are a relatively new addition to clear-span construction techniques. Courtesy of Coverall Building Systems.

covering material is not sturdy against horse abuse. Ventilation of hoop structures can be added as movable sidewall material. If the hoop covering material goes from ground to ground without any ventilation opening, then provide large endwall air exchange openings. Some designs can accommodate both ridge and sidewall ventilation at increased structural cost. See the "Additional Resources" section for information about a Ventilating Greenhouse Barns fact sheet.

ROOF SHAPE

Roof shape has a strong impact on the functional and aesthetic attributes of the stable. Some shapes offer adequate space for overhead hay storage, while others are better for enhanced ventilation or natural light entry. Simple roof shapes of good proportion can be equal in attractiveness to complicated shapes. Typical roof shapes are shown in Figure 3.6.

ROOFING MATERIALS

The most commonly used roofing materials for stables and riding arenas are metal, asphalt shingles, and wood shingles. Good roofing materials are essential to prevent water from damaging interior building materials. Selection of a roof material that fits desired durability and aesthetics is often a top priority, but cost is oftentimes the deciding factor. Direct any roof runoff water away from paddocks and the manure handling areas.

Metal

Metal is often the best buy for covering large-roofed areas (Fig. 3.7). Metal roofs offer easy and quick installation compared with other major materials. Use light insulation and a vapor retarder under a metal roof to minimize water condensation and associated dripping. Insulation also reduces the noise associated with metal roofs during rain and hail. The insulation will also moderate the radiant temperature effects on building occupants from a hot metal roof in summer and cold roof surface in winter. Metal roofing is available in a wide range of colors and manufacturer profiles with a long service life (20 years). Metal roofing is not combustible, but the insulation used with it may be. Some consider the metal roof material, with its rather industrial aesthetic, to be less attractive than other options.

Asphalt Shingles

The asphalt shingle is a popular roofing material with a relatively low cost and good life expectancy. Asphalt shingles are flammable, with class A shingles providing the greatest fire resistance. In high-wind locations, purchase shingles that carry a "wind resistance" label. Shingles are considered attractive by most people and provide a finished look to the building. They require skilled labor to install and require some upkeep. When installed over plywood sheathing, the shingle assembly provides enough insulation to reduce condensation under most conditions.

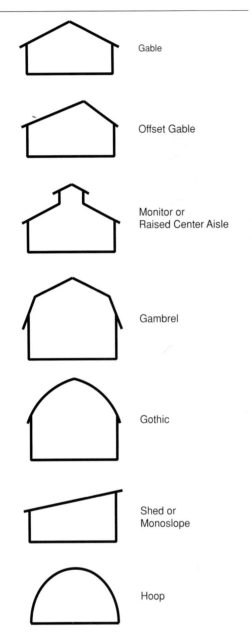

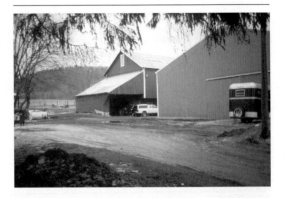

Figure 3.7. Metal-roofed and -sided indoor riding arena in foreground and wood-sided traditional bank barn in background.

Figure 3.6. Roof framing styles and typical uses. *Gable:* Most common stable and indoor arena roof with simple ventilation options. *Offset gable:* Good for extended roof over covered outside aisle. *Monitor or raised center aisle:* Enhanced natural ventilation and light entry at monitor. *Gambrel:* Traditional barn roof with upper story for storage. *Gothic:* Lots of upper-story storage space. *Shed:* Common on pasture shelters and small single-row stables. *Hoop:* Flexible material on metal frame.

Wood Shingles

Wood shingles are machine-sawn, while wood shakes are hand-hewn and rougher looking, but both add a quality rustic finish to the stable or arena. Fire preservative treatment is recommended, especially for people living in areas prone to brush fires. Most wood roofs are covered by warranties, but some local codes limit their use because of fire concerns. Skilled labor is needed for installation.

CONSTRUCTION MATERIALS

Horse stable construction materials need to be durable, easy to maintain, and satisfying in appearance. Horse facilities often emphasize marketing value and owner's pride in material selection and overall design (Fig. 3.8). High-quality materials are often more economical in the long term than cheaply constructed materials. The most common construction materials used in stables are wood, concrete, masonry, and metal, with some use of high-quality synthetic components.

Wood

Wood provides a natural appearance to exterior and interior of the stable. Wood is durable, provides some insulating value, and is considered attractive (Fig. 3.9). Wood products are available in many grades from purely functional plywood panels to finely finished oak panels. Wood requires some maintenance to maintain a finished appearance but with proper care has a long useful life. It is

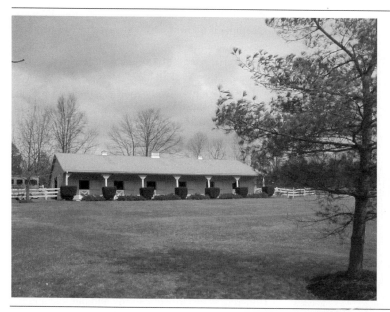

Figure 3.8. Horse stable construction often has a traditional style, with cupolas, Dutch doors, and white board fence being the favorite details with many farms. Materials need to be durable against horse activity and the moist, dusty environment. High-quality materials are often used for an attractive facility.

a relatively easy material for construction assembly. Wood is a porous material, so it will absorb water and can harbor microorganisms. It is flammable unless treated with a fire retarder.

Most stall walls are made of wood because it is resilient yet somewhat forgiving for horses' legs and feet when kicked (Fig. 3.10). Even when stall walls are made of other durable materials, such as masonry, stalls may be lined with wood to soften the impact of kicks. Sheet metal exterior paneling must

have an interior wood stall liner to prevent horses from damaging the metal and themselves on sharp edges. Horses can kick through unprotected sheet metal-siding material.

Hardwoods are preferred for strength and to discourage wood chewers. To resist kicking damage, 2-inch-thick boards are used in areas where horses will have contact. Fit boards or planks tightly together to reduce the number of chewable edges. Cover exposed wood edges with metal that is smooth

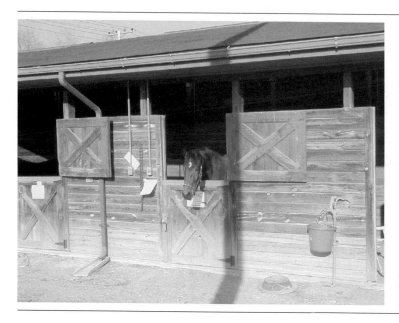

Figure 3.9. Wood is an attractive and strong material for horse stable construction.

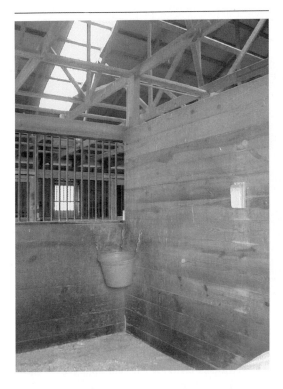

Figure 3.10. Wood is the most common material for stall wall construction. Wood is often used as a liner on the interior of masonry walls and is needed as a stall liner for metal-sided buildings.

and blunt, such as angle or channel iron. Plywood sheathing is a lower cost option than wood planking and can be stained for an attractive appearance. Plywood is very strong and requires less maintenance than wood planking.

Use exterior grade plywood sheathing on both interior and exterior of stable, because stable interiors can be at higher humidity levels than outdoor conditions. The glue used in manufacturing exterior grade plywood will withstand the high-humidity conditions. Use ¾-inch-thick plywood to resist damage from kicking; if installed over a solid backing, a reduced thickness can be used. Use preservative-treated wood and plywood in areas exposed to moisture, such as ground or soiled bedding contact, for longer material life.

Concrete

Concrete walls are very sturdy and durable and require little maintenance. Concrete is nearly fireproof and is vermin proof, so it is of value in areas where rodent exclusion is important. Poured concrete walls will need a poured foundation. Concrete works well in areas that require durability but has limited contact with horses. Horses may test concrete but will not persist in kicking or chewing it. Figure 3.11 shows a below-grade poured concrete exterior wall (bank-barn construction) with other stall walls constructed of wood. Wash areas, tack rooms, feed room, and office areas are locations that can make good use of

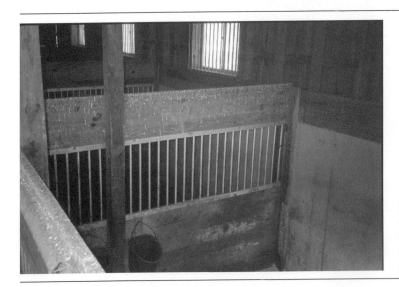

Figure 3.11. Poured concrete exterior wall of this stable is mainly below grade on this bank-barn construction.

concrete walls. Concrete will absorb moisture un-less sealed with paint treatment (see the section on masonry). The large mass of concrete will dampen temperature swings within a stable and will slowly heat and cool with seasonal temperature changes. Concrete walls are more difficult to insulate than wood or metal framing.

Poured concrete is a common and recommended floor material in tack and feed rooms for ease of cleanup and rodent exclusion. Chapter 7 contains more information on materials used in various floors around the stable.

Masonry

Masonry construction costs more than a frame build-ing, but its durability and low maintenance costs may make it more economical in the long run. It is nearly fireproof. Much of masonry cost is in the skilled labor required for proper construction, because the material cost is similar to wood. Masonry is often used in large horse operations because of its low maintenance, attractive appear-ance, and long life (Fig. 3.12). One popular option is a masonry outer wall (shell) with interior wooden stalls. Reinforce foundation and walls with steel rods and treat interior masonry walls with a fireproof paint sealer for a smooth, nonabrasive, and cleans-able surface (Fig. 3.13). Blocks with baked ceramic tile surface are desirable for laboratories, foaling stalls, and washing areas (Fig. 3.14). In stalls, ce-ramic tiles on the lower 5 feet can be combined with sealed block above. Consider wood wainscoting to

reduce impact damage to horses kicking or crashing into masonry walls. Masonry has many features sim-ilar to those of concrete, being vermin proof, requir-ing poured foundation and concrete slab, and having a large mass with associated temperature-stabilizing effects. Like concrete, masonry is more difficult to insulate than wood or steel frame construction.

Metal

Metal is expensive as a primary building material, but minimized labor costs may make total building costs lower than those of wood. Construction is simple and relatively fast. Sheet metal siding requires little main-tenance but is not durable if horses are allowed to contact. Fence horses away from metal-siding exteri-or to reduce dents and scratches in the siding and cuts to horses from sharp edges. The interior of a metal-sided building must be wood lined to keep horses safe from sharp edges and to decrease kicking damage.

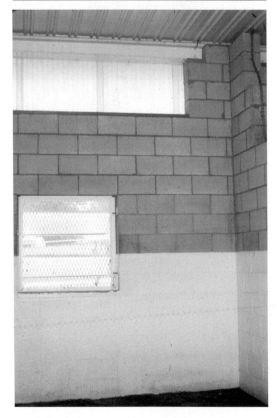

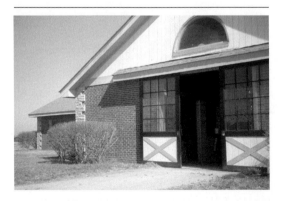

Figure 3.12. Brick is an attractive exterior construction material and may be used in aisle flooring.

Figure 3.13. Sealant is used on lower por-tions of masonry stall wall construction to as-sist in cleaning.

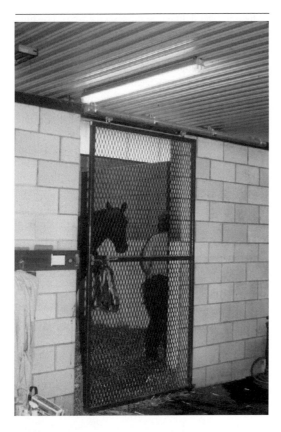

Figure 3.14. Concrete block masonry construction is more common as an exterior wall material but can also be used as stall partition.

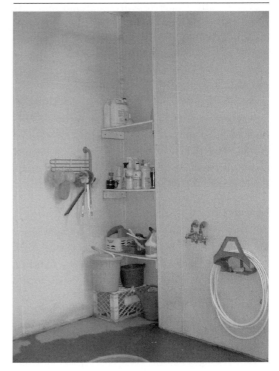

Figure 3.15. Fiberglass reinforced plastic (FRP) panels are a strong, waterproof material useful as wash stall walls.

Some people may not like the "industrial" look of steel-sided stables and arenas. Metal allows more noise echoes than wood or insulated interiors, which can be annoying to people and unnerving to horses. Metal conducts heat quickly, so building temperature will quickly match outdoor conditions. Steel frames with another material as exterior siding can combine some of the advantages of each material. Metal will contain a fire until hot enough to melt.

Specialty Building Materials

Fiberglass reinforced plastic (FRP) panels are used in wash stalls and other areas where water will be in contact with the building material and durability is required (Fig. 3.15). FRP is a strong, waterproof alternative to porous wood and easily damaged metal panels.

Translucent panels made of fiberglass, acrylic, or other materials are used along the upper portions of sidewalls to admit natural light into stables and indoor riding arenas (Fig. 3.16).

Curtain material, if translucent, may make up a portion of sidewall area to admit natural light and

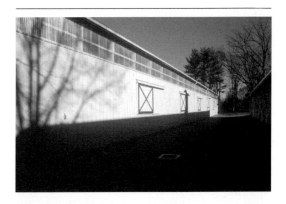

Figure 3.16. Translucent panels are popular as the upper portion of sidewall construction for admitting natural light to stables and indoor riding arenas.

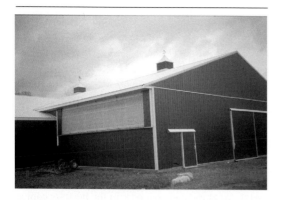

Figure 3.17. Curtain material along the top half of this riding arena's sidewalls is used for natural light entry and, when open, admits fresh air through the large openings.

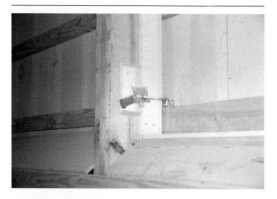

Figure 3.18. Durable latches provide tight closure of movable ventilation panels and large sliding doors.

fresh air when opened (Fig. 3.17). The curtain material is a strong, tarp-like, waterproof fabric that is commonly used in dairy and livestock housing ventilation applications. Similar strong fabric material is used to enclose hoop structures.

Insulation materials were mentioned briefly in relation to metal roofing applications where insulation is highly recommended as part of that roofing construction. See chapters 6 and 12 for more detail on insulation material properties and uses.

Surface treatments include paint and other coatings. Powdered coatings are often used on metal components, such as stall partition bars, for a durable finish. Use noncombustible paints on wood and other materials where practical. Combustible sealers will practically explode during a fire. Very light colors increase stable brightness inside and reflect some solar radiation outside.

HARDWARE

Metal hardware used around horses to secure items, such as doors and feed buckets, need to be durable, with smooth contours. When doors are open or buckets removed, the exposed hardware should not provide sharp projections that could injure a horse. Residential-style hardware is not strong enough for use in the horse-occupied area of the stable. Door latches, hinges, and sliding tracks need to withstand a 1000-pound animal leaning and kicking against them. Chose latches with one-handed operation so the other hand can carry things. It is particularly important that the feed room be secured with a horse-proof latch.

Doors and large panels that open for ventilation and natural light entry can be secured with a tight closure, with the hardware assembly shown in Figure 3.18.

Rodent Control and Stable Construction

Rodents are attracted to live in areas that provide them food, water, and shelter. A horse stable can be built and managed to discourage rodent invasion but will probably never eliminate all rodents. Deny rodents access to feed, water sources, and suitable nesting areas.

Many rodent control programs depend on physically keeping rodents from feed, water, and shelter. Advice to seal gaps in the structure to prevent rodent entry appears to be a good idea, but it is not practical for horse stables. Young mice can squeeze through a $1/4$-inch hole and young rats through a $1/2$-inch hole. Stables are managed with wide-open doors and stall windows; ventilation vents are open year -round; and many doors, even when closed, are not rodent proof in material or in the gaps that remain. Although the rodent access battle may be lost in the main horse housing areas, concentrate on securing the feed and tack storage and any human-occupied areas. These latter areas can be built to a more residential construction standard, which can physically exclude rodents.

The rodent control effort should concentrate on eliminating access to feed and, if possible, to water supply. Keep feed in containers that rodents cannot chew through. Rodents will chew through thin wood, soft plastic, and fiber materials. A metal trash can with a tight-fitting lid for individual feed bags should suffice for small stables. Once a feed bag is opened, it should be emptied into a rodent-proof container rather than feeding directly from the opened bag. Larger feed storage would be in a dedicated bin lined with sheet metal, fine wire mesh, concrete, or otherwise outfitted against rodents chewing through the container. Feed and tack rooms need concrete floors to prevent rodent tunneling. A concrete floor will facilitate cleanup of spilled feed, which should be disposed of in rodent-proof containers (metal can with lid).

In the stalls and paddocks, containers that provide feed without significant spilling will minimize the amount of discarded grain found in horse-feeding areas.

Materials of construction that are attractive nesting sites, such as loose fill and fiberglass insulation, can be eliminated from the stable design with other more suitable materials substituted, such as rigid board insulation (rigid insulation is also more suitable for the high-moisture environment found in stables). But even after eliminating unsuitable insulation, there will still remain tons of hay and bedding material, horse blankets, rags, and other rodent nesting materials in the barn. Exclude rodents from access to the horse tack storage area to minimize damage.

SUMMARY

Materials of construction used in horse stables and riding arenas are familiar ones, primarily wood, metal, masonry, and concrete. In the horse-occupied area, materials need to be very rugged to survive against horse abuse. Two-inch thick oak plank lining of horse stalls is typical construction. Indoor arenas and horse stables have more interior humidity and dust than found in human-occupied environments, so materials need to maintain integrity while resisting moisture and dust accumulation. Specialty materials, such as strong, waterproof FRP panels, are used in wash stalls and light-admitting translucent panels are used along the upper walls of arenas and stables. Most modern stables and all indoor riding arenas are constructed with clear-span framing using truss, rigid frame, or hoop style. The traditional barn framing using post-and-beam design remains functional and aesthetically pleasing for stable construction.

4
Horse Farm Site Planning

HORSE FARM SITE PLANNING

The overall appearance of a horse facility influences first impressions. Often a certain "look" is conveyed through design detail. Behind the detail is a functional, working layout of the site. Well-functioning site elements emphasize the blending of site features with a layout that facilitates daily horse care and is compatible with (or complements) surrounding environment. The objective of this chapter is to address horse farm site planning topics that emphasize functional layout of the facility. Topics are covered in order of importance, starting with the most essential. The emphasis is on features that are relevant to both private and commercial facilities.

The objective and scope of the horse enterprise determine how the site features fit together into a well-designed plan. Identify goals and set priorities. At a minimum, horse facilities will have the following basic features:

- Shelter for the horse
- Provision of feed and water
- Exercise area
- Manure management

In support of these basic features will be access to the site and storage for feed (bedding), tack, and other equipment. There is great variety in the scope of features found at horse facilities. For example, a backyard private facility will likely have a simple shelter with contiguous turnout (Fig. 4.1). Other private facilities have stables and riding arenas positioned near the residence (Fig. 4.2). In contrast, a commercial stable may have separate vehicle entrances for the owner's residence and the stable complex that contains several buildings. Both outdoor and indoor riding arenas are typically included in the plan.

Clear facility objectives are essential in the planning process. Often the objective will evolve as more information is obtained along with a clearer vision of where one is heading. A decision matrix is offered in Table 4.1 that can help in deciding what type of shelter or exercise area may meet facility objectives. Consider having compatible short- and long-term facility objectives to match anticipated growth of your horse interest and finances. Long-term objectives might be harder to define, but note the high cost of not thinking ahead. For a commercial facility, make the best estimate of farm size and scope by looking as far into the future as you comfortably can. Then double this estimate to allow for expansion. A good plan for twice the anticipated growth can be scaled down to fit current goals and finances while thoughtfully allowing space for appropriate expansion.

There are some general recommendations for how to approach site planning. First, plan on "paper" where mistakes are easy to correct. Developing a good thoughtful plan will be rewarding and cost effective, but time consuming. Second, develop a list of questions and ideas that need additional review. Start by preparing a scale map of the site showing slopes and drainage, utilities (underground and overhead), rights of way, current buildings and condition, traffic access points and major environmental features such as waterways. Try new site plans by overlay ideas using tracing paper or computer drawing layers on your farm scale map. Sketch the expansion facilities onto the site with dashed lines to assure they fit without undue disruption of short-term facilities. Once final ideas take shape, stake out the property with all proposed buildings and driveways, parking and lanes to see how they fit together. Make sure that the facility appearance fits with the surroundings.

Plan on paper where mistakes are easy to correct.

The discussion that follows assumes that the fundamental items that make the land useful as a horse

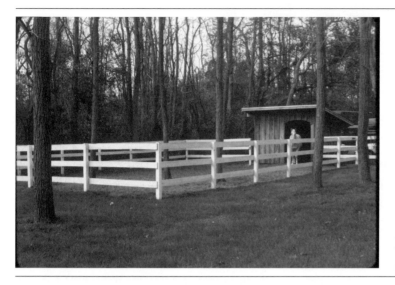

Figure 4.1. Horses may be successfully kept on full-time turnout with access to a simple shelter.

facility have already been satisfactorily established. These fundamental features include zoning and permits that allow horse facility development, acceptable utilities (water, electric, sewer, or septic) on site, sufficient operating labor, and site environment that can support the intended horse activity. Environment features include breezes for summer ventilation and topography with soils that can support buildings and horse activities. A short discussion of each of these items is included at the end of the chapter.

FEATURES OF HORSE FARM SITE LAYOUT

Essential Site Elements

DRAINAGE

Proper drainage considers both surface water flow and groundwater sources. Poor drainage causes more problems than any other farmstead planning factor. An otherwise successful and thoughtful layout can be ruined through lack of proper water

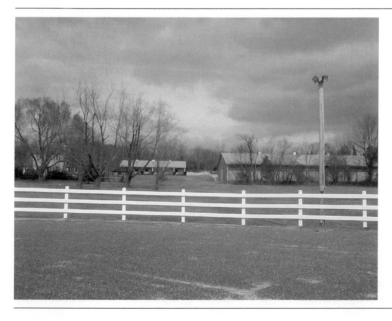

Figure 4.2. A well-thought-out farmstead layout places major buildings in suitable terrain with room for expansion. In this picture, showing an outdoor riding arena in the foreground, the stable (center, backgound) is surrounded by paddocks and placed behind the residence area. An indoor arena is close by on the right. Building locations avoided soils with poor drainage between the two arenas.

Table 4.1. Decision Matrix to Aid in Determining What Type of Shelter and Turnout Fit Facility Objectives

Horse Shelter	
Stable	Shelter in Turnout
Individual stall	Individual or group housing options
Controlled exercise	Self-exercise
Horses easily accessible	Horses less accessible
Cost variable	Less expensive
Labor intensive	Variable labor
Air quality variable	Fresh air quality
Combination of both possible	
Horse Turnout	
Exercise Lot	Pasture
Limited space	Plenty of acreage
Unvegetated	Grass surface
All-weather surface desirable	Grazing feed desirable
Pickup manure	Spread manure
Extra sturdy fencing	Sturdy perimeter and safe cross fences
Daily turnout labor	Pasture maintenance labor
Combination of both possible	

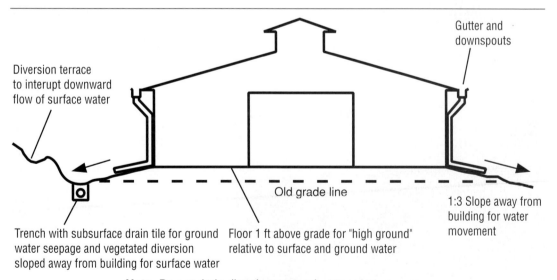

Gutter and downspouts

Diversion terrace to interupt downward flow of surface water

Old grade line

1:3 Slope away from building for water movement

Trench with subsurface drain tile for ground water seepage and vegetated diversion sloped away from building for surface water

Floor 1 ft above grade for "high ground" relative to surface and ground water

Note: Do not drain directly to natural waterways

Figure 4.3. Water handling and drainage features around the stable, indoor riding arena, manure storage, and other farm buildings. Similar features are used to keep excess water off of the outdoor riding arena.

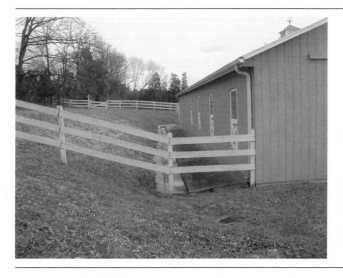

Figure 4.4. This stable was best positioned into a small slope because of drainage challenges at other more level, but lower, sites on the property. A shallow trench lined with concrete diverts surface water and downspout water away from the building foundation and discharges it on the downhill side of the structure via underground pipes.

drainage. Figure 4.3 shows aspects of water handling and drainage around a building site. Fortunately, small drainage problems can often be corrected with grading, ditching, and/or installation of subsurface drains. Improving an entire farm site that has extensive drainage problems is impractical and cost prohibitive. Driveways, parking, and lanes (or access) must be maintained during all types of weather; these are called "all-weather drives."

Poor drainage causes more problems than any other farmstead planning factor.

The best site for buildings and areas of high activity is on relatively high ground on well-drained soil. A well-drained site with reasonably level areas will allow buildings and outdoor arenas to be placed where they best belong, with minimal site preparation. Do not build in a low-lying area! Forego a level but low site with drainage problems for higher ground even if this means more excavation. Figure 4.4 shows improvements for water handling for a well-sited stable built near a small hill. Plan ahead to avoid costly drainage improvements after the building is in place. Even outdoor riding arenas, which are built to be "flat," need drainage considerations during site planning. Outdoor riding arenas need to shed water with a very slight slope and should be constructed so that they do not intercept surface water flow from nearby land (Fig. 4.5). For more detail, see chapter 18.

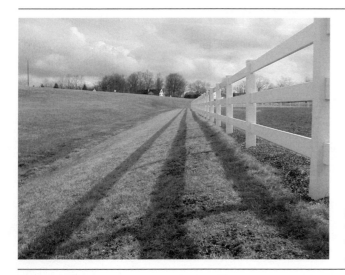

Figure 4.5. A vegetated diversion trench intercepts surface water from flooding an outdoor arena footing and saturating the base.

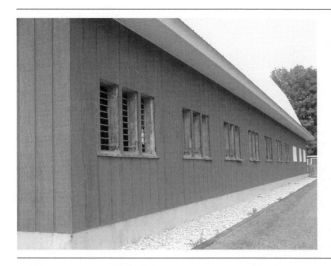

Figure 4.6. Rain run-off and snowmelt from large roofed areas can be handled without gutters and downspouts in cold climates with provision for capturing and diverting large amounts of water at the foundation base, as shown here with a wide swath of graveled French drain.

Periodic flooding around any building is intolerable and avoidable. Prevent water and snowmelt from ponding near buildings, manure storage, or driveways. Slope to shed water away from building sites and intercept incoming water from encroaching the building site. One of the least expensive and effective drainage control mechanisms is the use of gutters and downspouts on buildings. These become necessary on indoor riding arenas and large stables where roof areas shed large volumes of water that are best diverted away from the building pad. Alternatively, in climates with heavy snow and ice dam formation that compromise gutter use, construct so that roof runoff and snowmelt is captured and moved away from the building pad (Figs. 4.3 and 4.6). Consider that a relatively small, 60-foot by 120-foot indoor riding arena will shed more than 2200 gallons of water during a one-half-inch rain event. With an unguttered roof, more than a foot of water will fall on the 1-foot-wide by 120-foot-long ground area along each sidewall. It is best to divert all this water to where it can be handled than to allow it to pool at the building foundation or run off into an undesirable mass of mud.

Pavers for Mud Control

Buildings are located on high ground and additional drainage provided to assure a dry building site. This means that other parts of the farm may be less desirable in terms of water drainage. One way to maintain a grassed area to support horse and light vehicle traffic while accommodating periodic flooding (such as within a groundwater recharge area) or otherwise soggy ground conditions is to install paver blocks or a sturdy grid of rigid material within the grassed surface. The pavers or grid is installed and soil backfilled to be even with top surface of the pavers or grid.

Pavers come in many sizes and shapes that interlock (typical) to provide a porous surface that can support weight of pedestrian, horse, or vehicle traffic. Pavers are often of concrete construction. Grid material of UV-resistant fiber reinforced polyethylene is also available. Water can percolate vertically through spaces within and between pavers or grid material. Some designs have large spaces, while others have very small spaces. Choose a design with spaces small enough so that a horse hoof cannot become entrapped. Spaces within the paver surface need to be less than 4 inch round with a 1- to 2-inch gap preferred so horses can walk over the surface comfortably. Grid material is available that is made specifically for use in horse applications and has spaces small enough to minimize hoof entrapment.

Figure 4.7 shows paver blocks immediately after installation in part of a horse pasture used as a groundwater recharge basin. Grass was established within the spaces of the pavers (Fig. 4.8), while the concrete paver material holds the soil in place on sloped or high-traffic terrain. Figure 4.9 offers a close-up of the paver system selected for use in a horse pasture. The pavers have open spaces (most gaps about 1 inch, in this case) that are smaller than typical horse and foal hoof dimension.

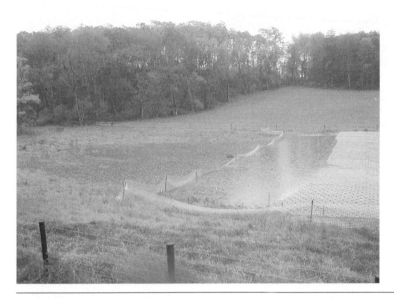

Figure 4.7. Paver blocks interlace for a strong, permeable surface (shown here) recently installed in a groundwater recharge basin in a horse pasture. The temporary fence was removed before horses were allowed back into the pasture. Courtesy of Larry Fennessey.

OFF-FARM FACTORS

Planning features will be influenced by factors other than just the land being developed. Off-farm regulations and consideration of neighboring facilities will play a role in how a horse farm site plan evolves. Legal restrictions and residential developments in the region must be considered. Anticipate growth of neighboring communities and housing developments. Locate building sites with some setback from property lines, even if not legally required, as a buffer for current or future neighbors.

Off-farm regulations and consideration of neighboring facilities will play a role in horse farm site planning.

Poor management may cause nuisances such as flies, odor, noise, and dust that affect neighbor and resident family use of the outdoors. The property line buffer, mentioned earlier, also plays a good management role in allowing some dilution and dispersion of nuisances before they travel out of the property. Good thoughtful layout of the site will

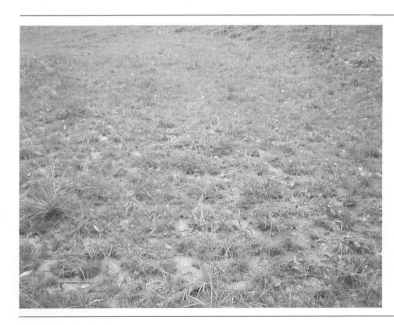

Figure 4.8. Grass will grow through the open spaces of the paver blocks (shown here) or grid material made for stabilizing high-traffic areas of horse paddocks. Courtesy of Larry Fennessey.

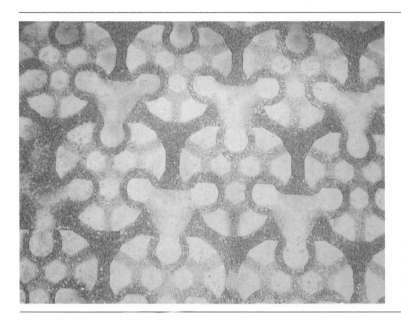

Figure 4.9. Close-up of interlocked paver blocks with small spaces to prevent horse hoof entrapment. Courtesy of Larry Fennessey.

streamline daily tasks to make them easier to properly manage with minimal nuisances. It is easier to avoid nuisance complaints from the start than to respond once a problem is chronic.

Loose horses are a nuisance related to horse facility impact on neighboring properties. Loose horses outside their fenced area are never desirable. In a location with frequent traffic, the consequences can be severe for the horse and owner with resultant liability concerns. Plan fencing construction (substantial horse fence materials on solid posts) and layout that will virtually eliminate the danger from uncontained horses (see chapters 14 and 15). Perimeter fencing, including an entry gate, around the horse complex is recommended so that loose horses are contained at stables with highly valuable animals or near high traffic roads. Even under the best management circumstances, horses may get loose from riders and handlers or escape fencing. The perimeter fencing provides some final containment to help keep the horse on the property.

ACCESSIBILITY

Vehicle traffic will need to get to the site year round. Road building can be expensive but is an excellent investment in the infrastructure of the site. Cars and pickups need at least an 8-foot-wide lane, while tractor-trailer trucks and commercial farm equipment need 12- to 16-foot-wide drives and gates. Good farm roads are necessary for emergency vehicles too. Bridges along main driveways are designed to support heavy vehicle traffic. Farm tractors pulling implements for pasture or manure management can require substantial room to make turns into buildings or fenced areas. Figure 4.10 shows distances needed for large trucks and tractors with implements to make an 180° turnaround. Likewise, large horse trailers and tow vehicles need plenty of firm terrain to safely negotiate turns. To help avoid backing maneuvers, provide a large courtyard or drive-through past stabling and storage areas for drivers towing large trailers. Even at a small private stable, consider where and how to provide convenient turnaround for your own and visiting horse trailers.

Road building can be expensive but is an excellent investment in the infrastructure of the site.

The vehicle entrance is usually a single drive for security of the stable site. Position the manager's house with visibility of the entry drive traffic. Position the entry drive at the municipal road with plenty of visibility of oncoming traffic for safe entry and exit of slow-moving horse trailers. When an entry gate is desired, place it no closer than 40 feet away from the road, with 60 feet preferred, to allow safe off-road parking of entering vehicles as they approach the gate (Fig. 4.11). The entry drive at a commercial property should be about 16 feet wide

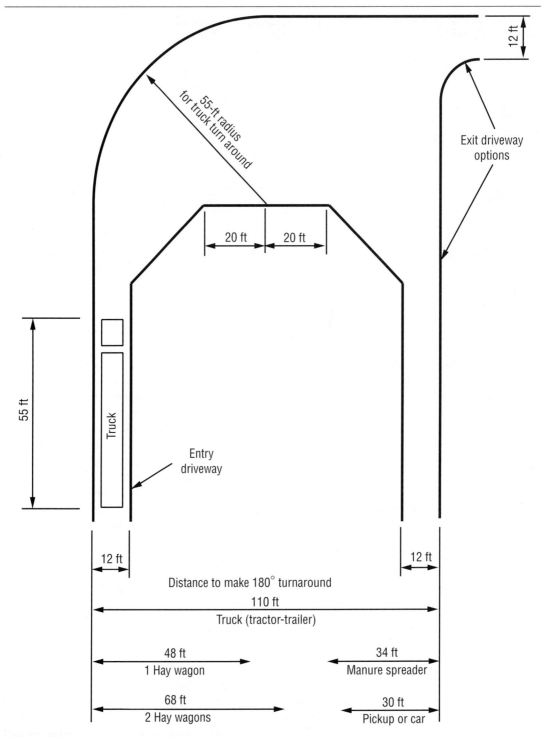

Figure 4.10. Practical 180° turning space for tractor-trailer truck is about 110 feet. Cars and pickups take 30 feet for 180° turn or 34 feet for tractor with manure spreader. Provide 48 feet for tractor with an implement the size of one hay wagon; add another 20 feet for a second hay wagon. Adapted from Fig. 411-6, MWPS-1.

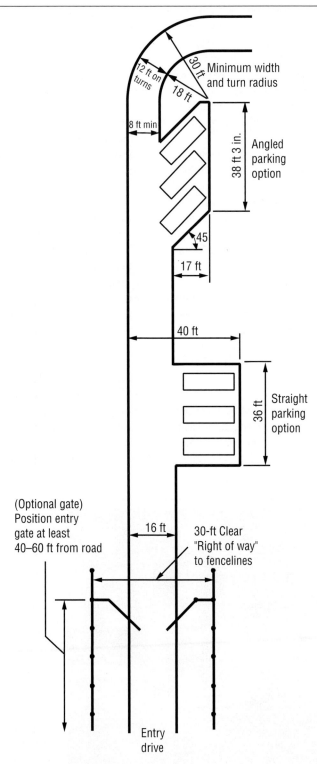

Figure 4.11. Entry driveway and farm lane dimensions, with angled and straight parking options shown. Adapted from Fig. 411-6, MWPS-1.

and allow 7 feet "right of way" on each side for drainage and snow storage. The farm driveway gate will need to be sufficiently wide to allow passage of large farm equipment that may overhang the roadway. For snow and drainage reasons, it is good practice to keep fences at least 5 feet away from other farm lane edges. Plan where to store snow that is plowed from lanes, courtyard, and parking areas (Fig. 4.12).

Provide lanes to storage areas and stable for convenient delivery of hay, feed, and bedding. Access lanes between buildings will allow mechanization of daily tasks and should also provide fire truck access for fire fighting. Fire safety guidelines require that farm drives and bridges need to support the weight of emergency vehicles (20-ton minimum capacity for fire trucks) for buildings to have a chance of being saved from destruction. Chapter 9 has more detail of site layout in relation to fire-fighting equipment access. Similar road and bridge capacities are needed if tractor-trailers are expected in delivery of hay and bedding or for horse transport.

Horse Farm Elements

Regardless of the type of horse facility, there are common attributes of a site plan. Horse farm basic elements include a site for shelter, an area for horse exercise, and storage of feed, bedding, and equip-ment. Manure management will require at least a short-term storage area for one day to four weeks of accumulation. Long-term manure storage of up to one year, composting, or land application sites may also be needed. Some sections of land will be used for driveways to the residence and buildings. Roadways within the farm property, even if informal, are needed to assist movement of hay, bedding, and manure between storage and stable buildings. Provision of feed and water are covered in Chapters 5 and 10.

Shelter

Provide horse shelter against the worst of winds and for some protection during fly season. Provide 100 to 150 square feet of sheltered space for an individually kept horse or 60 to 100 square foot per 1000 pounds for group-kept horses. More space is needed if aggressive horses are kept together. The shelter may be as simple as natural features (for example, a sunshade roof in warm climates) but is more typically a roofed, three-sided shed with an open front directed southward for sun penetration during winter. Consider site prevailing summer and winter wind directions to orient for sun entry but blockage of worst cold-weather winds. Simple shelters are often used in turnout areas so that the horse has free choice of being inside or outside the protection. Most owners relay stories of horses not often using the shelter, but it needs to be

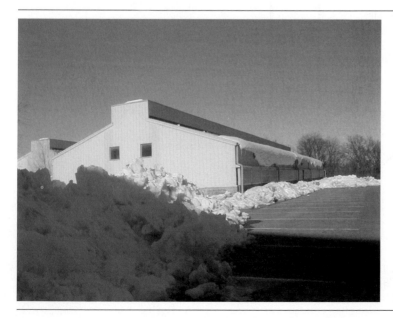

Figure 4.12. In cold climates, adequate space is needed for snow storage around buildings, parking areas, and driveways.

provided to protect animals during occasional periods of severe cold wind and precipitation. Horses also tend to frequent the shed's darkness as protection against flies. Horses with access to natural features such as forest or wind-blocking topography (for example, a large rock outcropping) may find shelter without need for a building.

The shelter may be a horse stable with individual stalls. The stable has long been the standard for horsekeeping but is not necessary for proper horse care. Horses are often healthier and happier in a turnout with simple shelter. However, many people prefer the stable environment for keeping a large number of horses in show or performance condition. Horses are typically housed in box stalls of 100 to 144 square feet with larger sizes provided in some cases, such as stallions, foaling mares, or larger breeds. Chapter 5 has more information on stall layout detail.

EXERCISE AREA

Most horses benefit from regular outdoor exercise at liberty. Turnout needs can be met with relatively small exercise lots. Horses kept on pasture are a common sight. Horse owners need to decide if a turnout area will function primarily as an exercise lot or if pasture forage production will also be expected.

Horses benefit from regular outdoor exercise at liberty.

There is tremendous variability in horse farm objectives and management styles, so that no common effective formula can be offered for turnout routines or the land needed. Some facilities keep horses outside full-time, with simple but effective free-access shelters. At the other extreme, some facilities keep horses indoors most of the time, with very limited and controlled time for turnout. As a sweeping generalization, private pleasure horse farms tend to follow the full-time turnout model, while commercial boarding facilities follow the limited turnout model. Contrary to popular impressions, most horses in the United States are kept in suburban settings rather than rural settings, and so abundant land for productive forage pasture is not always available.

The importance of pasture as the primary feed for horses has diminished with horses being kept on limited land. Turnout areas are often for exercise and are not managed or maintained for pasture grass production (Fig. 4.13). Unvegetated turnout should be designed and maintained as a dry, well-drained paddock, which means implementing a plan for drainage, mud control, and waste removal. See the "all weather paddock" sidebar in Chapter 14 for more information.

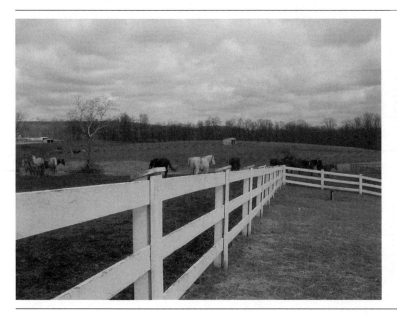

Figure 4.13. Many successful horse farm layouts incorporate a sacrifice paddock area (foreground). The paddock has use in all weather by more horses than vegetation can support in combination with more extensive pastures containing grazing forages and simple shelters (background). An all-weather surface and provision for water drainage from the sacrifice paddock are essential to avoid muck and off-site pollution.

Plan on at least 500 square feet of turnout area per horse. For a single horse, use 10 feet by 50 feet as the minimum size for a run and 20 feet by 25 feet as the minimum paddock size. These dimensions will provide a bit of liberty for the horse to stretch, roll, and romp at moderate speed. Larger paddock sizes are desirable. Fencing for these small turnouts needs to be extra safe and sturdy because horse contact with the fence will be frequent. Additional information on layout for fencing a horse turnout is available in Chapter 14.

> *There is tremendous variability in horse farm objectives and management styles, so that no common effective formula can be offered for turnout routines or the land needed.*

STORAGE FOR FEED, TACK, AND TOOLS

In addition to the building space occupied by horses, provide about 30% more area for storage of feed, tack, and tools (Fig. 4.14). This rule of thumb for storage area capacity is from observation of various facility layouts with good chore

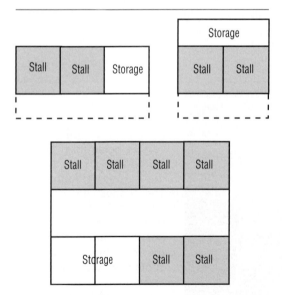

Figure 4.14. Stable storage "rule of thumb" is to provide about 30% of horse stall area as storage. Additional storage space is needed if bedding, large equipment (tractor), and hay will also be stored in the stable.

efficiency and suitable storage space. This storage is for the items used on a daily basis for horse care and recreation. It is far better to incorporate the storage needed in the original plan than to be tripping over tools and feed tubs in the working spaces of the facility. In a small, two-horse stable, all tack, feed, and tools may be kept in the equivalent of a "third" stall. Cabinets and shelving will organize the various supplies and grooming tools used in horse care. In larger facilities the storage for the feed, tack, and tools have evolved into separate specialized rooms. A large amount of additional storage space is needed for an annual supply of hay or bedding (more detail in later section of this chapter).

MANURE MANAGEMENT

Manure management and use have become critical factors for horse owners. Regulations that protect the environment from poor manure management practices are common. Plan a dedicated site for manure storage, and have options for manure removal or use on site. Short-term manure storage will always be needed for several days or for monthly removal, and long-term manure storage of up to one year may need to be part of the manure management plan.

For labor efficiency, locate the short-term manure storage with convenient, year-round accessibility to the stable and paddocks. Manure is removed frequently (often daily) from stalls and heavily used paddocks. Horse manure production is about 1 cubic feet per day per horse. There is great variability in horse stall bedding use and soiled bedding removal, but figure on about 2.5 cubic feet per day per horse of stall waste (manure and bedding). The annual amount of stall waste from one horse is likely to be about 12 foot by 12 foot by 6 foot high.

> *For labor efficiency, locate the manure storage with convenient, year-round accessibility to the stable and paddocks.*

Manure storage must be located on a relatively high, well-drained site where manure pile leachate can be diverted away from nearby water sources. Visual screening, such as a solid fence or tree and shrub plantings, around the manure storage is beneficial from an aesthetic standpoint and can dilute potential dust and odor. Chapter 8 has more detailed information on manure storage placement and design.

Options for manure use include land fertilization and composting. Land application requires access to machinery for spreading manure on suitable acreage and a crop with a nutrient management plan. Composting is a separate operation in addition to traditional horse farm activities, and it provides an opportunity for marketing a manure by-product.

Many horse farms stockpile manure for future handling or arrange for frequent removal from the site. Removal from the site may be via dumpster or truck on a daily or weekly basis. Commercial compost producers may be interested in purchasing horse stall waste if quality and quantity meet their needs. A seasonal stockpile of horse manure may be handled by others who have suitable machinery and cropland.

Because manure can be a site of fly breeding, nutrient runoff, and odor generation, its management is critical to good neighbor relations and environment health. Be sure to plan manure management as one of the first and important steps in the site plan. Have a backup plan. When the local manure hauler goes out of business or his equipment is unavailable for six months, have a backup plan for use and storage of the manure. Even if not yet required by regulation in your location, compose a brief written manure management plan to demonstrate good environmental stewardship.

Include manure management as one of the first important features of the site plan.

Optional Elements

Many horse farm sites incorporate useful facilities in addition to a shelter, which may include a riding arena; bedding and hay storage; machinery, trailer, and equipment storage;, office; and a manager's residence. Specialty farms will have facilities particular to their function, such as breeding and foaling facilities, training track, and veterinary facilities. The more common elements will be briefly discussed. There is a long list of other facilities that may be incorporated into a stable plan including wash stall or trophy display. Amenities such as kitchenettes and laundry offer convenience but are of concern as a source of fire ignition.

Pasture

Pastures with healthy productive grass for grazing will need 2 to 5 acres per horse (in temperate regions of the United States) and effective pasture management for forage production. Management requires knowledge of forage production along with time, equipment, and money. The benefit of pasture can be an economical, high-quality horse feed combined with a healthy exercise area. The pasture acreage needed per horse will depend on the type of soil and its fertility, rainfall and drainage at the site, forage species used for pasture grazing, and the season of the year. Pasture forages are not uniformly productive all year round. Thus, there is a need to provide for hay storage in addition to pasture management. Pastures that are more than 70% grass species will need annual nitrogen fertilization. Legumes, such as clover and alfalfa, fix atmospheric nitrogen into the soil for grass use.

Successful pasture management requires knowledge of forage production along with time, equipment, and money.

Pasture management systems benefit from rotational grazing to allow forage regrowth and improve plant vigor. Divide the pasture acreage into at least three sections so that horses can be kept off each section for about 4 weeks. The regrowth period depends on forage species and rainfall. Move horses off a pasture section into the next section when grass is grazed to a 3- to 4-inch height. Kentucky bluegrass may be grazed down to a 2-inch height. Overgrazing will subdue legume growth and increase weed invasion, while undergrazing allows forage to mature into a relatively unpalatable stage.

Timely mowing of horse pastures is usually required for maintaining good forage quality and quantity. Mowing interval will be similar to that used for residential lawns. Horses are notorious as selective grazers and overconsume the favored grasses while allowing the rest of the pasture to grow into unproductive plants. Overgrazing of preferred sites and inadequate fertilization result in weed and brush infestation in poorly managed pastures.

The intent of this section was to provide an outline of the acreage and management effort needed for successful pasture systems in relation to horse farm site planning. Two sources with more detailed information on pastures for horses are listed in the "Additional Resources" section.

RIDING ARENA

Often a riding area is desirable. The minimum size for most riding arenas is about 60 feet by 120 feet, which allows most cantering horses enough room to safely round the corners. Many outdoor riding arenas are considerably larger than this, as are arenas used for driving horses. The arena site must have a graded pad 2 to 10 feet larger, in all directions, than the actual riding area. Public horse farms often have more than one riding area with indoor and outdoor riding arenas, trails, and training pen. Outdoor riding arenas may have a nearby structure for spectators. For more detail see Chapters 16 and 18, which feature design and construction of indoor and outdoor arenas.

LONG-TERM HAY AND BEDDING STORAGE

Particularly for public stables, it is strongly recommended that long-term hay storage be separate from the horse stabling facilities. With visitors on site who may not be aware of the danger of smoking near hay storage, the potential for accidental hay ignition increases. Post signs and enforce a no smoking policy. Private horse farms should likewise consider separate hay storage, particularly if horses are kept in the stalls more than they are kept outside. A separation of at least 75 feet between hay storage and other buildings is recommended to minimize fire spread from the storage structure to surrounding buildings. Plan on having a few day's worth of hay and bedding short-term storage in the stable or shelter for convenient daily use.

Long-term hay storage should be separate from the horse stable.

Hay storage space requirements are about 200 to 330 cubic feet per ton. Provide straw storage at about 400 to 500 cubic feet per ton. Hay and bedding storage can be of simple construction, with only a roof for moderate protection or enclosed with three or four sides for better protection from precipitation (see Chapter 13 for more detail of long-term hay storage design). However, it must have enough openings to be well ventilated for dissipation of hay curing heat to diminish the risk of spontaneous combustion (for more information on combustion, see Chapter 9). Provide year-round suitable road base to accommodate large delivery trucks (and potentially a fire truck) and convenient access to the storage for easy unloading.

The fire hazard from stored hay should not be underestimated. The fire department is rarely able to save the hay or storage structure once ignited, because forage fires offer intense heat and burn at a very fast rate. Fire departments work to contain the fire but have little chance of putting it out or saving the structure. If the hay storage is your stable, understand the risk.

Hay storage within horse stables rather than in a separate building has strong supporters. The daily convenience of tossing bales down from a haymow into the stalls is undeniable, but at issue is whether this can outweigh the dust, mold, and fire hazard of hay storage in the horse stable. Consider that the overall labor savings may actually be small because a considerable amount of labor (or machinery) may be used to get the hay up into the mow.

For small private stables where horses are outside most of the time, in-stable hay and bedding storage can be tolerated and may be desirable than building another separate hay and bedding storage structure. Recognize that there will be more dust and mold in the stable with overhead stored hay and bedding. At a small stable, a separate hay and bedding storage may be combined with equipment storage as long as care is taken in not allowing hot engine or exhaust components to ignite chaff.

EQUIPMENT STORAGE

Equipment needs on horse farms are minimal compared with other agricultural operations. A small farm tractor or large garden tractor is useful for a variety of tasks at a private stable. Equipment will be needed for managing the pasture and manure, bedding and hay movement, and riding arena footing. Tractor attachments are available for most of these tasks. Particularly for pasture and manure management tasks, outside contractors may be employed rather than investing in all the necessary equipment. Pasture management involves mowing and fertilization equipment. Land application of manure can offset some pasture fertilization needs. Manure handling equipment will be needed for movement and use or disposal of manure. Hay and bedding transport might include overhead conveyors to load a haymow or cart to transport from long-term storage to the stable. Riding arena management involves conditioning, redistribution, and leveling of footing material that are often done by dragging a device over the footing and watering for dust control.

A covered storage area or building for the equipment will prolong equipment life. A dedicated storage also allows for increased security and neat appearance than equipment scattered around the farmstead. Horse trailers will need a dedicated parking area that is convenient for tow vehicle hookup yet out of the way of daily chores.

Horse management still depends on a lot of daily hand labor, and so storage will be needed within the horse shelter for rakes, shovels, and brooms. These are dirty tools and not typically welcome in cleaner places such as the tack room, office, or lounge; so dedicating a space for them is desirable.

LONG-TERM MANURE STORAGE

Annual storage for stall waste (manure with bedding) is approximately 800 to 900 cubic feet per horse. This volume has considerable variation among farms, so use actual numbers from current management style when available. Short-term manure storage is needed on all horse farms, whereas long-term storage may not be needed if the manure is moved off site or used frequently. The long-term storage site needs the same features in relation to location, drainage, leachate control, nuisance management, and environmental protection as discussed earlier in the "Manure Management" section. Often the long-term manure storage is kept distant from the main stabling area for site aesthetics. Manure may be transported on a daily or weekly basis from the short-term storage near the stable to the more remote long-term storage. More information on manure storage design is available in Chapter 8.

PEOPLE AMENITIES

Farms that are open to the public need accessible land for participant and spectator (family member) parking. Plan for access and parking for three potential types of visitors: family guests, business visitors, and heavy delivery trucks (Fig. 4.11). Even a private stable will benefit from extra space for maneuvering horse trailers. For commercial stables, parking should have safe footing and convenient access to the horse housing and riding areas even during darkness. Provide outdoor lighting for visitor safety and for nighttime activities that involve trips to the hay and bedding and manure storage (Chapter 11 has guidelines).

Social functions are often informal at horse facilities, but an area or nook with seating is often well used by patrons and employees. Viewing areas for indoor arenas and lounges are incorporated into some stable facilities. Parents paying the horse board and lesson bills will be well served with a clean, comfortable place to safely view their child's horse activities.

Provide bathroom facilities (sometimes a portable toilet will do) at a public stable or at a horse facility with employees. Otherwise, be ready to open your house bathroom to guests. Potable water for human consumption and water for cleanup are also necessary in a commercial facility. A sink or tap for hand washing and tack cleaning is welcome in any facility. See Chapter 10 for more detail.

Your veterinarian and farrier need bright, comfortable places to work where the horse can be reasonably confined on a nonslip surface. Provide an extra well-lit grooming bay or portion of the work aisle for vet and farrier work, and locate this near a suitable parking area for their vehicle that contains supplies (Fig. 4.15). Some farms install stocks when a lot of routine veterinary care is done, such as with breeding facilities and farms with many horses.

> *Provide the veterinarian and farrier with a bright, comfortable place to work where the horse can be reasonably confined on a nonslip surface.*

Consider an office area for keeping paperwork, conducting business management, and greeting guests. In smaller facilities a portion of the tack room may suffice as an office, while in a commercial facility a dedicated room(s) may be necessary. Offices and lounges are often heated, possibly air-conditioned, for comfort. Tack rooms are often slightly heated for better leather condition during cold, humid conditions. Construction of the office, tack, and lounge areas may be to a residential standard rather than the "barn" construction used in the horse-occupied areas. Even so, the residential-type construction must withstand the rigors of the humid and dusty stable environment. These human-occupied areas have a greater fire hazard and attractiveness to rodents, with the increased use of electric appliances, heaters, and insulation.

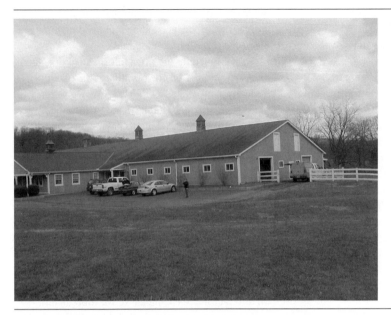

Figure 4.15. Adequate, safe, and convenient parking accessible year round is needed near the stable for staff, guests, and farrier and veterinary care. Driveways also provide delivery and emergency access to buildings.

Most horse farms have a residence for the owner and/or manager. Some have additional residences for workers. Decide what level of interaction is needed between the residence and the horse facility. Consider privacy on "days off" at a public facility balanced with accessibility for routine and emergency horse care. Separate driveways to the residence and horse facility increase separation of private and work functions but can add security risk with an unattended driveway at the horse facility.

FARMSTEAD PLANNING

An affinity diagram can help sort through the many decisions about where farm components need to be located. "Affinity" helps define relationships that farm features have to each other and sets the context for the plan. For example, what needs to be near the stable? Close-by turnout paddocks and short-term manure storage will improve chore efficiency. Long-term hay storage can be farther away, with long-term manure storage even farther. Accessibility can be improved by planning material and horses movement distances.

Versatility

For home-based enterprises, consider construction that can be easily converted to another use should you outgrow your horse interest or decide to sell the property. Clear-span (no interior posts) construction stables can often be easily converted to garage, workshop, or office.

Expansion

Leave room to add onto your facility without major disruption of surrounding buildings or functions. Consider and plan where you would put another stable or indoor arena or add an office wing to the current facility. Leave at least one side of the stable that has open expansion potential.

Livability

You and the neighbors will interact with the environment surrounding your stable layout. Plan for prevailing breezes to move any odor away from activity areas, especially during seasons when people are outdoors more often. Consider the views that you and your neighbors have of the facility and each other, so that privacy is preserved and nuisances are kept to a minimum.

Chore Efficiency

Layout of buildings in relation to material storages (hay, bedding, manure, etc.) will have a long-term impact on daily chore efficiency. Make travel lanes convenient and accessible even during mud and snow seasons.

Example Site Plan

Figure 4.16 (a set of nine figures) shows the development of a site plan that serves as a simple example to demonstrate the use of a scale drawing and affinity diagram that incorporates the above

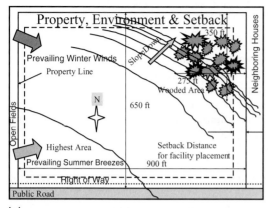

(a)

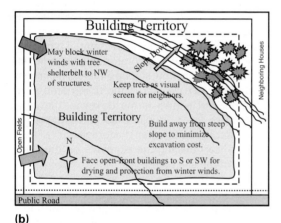

(b)

Site Elements

Turnout & Pasture

Hay & Bedding Storage

Manure storage

Access Drive

Residential Area

House

Stable

Riding
Area

(c)

Figure 4.16. This set of drawings serves as a simple example site plan preparation that demonstrates the use of a scale drawing and affinity diagram. This example is a private farm for six pleasure horses where the facility goal is to have an attractive property with efficient daily chore setup for a busy dual-career family.

(a) First, prepare a scale drawing that shows distances to important features. Include property lines and environmental site features that include prevailing winds, topography, and natural site features such as the wooded area. Note any current buildings and adjoining features that may influence the site plan, such as the public road, neighboring houses, and open fields shown here. Show any legal requirements and utility access that influence the property. Even if not legally required, decide on a setback distance, which may be different on each side, to provide a buffer between your site and neighbor activities. In this case, a larger setback would be considerate on the side with neighboring houses with a smaller setback on the side adjacent to the fields. Plan on the fields being developed and develop this site accordingly. Note the location of high ground at the southwest quadrant of the site.

(b) Start making decisions about where stabling and residential facilities can be built. To minimize excavation and construction cost, build on the more level land at the site. Block out this "building territory" with a layover on the scale map. Decide to keep the wooded area as a visual and sound screen for the neighbors; this is also the least desirable section of land to build on because of the steeper slope. Additional tree windbreak may be added to the northwest section of the property to reduce wind speed and snow blowing onto the site during winter. Attempt to keep the southwest side open for cooling summer breezes.

(c) Here are the basic residential and stabling elements that will be located on the example site. At this stage, some elements may be rough estimates, while others are fairly well designed. For example, the owners have decided on a residential yard area and the basic square footage of house and stable. But they only have rough estimates of desirable turnout acreage and material storage capacities. All areas are simply placeholding shapes for the affinity diagram of how site elements interact with each other. No architectural detail is necessary at this stage but could be included. For example, the stable might end up

Continues on the next page

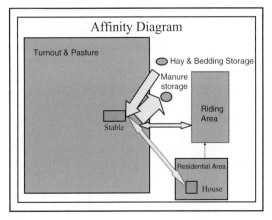

(d)

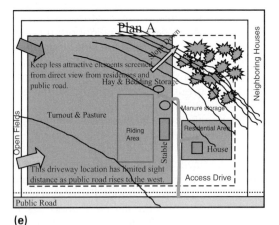

(e)

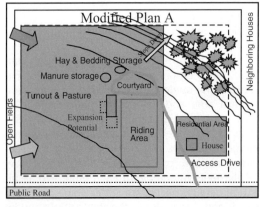

(f)

being more of an "L" shape. The turnout area is not likely to be a large rectangular area in the final design. Subtle differences in shapes and areas should not affect the rough layout of farmstead elements but will be important when the final detailed plan is developed. Whether working on paper or computer, create shapes to scale for the basic site elements. The next step is to create an affinity diagram of how the elements should relate to one another.

(d) Create the affinity diagram. Take the basic site elements, and note which ones need to be near each other and how much activity circulates among them. The stable will have efficient turnout routine if it is virtually surrounded by the turnout paddocks. The manure storage should be close with a one-way flow of a lot of material from stable to storage. Position the manure storage out of sight of homes and the public road. The hay/bedding storage needs to be close to the stable but at a safe distance with one-way flow of material into the stable. The riding arena is usually close to the stable but has less activity than material handling. The house is placed at a comfortable yet convenient distance from the stabling area. The family would like to see activity in the riding area from the home. Not shown is the driveway that provides access to the public road and among the house, stable, and material storages. The next step is to start placing the elements on the scale drawing of the site plan.

(e) Plan A. Try an idea such as locating the residence near the neighboring homes for compatible use and to feel part of the "neighborhood." Locate the stable near the house. Put the manure storage behind the stable so it is out of view of houses and the public road. Site the long-term hay and bedding storage at least 75 feet from the stable for fire safety. Relatively flat terrain is available to the west of the stable for the riding area. Paddocks can surround the stable. The access drive is troublesome. One problem is that it enters the public road with a sight-limiting rise to the west. A second problem is the dead end at the material storages that will require delivery trucks to back up. There is no good place to turn around a horse trailer either. The family would not be able to see most activity in the riding area from the residence. Modifications to Plan A are shown on the next diagram.

(f) Plan A is modified so that riding arena activity can be seen from the house by swapping the locations of the stable and riding area. The access drive is improved by moving it farther from the sight-limiting hill and a courtyard is added for de-

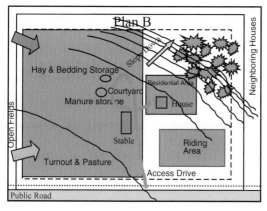

(g)

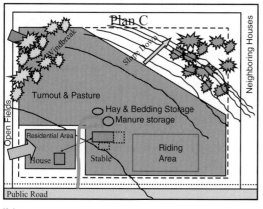

(h)

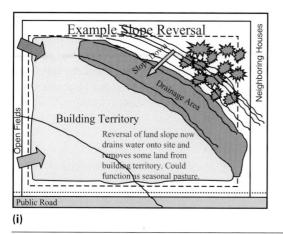

(i)

livery truck and trailer turnaround. Note that the stable will have more expansion potential in its new location. But now the stable is no longer conveniently close to the house and the layout is spreading out at the expense of turnout acreage. The design could be tightened up a bit by placing things closer together. Instead the family opts to move the residence area.

(g) Plan B. The residential yard does not need to be flat for this family's enjoyment and, in fact, there is a nice view into the wooded area; so the house is moved back toward the wooded hillside. This increases the privacy from the neighboring houses too. The riding area may be located in the front part of the property and in view from the house and the stable is again closer to the residence. But more things seem wrong now. The access drive is back in a poor location along the public road and now the house has full view of the manure storage. In addition, prevailing summer breezes put the residential area at risk of nuisance odor.

(h) Plan C. The family decides to locate the house upwind of the stabling complex. They keep the stable about 100 to 200 feet from the house and place the riding area near the stable but in view of the house. The stable has room for expansion around it. The material storages are shielded from resident and public view behind the stable. The manure storage is separated further from the neighboring houses than in the previous plans and has the wooded area as a buffer against nuisances. A windbreak is added for winter wind reduction. A shorter access road is proposed that incorporates a courtyard for delivery truck and trailer turnaround and the drive enters the pubic road at a high point for improved visibility compared with the previous plans. Turnout surrounds the stable. The stable is set back far enough from the road to allow enough room for paddocks along the front of the property. At this point, the planning moves into a more detailed phase where more exact locations and dimensions make the plan even better. Functionally, this plan will allow efficient handling of manure and bedding and provide a tidy, pleasant-looking stabling facility.

(i) To make a point about site drainage, consider the impact of a similar site where the only difference is the direction of the steepest slope of land at the site. If the steep section sloped down to the building territory, some potential building sites are removed from consideration in order to manage surface and subsurface water draining off the high land.

features. This figure offers a series of farmstead planning ideas, with good and bad features noted, in an effort to create a rough working plan that meets the stated goal of the facility.

FUNDAMENTAL FEATURES

The following features all need to be thoroughly explored and thoughtfully approved before a site plan gets any detailed attention.

Regulations

Even the best-laid plans and dreams can go awry if the property cannot be legally used for the intended purpose. Before land is purchased, be sure that horse farm plans are compatible with land restrictions in the area. Before construction starts, plans may need to be approved by local authorities to be sure that zoning and building requirements are met. Be clear about whether your facility is considered an agricultural property, residential with limited livestock (such as horses), or commercial. Know the limits of commercial use if you are boarding someone else's horse on your personal property. There may be lot size restrictions on keeping livestock or regulations on animal density in relation to land area.

Utilities

Sufficient water is essential for horse facilities. Potable drinking water is needed if human consumption is planned; otherwise good-quality water may be used for other purposes such as horse drinking, cleaning, horse bathing, and bathroom use. Ponds are often incorporated into farmsteads for fire-fighting use. Electricity will be needed in commercial facilities but can be a simple convenience, rather than necessity, for small shelters. A means for sewage handling will be needed if a bathroom is included in the horse facility.

Environment

Cooling summer breezes will be welcome at the site. Locate stables and shelters to capture the prevailing summer breezes, and attempt to block the prevailing winter winds with tree shelterbelts. Sunlight penetration and ground slope can aid in dry ground management around buildings. Soil type will not be a dominant feature in a horse enterprise as it is in a farm plan that includes crop production. Nonetheless, suitable soil and gentle topography are desirable for building support and pasture forage production.

Labor

Horse facilities are still quite labor intensive compared with other commercial livestock enterprises. Virtually all horse-feeding and waste removal chores are done by hand. Plan for both availability and timing (daily and seasonal) of labor. The importance of site planning and use of affinity diagrams is primarily in creating efficient labor patterns. Mechanization of water supply to stalls and paddocks is becoming more common with automatic waterers. In stables with limited turnout times, horses are usually individually led to and from paddocks. For large stables, it is not uncommon for a manager's or groom's residence to be included as part of the farmstead plan.

Business Matters

The appeal of many horse enterprises is in the detailed attention to the aesthetics of the farm plan. This image is an important part of the marketing and strategic plan for making a favorable impression on farm visitors. Proximity to customers or a horse industry center may be important to certain commercial facilities. Industry centers have the veterinarians, facilities, and various professionals who support the horse specialties in their area. Consider the commuting convenience of horse owners who would board horses at your facility. There may be an advertising benefit or customer convenience to being located along a well-traveled route.

Existing Buildings

Some proposed horse farm sites may contain farmsteads that were previously used for other purposes. Try to keep the most functional buildings and work the new plan around them. It is expensive to move or demolish buildings. Balance this expense with the compromises in working around a building not suitable to horse facilities. The tendency is to overvalue old buildings. Certainly there is value in preservation of old or historic structures that are in good repair when these can be put to good use for more general purpose, such as machinery or hay and bedding storage.

SUMMARY

Once the scope of the horse enterprise is determined, then short- and long-term goals will evolve for site development. Fundamental features, such as regulations permitting horses, access to utilities, and suitable environment of the site, will need to be determined before any detailed planning can occur. The basic needs of the horse include a shelter, access to clean water and feed, and a fenced turnout area. Manure management will be necessary for proper storage and use of the stall and paddock waste. Storage will be needed for tack and tools, in addition to feed and bedding storage. Consideration of neighbors and other off-farm features often influence plan details. Accessibility among buildings within the site improves labor efficiency.

Once the essential features for horse care are provided, then one can consider the features that make a horse enterprise more livable. Most people picture horses on lush pasture for feed and exercise, although this may not be a reasonable design for many horse facilities. An outline of the management needed in order to maintain productive forage pasture includes mowing, fertilization, and rotation of grazing spaces. Many horse owners will be interested in a place to ride or drive their horse on trails or in arenas. For some horse farms, long-term manure storage and hay and bedding storage will be needed to manage the large quantities of these materials. Likewise, storage for material handling equipment will be necessary. Finally, amenities for the people who work and enjoy the horses at the facility would include an office, lounge, ample parking, and bathroom facilities. Horse farms are quite variable in their scope and objectives; thus no common formula, other than the basic needs, can be offered.

A site plan should be developed through the use of affinity diagrams to make sure that elements of the site that need to be near each other are located properly. The farmstead planning should consider the versatility and expansion possibilities of the buildings and turnout areas. Care in determining chore efficiency will be rewarded in daily time savings. A thoughtful plan will put all the features together in a livable package for you and neighboring properties.

5
Stall Design

The stall is the basic functional unit of a horse stable or shelter. A simple backyard pleasure horse stall may at first appear different from a stall in a full-feature boarding operation, but they both provide a suitable environment for the horse and handler. Safety for handlers and horses should be a primary consideration in stall design. Comfort for the horse is very important, as is convenience for the handler in performing chores associated with good horse care (Fig. 5.1). No matter what your management style or needs, the basics of a safe horse stall are the same. Many options that affect function and cost are available for horse stall features.

This chapter provides an overview of some basic stall features for a typical 1000-pound horse. You should adjust the dimensions for significantly larger stall occupants.

DIMENSIONS

The size of the horse and the amount of time the horse spends in the stall help determine stall size. Larger horses require more square footage than do smaller ponies to be able to turn around, lie down, and get up comfortably. A 12-foot by 12-foot stall is the standard recommendation for a 1000-pound horse. Many stables are successful with stalls slightly smaller than this, but walls less than 10 feet in length are not recommended. Generally, the stall wall length is 1.5 times the horse's length. The more time a horse spends in a stall or the more active it is, a larger stall size is justified. A divider between two standard stalls may be removed to allow more space for a mare and foal or a stall-bound horse (Fig. 5.2).

An 8-foot-high stall partition is standard. Partition height needs to be at least 7½ feet to prevent horses from getting legs over the wall (Fig. 5.3). Most horses can kick as high as 7 feet. An 8-foot-tall by 4-foot-wide stall doorway opening has been the recommendation for years, although this is not often seen in stables. Stall door manufacturers typically supply a doorway opening of slightly over 7 feet with a 42- to 45-inch width. These are the dimensions of the actual open area that the horse can pass through. These smaller doorway openings are adequate for horse and handler safety.

Horse barns are commonly built with a ceiling height of 10 to 12 feet, with 8 feet being the minimum (Fig. 5.4). A low ceiling not only inhibits air circulation but also increases the chance of a horse striking its head. In fact, many stables have open truss or rafter construction with no ceiling. In this case, the minimum height is the clearance to the lowest item on which a horse may strike its head, such as a light fixture or truss bottom chord.

DOORS

Doors come in a wide variety of materials and configurations, although swinging and sliding doors are common (Fig. 5.5). Doors can cover the full length of the doorway opening, be divided into two panels (Dutch door; Fig. 5.6), or can partially cover half to three-quarters of the opening, which is more common with metal mesh doors (Fig. 5.7).

Swing doors should open into the aisle rather than into the stall. Open swing doors decrease aisle workspace but may be latched open to alleviate this problem. They also require less hardware to function properly, but heavy-duty hinges are needed to prevent sagging. Sliding doors, in addition to the overhead track, need a stop to prevent the door from opening too far and falling off the track. They also need floor-level guides to keep the lower portion in place when the horse is pawing, leaning, or kicking at the door. Full-length doors should have less than 3 inches of clearance under them to prevent the horse from getting a hoof or leg stuck (Fig. 5.8).

All doors and doorjambs need to be durable, with secure latches, and free of sharp edges or protrusions. For example, door guides on sliding doors should be rounded and out of the traffic path. Door

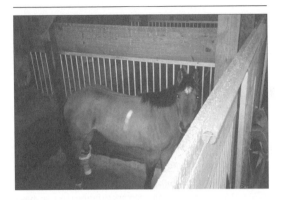

Figure 5.1. The stall is the basic functional unit of a horse stable offering a safe and secure environment that is comfortable for the horse and convenient for the handler.

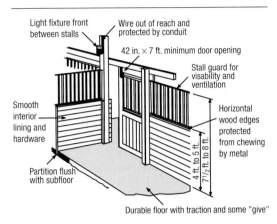

Figure 5.3. Typical box stall construction. Adapted from *Horse Facilities Handbook*.

latches and other clasps that can be operated with one hand are an advantage at chore time (Fig. 5.9). Position door latches out of reach of horses that may find pleasure in learning how to operate them. Horses may try to jump over doors that are half height (such as a Dutch door); however, options are available that allow a horse to hang its head out yet discourage jumping.

LIGHTING AND VENTILATION

Lighting is important for proper care and observation of stalled horses. Shadows and poorly lit areas make stall cleaning cumbersome and inhibit observation and care. For natural lighting, provide a minimum of 4 square feet of window space in each stall. Glass windows should be either out of reach (generally above 7 feet) or protected by sturdy bars or mesh (Fig. 5.10). Plexiglas is a good option for window glazing.

Place electric lighting fixtures along the front or sidewalls to decrease shadows in the stall (Fig. 5.3). One fixture above the center creates shadows as the horse comes to the front of the stall for observation. A 100-watt incandescent or 20-watt fluorescent are suitable electric fixtures. Position fixtures at least

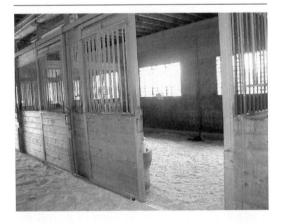

Figure 5.2. Interior partition removed to make one large stall from two regular-sized stalls. Large windows for plenty of natural light. Window glazing is removed for good air movement in warm weather.

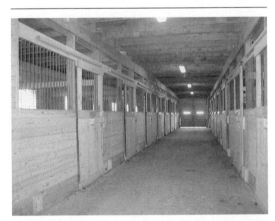

Figure 5.4. Large stable with hay storage in closed loft above a high ceiling. Windows for light and fresh air are provided in each stall. An overhead door provides access to the aisle while sliding doors access each stall.

Exterior Stall Doors

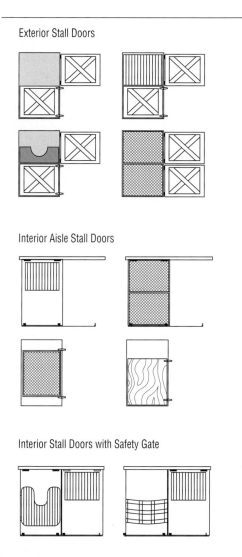

Interior Aisle Stall Doors

Interior Stall Doors with Safety Gate

Figure 5.5. Examples of stall door designs.

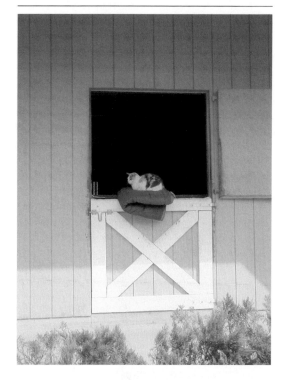

Figure 5.6. Dutch doors are popular horse stable door construction because horses are able to look or reach outside while contained by the lower door partition.

8 feet high to minimize contact with the horse. For further protection, provide a shatterproof cage, which is available at most lighting supply stores.

All electrical wiring in the barn should be housed in metal or hard plastic conduit where horses have access.

Rodents may chew unprotected wires, creating a fire hazard. Metal conduit can be used but has the tendency to rust. Position electrical fixtures out of reach of horses (where possible), children, and pets. More specifications are available in Chapter 10.

Fresh air should be available to every horse for good respiratory health (Fig. 5.11). A window (which opens for each stall), eave and ridge vents, and no ceiling (or at least a high ceiling) will enhance fresh air exchange. Storing hay and bedding over the top of the stalls, where they share the same air space as the horses, is not recommended. Not only are these substances a fire hazard, but they also carry dust and allergens and inhibit air circulation.

Open panels on the tops of stall dividers and open mesh doors help the air circulate within the stall interior. Stalls with solid walls are outfitted with mesh doors to encourage air circulation into the stall (Fig. 5.12). Often, the stable aisles are well ventilated, while the stalls suffer from stagnant air caused by poor air circulation. More information is available in Chapters 6, 10, and 11.

PARTITION DESIGN

Stall dividers are commonly 2-inch-thick rough-cut oak or tongue-and-groove pine. Kicking and

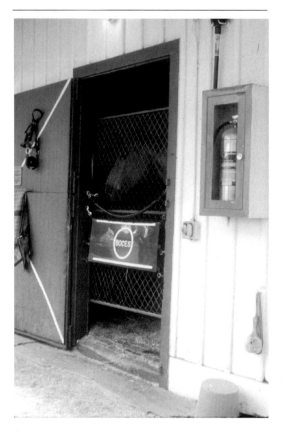

Figure 5.7. Screen stall door with additional solid door. Fire extinguisher is handy.

chewing damage is more obvious with softwoods, with most kicking damage in the lower 5 feet of the partition. Use pressure-treated lumber for the bottom boards in contact with the ground (Fig. 5.13).

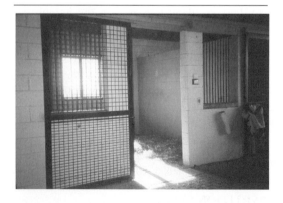

Figure 5.8. Concrete block stall wall construction with full screen sliding door.

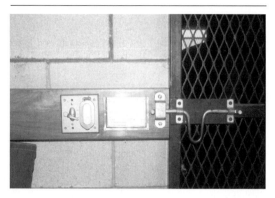

Figure 5.9. Strong secure hardware and protected electrical components are needed around horse stables. Many facilities provide information about horse identity and care conveniently located near each stall door.

Plywood (¾-inch minimum thickness) is a sturdy alternative to boards. Unlike boards, which may shrink, warp, or crack, plywood dissipates kicks, giving it a better strength-to-weight ratio. For a more fire-resistant alternative to wood, concrete and masonry may be used. Concrete and masonry provide strength and durability but have been criticized for thermal characteristics, high construction cost, and unyielding nature against kicks (see Chapter 3).

Stall partitions should be about 8 feet high and be flush with the stall subfloor to prevent hooves from getting caught underneath. Boards can be spaced up to 1½ inches apart to enhance air movement between stalls while discouraging encounters between stall occupants (Fig. 5.14). With spaced boards, use

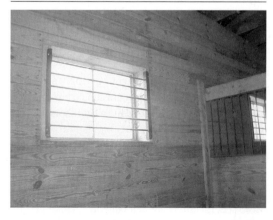

Figure 5.10. Protective bars on stall window.

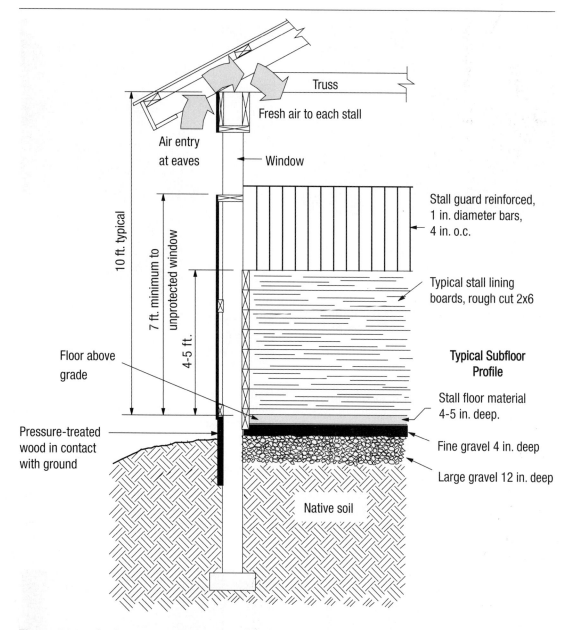

Figure 5.11. Stall cross-section showing typical dimensions and components.

vertical center bracing to stabilize the 12-foot-long wall and prevent the boards from breaking if kicked. Horizontal wooden edges are vulnerable to being chewed by horses unless capped with metal.

Stall walls do not have to be solid all the way to the top (Fig. 5.15). An open panel design at the top allows for better ventilation and easy observation of the horse. It also allows horses to see their compan-

ions and other barn activities to decrease boredom and stereotypie behaviors. An open panel partition has solid materials along the bottom 48 to 60 inches with an open panel on top. Bars of ¾- to 1-inch diameter pipe, or equivalent, are common. Place bars no more than 3 inches apart or use a heavy-gauge wire mesh with approximately 2-inch openings. Metal electrical conduit is not strong enough

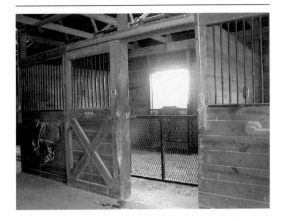

Figure 5.12. Stall with both interior and exterior doors, both of which have two doors. The primary exterior door is a Dutch door and the primary interior door is a sliding wooden door with bars on top portion. A half-screen door is provided at each location for increased airflow. Eave inlet allows fresh air exchange at back wall of stall.

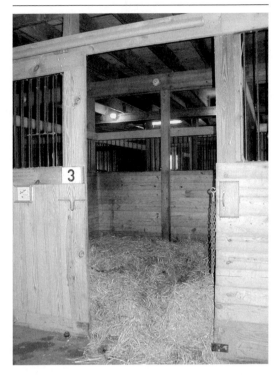

Figure 5.13. Rugged construction for horse stall is needed in material for walls and hardware for securing door. Pressure-treated bottom boards of wall are in contact with ground and manure. Open partition design allows enhanced visibility and ventilation air movement in this stable with two central aisles and four stalls across its width. Note smoke detector above back wall of stall.

for bars. To keep hooves from getting stuck between the openings, be sure the bar material is strong enough so it will not bend when kicked and allow the hoof to go through and be trapped. Table 5.1 provides recommended dimensions for stall bar lengths from 30 to 60 inches that offer enough strength to prevent most horse kicks from bending the bars. Some horses behave better if they cannot see their neighbors, in which case, a temporary solid panel (plywood, for example) can be installed over the bars or mesh.

FIXTURES

Horse stall interiors, including hardware, need to be smooth, rugged, and free of projections. Typical stall fixtures include a water bucket or automatic drinker, feed tub, a ring for tying the horse (Fig. 5.16), and optional items such as a hay rack or ring for a hay net or bag, and environmental enrichment devices (toys). When purchasing stall fixtures, consider cost, durability, ease of replacement, and ease of cleaning, especially for feed and water buckets. Horses are fast, strong animals that have all day to work on the stall components. Choose high-quality, durable hardware for long-term and trouble-free use.

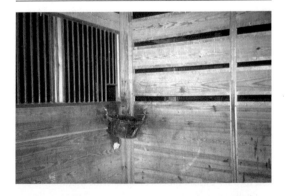

Figure 5.14. Gaps for enhanced airflow formed by spaced boards on stall wall. Boards protected from chewing with metal edges.

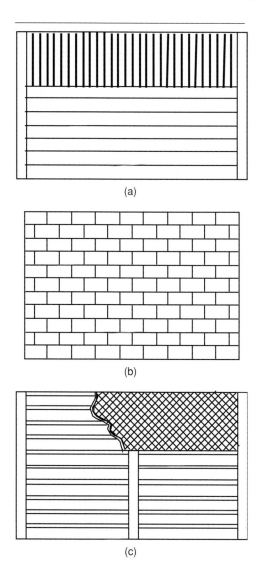

(a)

(b)

(c)

Figure 5.15. Partition design. (a) Solid panel (boards shown) below with stall guard (vertical bars shown) above. (b) Solid panel may be 2 × 6 boards, tongue-and-groove lumber, ¾-inch plywood, or concrete block (shown). (c) Spaced board panel with 1.5-inch air gaps between boards. Panel may be totally solid (shown on left) or with stall guard (wire mesh shown on right). Center wall board support is needed.

Grain and Water

Be sure to separate feed and water stations in the stall (Fig. 5.17). A horse will drop grain into the water bucket as he chews his ration if it is within reach of the feed tub. Water and feed buckets should be fastened to the wall rather than placed on the floor, where they can be tipped over. The bucket rim should be positioned just above horse chest height at nose level. This is low enough to allow the horse to reach it comfortably, yet reduce the chance of the horse stepping in it. Unfortunately, the correct placement of buckets is the ideal height for manure to be deposited in them. Fixtures to hang buckets should be smooth, free of gaps, and fastened securely to the wall. An eyehook and double-ended snap work well for buckets with a bail handle. Some manufacturers provide feed tubs and buckets with hardware for safe and secure wall attachment. The hardware should be equally safe whether the bucket is present or not. Be sure that fasteners allow easy bucket removal for frequent cleaning.

The decision to provide water in buckets or by using automatic watering devices is usually based on cost and management preferences. An automatic drinker is more expensive than a bucket to purchase and install (Fig. 5.18). Drinkers reduce the time needed to complete daily activities but are not a watering "cure-all." Drinkers, like buckets, need to be checked daily to ensure that they are free of manure and contain fresh water. Any watering device needs to be cleaned of algae and debris on a regular basis. Horses will drink more water if they have a clean container with fresh water. Buckets allow water to be easily removed from the stall for post-exercise or treatment purposes and allow you to monitor the horse's water intake. Proper drinker placement is similar to water bucket placement in height and separation from feed tub. Some models allow two stalls to share one drinker.

Select an automatic drinker by considering the strength and maintenance requirements of the materials that will come in contact with the horse, the smoothness of these surfaces, water refill mechanism, and ease of cleaning. Some drinkers require the horse to lower the level of the water to refill it, whereas a refill mechanism that requires the horse nose to open a valve can be difficult or frightening for some horses to use. Valve mechanisms can also become a "toy," and some horses delight in holding the valve open and flooding the stall. In colder climates, protection is needed to prevent waterlines from freezing and breaking. Methods to guarantee against freezing include burying the water lines and providing access to ground heat below the frostline. Heating the barn and/or using electrical heat tape on exposed waterlines

Table 5.1. Recommended Dimensions for Firmly Braced Stall Bars That Resist a Horse Kicking Through

Maximum Span (in.)	Minimum Pipe Dimension		
	Standard pipe size	Outer diameter $\varnothing \times T$, (in.)	Minimum Solid $\varnothing$ (in.)
30	$\frac{3}{8}$	$\frac{3}{4} \times \frac{1}{10}$	$\frac{5}{8}$
40	$\frac{1}{2}$	$\frac{7}{8} \times \frac{1}{8}$	$\frac{3}{4}$
50	$\frac{3}{4}$	$1\frac{1}{8} \times \frac{1}{8}$	1
60	1	$1\frac{3}{8} \times \frac{1}{8}$	$1\frac{1}{8}$

Source: Att Bygga Häststall, en idéhandbok.

Note: Span is bar length above solid stall wall. "Kick safety" of bars depends on more than just the dimensions listed. It also depends on steel quality (modulus of elasticity), free space between bars, how bar is fixed to frame with fastened/welded bars (shown here) four times stronger than loose bars, and height of the wall underneath the bars.

$\varnothing$, diameter; T, thickness.

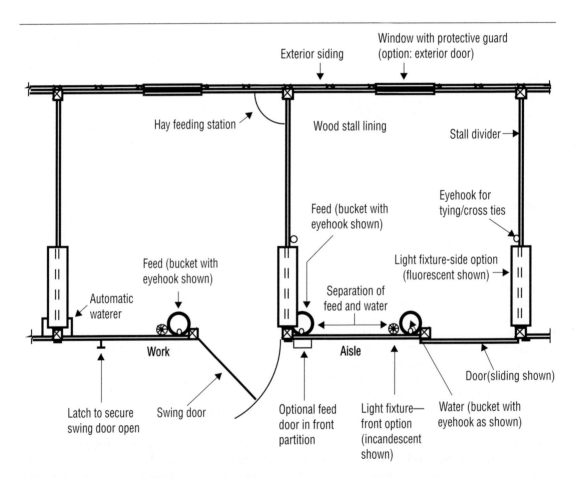

Figure 5.16. Overhead view of horse stall features including options for doors, feed and waterer locations, and lighting fixtures.

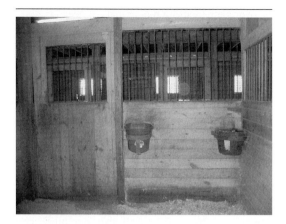

Figure 5.17. Stall with sliding door and separation of feed and water buckets. Water bucket is supplied by an overhead heated and insulated water line with individual valve to fill individual stall bucket.

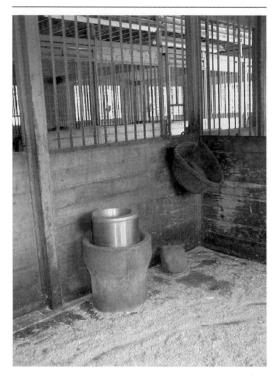

Figure 5.18. Automatic waterer, salt block, and feed bucket at front wall of stall.

are suitable in most circumstances but are subject to failure with utility or equipment malfunction (more information is available in Chapters 10 and 12).

Hay Feeding

The ideal way to feed forage (hay) varies among owners. Hay can be fed directly off the ground, but this method allows the forage to come in contact with waste, dirt, and to be mixed with the bedding. A corner apron of concrete can minimize forage contact with a dirty floor. A primary advantage of floor feeding is that it allows the horse to eat in a natural position.

Hay racks, hay bags, and hay nets can keep forages off the ground. Hay fixtures should be used with extreme caution since a horse's leg may become caught if the horse kicks or rears near the rack or net. Consider the horse's habits, personality, and behavior before selecting a fixture. When a hay rack, net, or bag is used, the bottom end should be at wither height for the horse—too high, and hay dust falls into the horse's eyes and nostrils; too low, and the horse may become tangled. All weld joints on racks need to be strong and smooth with rounded corners.

There is much disagreement over the proper hay feeding station. A hay rack or net is disliked by some owners because of the inhalation and irritation of hay dust and its unnatural position for a horse to eat. An alternative to a rack or net is a hay manger. Mangers let the horse eat in a more natural position, are less prone to trap the horse, and reduce dust fall. A well-designed manger is usually made of wood, starts flush with the floor, and ends above horse chest height. Hay chaff and dust can accumulate in the bottom of the manger and must be removed regularly.

Tie Ring

A ring for tying the horse is often placed at or above horse wither height. Place the ring away from the feed and water buckets and toward the back on one of the sidewalls. This keeps the horse secure when cleaning the stall or grooming and tacking. Be sure the wall is strong enough to withstand resistance from a horse, and fasteners are smooth on both sides of the wall.

FLOORING

Many stall floor options are available and should meet most of the following requirements. Horses are hard on flooring, so it must be durable against pawing and use by a 1000-pound occupant. A good floor has some "give." A floor that absorbs some of the impact and weight of a horse will reduce stress on the horse's legs and ease foot problems. The floor should be nonslip to prevent injuries, especially muscle pulls when the horse tries to stand from a lying position. Slippery floors can inhibit the horse from even trying to lie down.

Since horses have their heads close to the ground for most of the day, a non-odor (ammonia) retentive and nonabsorbent floor is beneficial. Minimize the time needed to clean and maintain the stall floor by choosing a low-maintenance material. No single flooring material seems to have all the desirable attributes. Dirt has "give" but is not durable; concrete is durable but has no "give." Some of the hardness of concrete and other unyielding materials can be overcome by using rubber mats or deep bedding. Sufficient bedding helps prevent sores or abrasions. Rubber mats and clay can be slippery when wet. For more information on flooring, see Chapter 7.

SUMMARY

By following simple guidelines that consider both handler and horse needs, you can provide a pleasant and safe stall environment. Fortunately, there are many good options for horse stall components. For example, doors and flooring materials are quite variable among successful stables. Good, safe, and easily managed stables incorporate the features presented here that address stall size, durability, and horse care. Providing a stall of proper dimensions with a good environment is essential.

6
Ventilation

Although horse enthusiasts have a wide variety of riding and driving disciplines, breeds, and interests, all agree that good air quality inside their horse's stable is important. Veterinarians and professional horse handlers recommend good ventilation for stabled horses to maintain respiratory health. We know that the stable should smell like fresh hay and clean horses rather than manure or ammonia. Yet, failure to provide adequate ventilation is the most common mistake made in construction and management of modern horse facilities. Why would such a universally agreed upon feature be overlooked in stable design? Are we placing human needs over horse comfort? Have building designers and owners lost perspective of the features of a well-ventilated stable? There is a trend toward residential construction practices in horse housing. Horses are considered livestock when it comes to housing design, despite the fact that they are our companions and pets. This chapter outlines proven practices of ventilation that have been successfully used in maintaining good air quality in horse facilities. Although the emphasis is on stables with box stalls to each side of a central aisle, the principles are equally effective in maintaining good air quality in other stable layouts and in run-in sheds or indoor riding arenas.

Inadequate ventilation is the most common mistake made in modern horse facilities.

WHAT IS VENTILATION?

The objective of ventilation is to provide fresh air to the horse. Ventilation is achieved by simply providing sufficient openings in the building so that fresh air can enter and stale air will exit. There are ways to provide each stabled horse with access to fresh air all the time (Fig. 6.1). The stable will have "holes" in it to admit air; it cannot be constructed tight as a thermos bottle like our own homes. Compared with our homes, stables have much more moisture, odor,

mold, and dust being added to the air, not to mention manure being deposited within the facility.

Ventilation is needed to remove heat from the stable in hot weather. It is beneficial to provide a cooling breeze over the horse, which is more comfortable than hot, still air. During warm weather the stable doors and windows are usually open to aid in moving air through the stable. During cold weather the stable is often managed with closed windows and doors to keep chilling winter winds off the horse. In winter, the ventilation goal changes from heat removal to controlling moisture, odor, and ammonia that have built up in the more closed environment of the stable. Moisture comes from horse respiration and other stable activities such as horse bathing and facility cleaning. With moisture buildup comes increased risk of condensation, intense odor, more ammonia release, and pathogen viability, which contributes to respiratory infection.

The objective of ventilation is to get fresh air to the horse.

Ventilation involves two simple processes (Fig. 6.2). One is "air exchange," where stale air is replaced with fresh air, and the second is "air distribution," where fresh air is available throughout the stable. Proper ventilation provides both; one without the other is not adequate ventilation. For example, it is not good enough to let fresh air into the stable through an open door at one end of the building if that fresh air is not distributed throughout the horse stalls. Nor is proper ventilation satisfied if a tightly closed stable uses interior circulation fans to move stale air around the facility.

COMMON VENTILATION QUESTIONS

What Are Comfortable Conditions?

A horse's most comfortable temperature range is between 45 and 75°F. Our most comfortable human

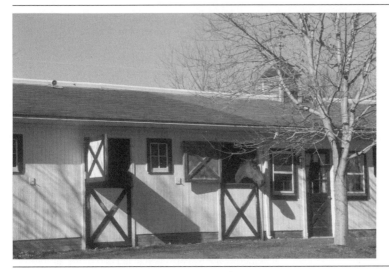

Figure 6.1. Horse stables have obvious door and window openings to maintain fresh-air conditions during most weather. This stable also provides openings that are always open at the ridge vent and cupola and along the eaves of the building so that even during the coldest weather, when doors and windows are closed, there is still some fresh air exchange.

temperature is at the upper end of the horse comfort zone. Clearly, horses tolerate cold very well and adapt to chilling breezes when housed outside. If conditioned to cold weather, horses with a long-hair coat and adequate nutrition can withstand temperatures below 0°F. Even show horses with a short-hair coat can be maintained in a cold but dry indoor facility when provided with blankets and hoods. Within a box stall, horses have the freedom to move away from uncomfortable conditions.

What Is a Well-Ventilated Stable Going to Feel Like?

The stable environment in winter is almost as cold as outdoors but comfortably dry with no condensation dripping from the structure. Cold and humid conditions are uncomfortable for both horse and human and lead to a stuffy, dank environment within the stall. On first entering a stable, make an objective evaluation about its air quality before you have adapted to those conditions. In hot weather, the stable temperature will be within a few degrees of the outdoor temperature and more comfortable because of shading from the sun.

During winter, horse stables should be kept no more than 5 to 10°F warmer than the outside temperature. This guideline helps assure fresh air conditions, but it also means freezing will occur inside stables in northern climates. It is a management mistake with regards to air quality and to your

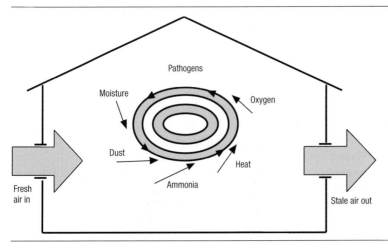

Figure 6.2. Air exchange (fresh air in and stale air out) and air distribution (movement of fresh air to all portions of the stable) are the two ventilation processes.

horses' health to close the barn tight just to keep conditions above freezing in cold weather. If condensation is chronic on interior surfaces, then the stable is too closed off for proper ventilation.

Horse owners often want warm stable conditions for their comfort during horse care activities. Instead of heating the whole barn or cutting off ventilation to trap horse body heat, provide a heated grooming and tacking area. If freezing conditions cannot be tolerated, then supplemental heat will be needed in susceptible areas, such as the tack room or washing and grooming areas. Frost-proof, self-draining hydrants (Fig. 6.3) and freeze-proof automatic waterers are available. Water pipes within the stable need to be buried to the same depth as supply plumbing to the stable site.

What about Drafts?

A draft occurs when cold air blows on a horse. Warm air blowing over a horse is not a draft. Since horses tolerate colder conditions than humans, what we consider drafty is not necessarily uncomfortable to the horse. Be sure to differentiate between cold temperature and draft. A main principle of ventilation is

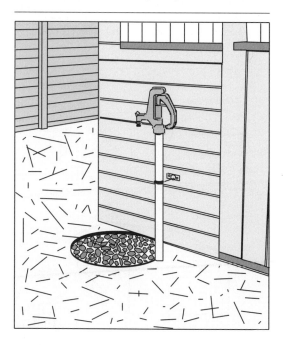

Figure 6.3. Design detail for freezing conditions, such as the self-draining water hydrant, will be needed in most horse stables located in cold climates.

that even very cold fresh air can be introduced into a horse stall, so that when mixed and tempered with stable air, it no longer has the air speed and chill of a draft. Consider a horse outside and the amount of wind speed it comfortably tolerates, and realize that normal air currents of good ventilation in a stable are of little consequence.

What about Air Distribution within the Stable?

An open, unobstructed interior helps move air around the stable. Provide airflow between the openings in the stable where fresh air enters and stale air exits. Fresh air is brought into the horse stalls where it picks up moisture, heat, dust, and ammonia and can exit out another opening. Stuffy stables, and their poor air quality, are the product of limited air exchange and/or obstructions to getting the fresh air to where the horses are stalled.

> *An open, unobstructed interior gets fresh air to the horses and provides an exit path for stale air.*

> *Go into the horse stall to determine the air quality of a stable.*

Go into the horse stall to determine the air quality of the stable. Moisture, odor, and ammonia are generated primarily in the stalls, where fresh air is needed for horse respiration and to dilute air contaminants. Since most dust and ammonia are down near the bedding and manure, check air quality near the floor as well as at horse-head height (Fig. 6.4). Floor-level air quality is particularly important for foals or when horses eat at ground level and spend time lying in the stall. It is not uncommon for the stable's working aisle to be breezy and well ventilated while the stalls suffer from stuffy conditions.

How Much Ventilation Should Be Provided?

Natural ventilation is often expressed in "air changes per hour." An air change per hour (ACH) means that the total volume of air in the stable is replaced in an hour's time. Six air changes per hour means a complete air change every 10 minutes. Horse stable resources interested in good stable air quality suggest that 4 to 8 air changes per hour be provided to reduce mold spore contamination,

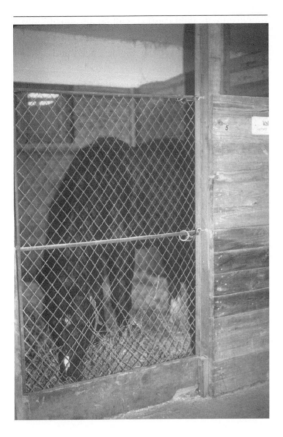

Figure 6.4. Getting fresh air to where the horse is located is the primary objective of ventilation. Go into the horse stall to evaluate air quality in the horse stable.

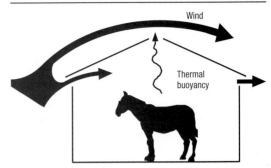

Figure 6.5. Horse stable ventilation uses architecture with openings along both sidewalls and ridge to accommodate the two forces behind natural ventilation: thermal buoyancy and wind.

minimize condensation, and reduce moisture, odor, and ammonia accumulation. For comparison, the modern home has ½ air changes per hour from infiltration through various cracks, such as around doors and windows. This recommendation for stable ventilation is substantially more than the average residential air exchange rate to maintain fresh air conditions and good air quality in the more challenging stable environment.

How is Ventilation Provided to the Structure?

Natural ventilation is used in horse stables and riding arenas. Wind and thermal buoyancy (hot air rises) are the natural forces that drive this type of ventilation (Fig. 6.5). Natural ventilation uses openings located along both sidewalls and ridge (roof peak) to accommodate these air movement forces. At least two openings are needed; one is not enough. (Fig. 6.6

shows the building terminology used in this book.) Openings along both sidewalls are more important than the ridge opening if stable design cannot accommodate both ridge and sidewall openings. Interestingly, even open front-shelters need an opening on the back sidewall to effectively distribute fresh air throughout that seemingly very open structure design (Fig. 6.7). The stable ventilation system will work better when both ridge and sidewall openings

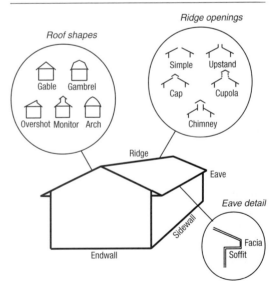

Figure 6.6. Building terminology used for describing ventilation system design and functions.

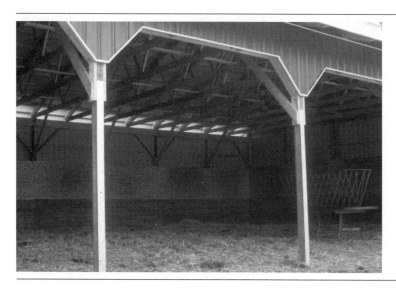

Figure 6.7. Sidewall openings on both sides of a building are key for natural ventilation function. Even an open-front shelter, with the whole front area opened, needs a back eave opening to ventilate properly.

are provided. The ridge opening allows warm and moist air, which accumulates near the roof peak, to escape. The ridge opening is also a very effective mechanism for wind-driven air exchange, because wind moves faster higher off the ground.

Wind is the dominant force in horse stable natural ventilation. With the variability in wind speed and direction, openings on the stable will frequently alternate between being an inlet for fresh air and an outlet for stale air. Wind will push air into the stable through openings on the windward side of the building while drawing air out of the stable on the leeward, or downwind, side. Once the wind speed is more than about 1 mph, wind-driven ventilation will dissipate the effects of thermal buoyancy in horse stables.

Since horse stables are typically unheated, they are considered "cold" housing. Thermal buoyancy (hot air rises) is dependent on a temperature difference between the warmer stable interior, where the horses' body heat will slightly warm the surroundings, and the cooler outside conditions. Because a properly ventilated stable has less than a 10°F difference between the stable interior and outside conditions, there is not a large temperature difference as a driving force for buoyant air movement.

What about Using Fans?

The other major type of ventilation is mechanical ventilation, which uses fans, inlets, and controls in a pressure-controlled structure. Mechanical ventilation is typical in some types of livestock housing (poultry and swine housing of young animals) where barns are heated to high temperatures (70 to 90°F) for animal well-being. Tight control of ventilation rate is needed in these heated livestock buildings to maintain constant and uniform temperature. Mechanical ventilation is not commonly needed in horse stables. Natural ventilation is adequate for housing animals, such as horses and cattle, which are tolerant of a wide range of temperature conditions. Mechanical ventilation is more expensive to install and maintain but offers control over the air exchange rate. Heated stables benefit from the controlled mechanical ventilation exchange rate during the heating season. Each fan has a known capacity in cubic feet per minute (cfm) and provides a uniform air exchange rate.

Minimum mechanical ventilation recommendations for each 1000-pound horse are 50 cfm for moisture and air quality control in cold weather, 100 to 200 cfm for heat removal during mild weather, and at least 350 cfm during hot weather. Inlets are sized at 1.7 square foot per 1000 cfm of fan capacity; expressed another way, this inlet sizing is 24 square inch per 100 cfm. Mechanical ventilation operates as a system with a fan(s) creating a static pressure difference between the interior environment and outside conditions. This pressure difference is the driving force for air movement and is maintained around 0.05-inch water gage for a

Table 6.1. Mechanical Ventilation Fan Capacity and Inlet Size per Horse Compared with Natural Ventilation Objectives[a]

Ventilation Rate		Inlet Area Needed
ACH	cfm/horse	in.[2]/horse
1	25	6
2	50	12
4	100	24
8	200	48
16	400	96

ACH, air change per hour; cfm, cubic feet per minute.

Note: 1 ACH of a 12 × 12 ft^2 floor area × 10 ft ceiling height stall volume = 1440 ft^3/stall/hr = 24 cfm/stall.

[a]Mechanical ventilation inlet sized at 24-in.^{2} opening per 100-cfm fan capacity; static pressure difference of 0.05-in. water; inlet air speed 800 fpm for mixing.

ventilation system suitable for a horse stable or riding arena. Air enters the building in a properly designed mechanical ventilation system at about 800-fpm (feet per minute) velocity for good air mixing and distribution into the stable. The stable must be managed so that air will enter the building only through the inlets designed to provide fresh air. In most cases this means all doors and windows are closed when the fans are operating.

Inlets are sized as shown in Table 6.1. Table 6.2 provides fan capacity and inlet sizing for an example six-horse stable. Inlets are best positioned throughout the structure for more even distribution of fresh air than providing one large inlet. Locate an inlet within each stall at the eave so all horses get some fresh air. When the fan is operated continuously, then the inlets can be simple holes left permanently open. Self-adjusting inlets will be needed if the fan will cycle on and off (on a timer with two minutes of ventilation and three minutes off, for example) or when there is variation in the amount of air exchange (variable speed fan or more than one fan stage). See the "Additional Resources" section for sources of more information on mechanical ventilation equipment and system design. Larger openings are provided on naturally ventilated buildings because the air is not typically entering at as fast an air speed as needed by a mechanical ventilation system.

An older recommendation of 25 cfm per 1000-pound horse for air quality in cold conditions is a very low ventilation rate resulting in just 1 ACH for a single stall (Table 6.1). To put this previous cold weather ventilation rate into perspective, it has been determined that 15 cfm per person is enough to keep a house from smelling stale or stuffy. This recommendation has been developed as houses are built to

Table 6.2. Example Mechanical Ventilation Fan and Inlet Design for Six-Horse Stable[a]

		Six-Horse Stable Example				
Ventilation Rate		Total		Slot Inlet Area		
ACH	cfm/horse	Ventilation (cfm)	Inlet Area (ft^2)	Total (in. × in.)	Each Stall (2 in. × in.)	Each Stall (1 in. × in.)
1	25	150	0.26	2 × 18	2 × 3	1 × 6
2	50	200	0.51	2 × 36	2 × 6	1 × 12
4	100	600	1.0	2 × 72	2 × 12	1 × 24
8	200	1200	2.0	2 × 144	2 × 24	1 × 48
16	400	2400	4.0	2 × 288	2 × 48	1 × 96

ACH, air change per hour; cfm = cubic feet per minute.

Note: 1 ACH of a 12 × 12 ft^2 floor area × 10 ft ceiling height stall volume = 1440 ft^3/stall/hr = 24 cfm/stall.

[a]Mechanical ventilation inlet sized at 1.7-ft^2 opening per 1000 cfm fan capacity; static pressure difference of 0.05-in. water; inlet air speed 800 fpm for mixing.

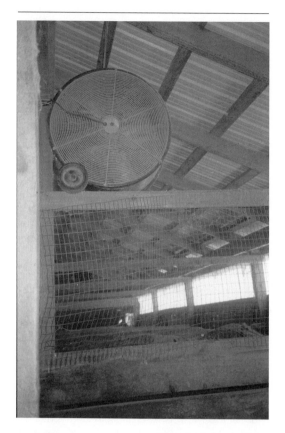

Figure 6.8. Stables without adequate air movement can use circulation fans to supply wind speed over horses in key locations. Choose fans that have motors and components that can tolerate the dust and humidity of horse stables. Fans, such as the one shown, are marketed to the agricultural and horticultural markets.

tighter construction standards and natural air leakage has been virtually eliminated. The 25 cfm per horse recommendation is not even double the residential human ventilation rate. The 25 cfm per horse minimum rate is too low to truly maintain fresh stable conditions considering that daily each horse respires the moisture (2 gallons per day) created by a typical residential family of four (respiration, showers, cooking, etc.). In horse stables, additional moisture and gases from feces and urine need to be removed. Proponents of natural ventilation suggest a minimum of 4 ACH to maintain good air quality in horse stabling; this would be an excessive rate for a heated barn (fuel expense in heating incoming air)

but not unrealistic for unheated, mechanically ventilated stables.

What about Using Fans to Move Air around the Stable?

Circulation fans may be used in stables for temporary relief to disrupt warm, stale areas or to provide a cooling breeze over the horse's body (Fig. 6.8). These fans move air already in the stable so they do not provide more fresh air to the horse. A properly designed stable ventilation system (natural or mechanical system) should virtually eliminate the need for circulation fans.

Another application of mechanical ventilation uses a fan blowing air into a duct to distribute fresh air throughout a part of a stable where direct access to outside air is difficult (Fig. 6.9). This duct system can be used in retrofitting older barns and is particularly effective in the underground portions of bank barns where access to fresh air is limited. Ducts can also effectively distribute supplemental heat in a barn. Chapter 12 provides duct design details.

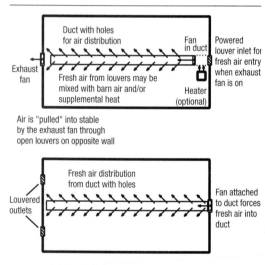

Figure 6.9. Overhead view of two mechanical ventilation systems with fan and duct used to distribute air. Top diagram shows distribution duct for a combination of fresh, heated, and/or recirculated air. Exhaust fan system draws air into stable through louvered inlet on one wall and discharges stale air on the opposite wall. Bottom diagram shows fresh air distribution with no recirculation. Louvered outlets provide stale air exit.

RECOMMENDATIONS FOR PROVIDING EFFECTIVE NATURAL VENTILATION

Permanent Openings

Furnish stalls with some sidewall openings that are permanently open year round. Each stall should have direct access to fresh air openings. A guideline is to supply each stabled horse the equivalent of at least 1 square foot of opening into its stall to allow ventilation even during the coldest weather. The best location for this permanent opening is at the eave (where sidewall meets roof). A slot opening along the eave that runs the entire length of the stable is often used (Figs. 6.10 and 6.11).

There are several benefits of a continuous slot opening at the eaves. The slot opening provides equal distribution of fresh air down the length and on both sides of the stable, providing every stall with fresh air. The opening's position at the eave, 10 to 12 feet above the floor, allows the incoming cold air to be mixed and tempered a bit with stable air before reaching the horse. The long slot inlet is desirable during cold weather, because air enters the stable through a relatively narrow opening as a thin,

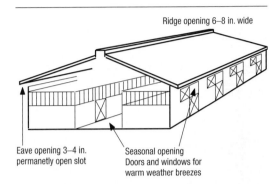

Ridge opening 6–8 in. wide

Eave opening 3–4 in. permanetly open slot

Seasonal opening Doors and windows for warm weather breezes

Figure 6.11. Perspective view of ventilation openings on a central-aisle stable. Eave inlet slot runs entire length of sidewall. Ridge vent shown has simple opening with upstand.

cold, and fresh sheet rather than as a large, drafty mass as provided by an open window or door.

Each stall should have direct access to fresh air openings that are open year round.

A minimum guideline for cold climates is to provide at least 1 inch of continuous-slot, permanent opening for each 10 feet of building width. For a 12-foot-wide stall, a 1-inch-wide continuous slot will supply 144 square inch, or 1 square foot, of permanent opening. This 1-inch opening per 10-foot building width is one-half that recommended for successful natural ventilation of livestock housing, which uses a minimum 2-inch opening per 10-foot building width. Typical livestock barns (freestall dairy housing, for example) have about three times the amount of animal body weight per floor area and similar increases in moisture and manure gas as found in horse housing. Therefore the above recommended minimum opening for horse stables (1 inch per 10-foot width) provides greater opportunity for fresh air quality in the stable than that found in typical livestock housing.

One functional and recommended inlet design, shown in Figures 6.11 and 6.12, incorporates 3 to 4 inches of permanent opening at the eave on each sidewall of a center aisle stable (36 feet wide). This is slightly above the minimum recommendation and works well to ensure a well-ventilated stable during cold and cool conditions when other stable openings (doors and windows) are often kept closed. Figure 6.13 shows an indoor riding arena

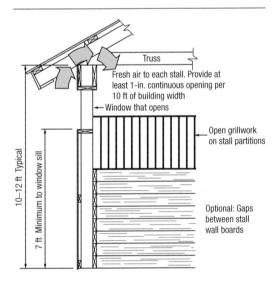

Truss

Fresh air to each stall. Provide at least 1-in. continuous opening per 10 ft of building width

Window that opens

Open grillwork on stall partitions

10–12 ft Typical

7 ft Minimum to window sill

Optional: Gaps between stall wall boards

Figure 6.10. The best way to provide draft-free fresh air to each horse stall is through an opening at the eave. Figure shows a cut-away view of stall components and eave opening. The eave is open year round with additional, large warm weather openings provided by opening windows and doors.

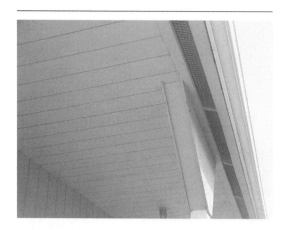

Figure 6.12. Eave vents protected with wire mesh of large openings are a good option to provide for fresh air into stables during all weather. Here the 4-inch opening on the breezeway soffit is matched by an equal-sized opening on the opposite sidewall eave.

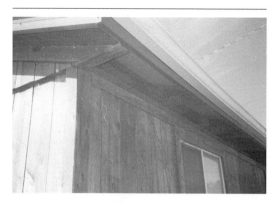

Figure 6.14. Do not be afraid to provide plenty of permanently open fresh air vents to the stable. This eave inlet is 13 inches wide, on a 16-inch overhang, on a 32-foot-wide stable in a cold climate. Ridge opening is also provided and the stable environment has excellent fresh air quality year round.

eave equipped with a permanently open 4-inch-wide vent for year-round air exchange and fresh air distribution throughout the arena. Some stables and arenas have larger permanent openings, sporting a 13-inch eave vent opening on a 16-inch eave overhang and a 6-inch opening at the ridge (Fig. 6.14). These vents are open all year.

Other stables outfit the eave opening with a hinged panel so that the opening size may be partially closed during extreme cold weather (Fig. 6.15). It is open the full 6 inches all summer and reduced to a 2-inch

slot in the winter by swinging a 1 × 4 board over part of the opening. Do not cover more than 75% of the eave opening and only do so during severe weather. In foaling stalls, during moderate climates, a 2-inch by 7-foot-long slot may be installed about

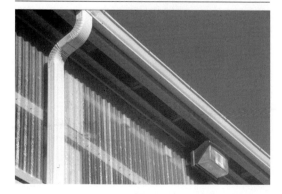

Figure 6.13. Riding arenas also need fresh air exchange year round, which is easily provided by eave inlet openings.

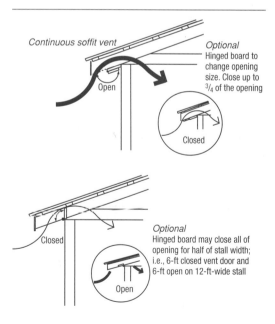

Figure 6.15. Options for eave inlet openings where variable opening size is desired.

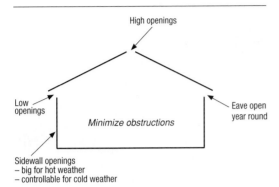

Figure 6.16. Natural ventilation construction features include high and low openings, some of which are open year round. Larger openings provide hot weather air movement.

20 inches above the floor to guarantee fresh air at foal level. This gets the foal off to a good start.

Seasonal Openings

In addition to the permanent openings for cold weather, another set of large openings allow cooling breezes to enter the stable during warmer weather (Fig. 6.16). Stables with interior central aisles have large endwall doors that are opened for this function. When horses are kept indoors during warm weather, allow breezes to enter the horse stall through windows or doors that open from the stall to the outside (Fig. 6.17). Provide openings

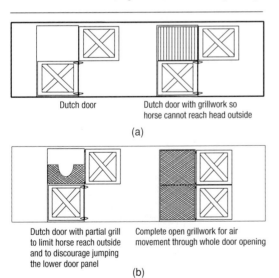

Figure 6.17. Options on exterior stall doors to provide warm weather ventilation openings.

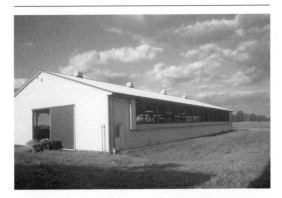

Figure 6.18. Stable with island design of stalls with exercise aisle around perimeter. Stable has sidewall curtains for air and light entry.

equivalent to at least 5% to 10% of the floor area in each stall. For a 12-foot by 12-foot box stall, sufficient openings would be a 3-foot by 2½-foot open window for 5% opening or 4-foot by 3½-foot open window (or top of Dutch door) for 10% opening.

Figures 6.18 to 6.21 show a movable curtain for providing large sidewall openings to stables or riding arenas. The curtain is a strong tarp-like material that is moved with a manual winch, although it could be easily automated. When translucent curtain material is used, there will be natural light addition to the stable or arena interior. The curtain material

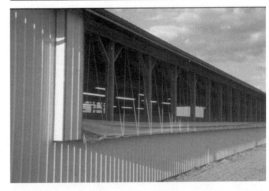

Figure 6.19. Strong, translucent curtain material is raised and lowered over the top portion of the sidewall. Permanently open eave vents on top of curtain provide ventilation even when curtains are fully closed during colder weather.

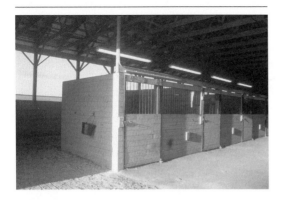

Figure 6.20. Interior view of a racehorse stable that has stalls set up in an island configuration but with central work aisle. Sidewall curtain opening admits plenty of light and fresh air to the facility.

can be solid, as shown, or a porous mesh (similar to shade cloth used in greenhouse applications) that buffers wind velocity but allows fresh air entry. The curtain is often installed on the top third or half of the sidewall height in horse facilities although it could provide an opening as large as the entire sidewall height. The curtain material is not horse sturdy and needs to be protected from horse contact. An open curtain allows for great air exchange and essentially allows the building roof to act as a sunshade during hot weather.

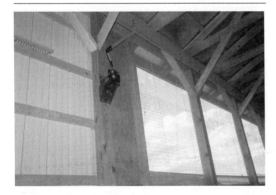

Figure 6.21. A hand-activated winch moves curtain up and down for less or more fresh air entry, respectively. Even with curtain closed, a 5-inch opening at eave admits fresh air during all weather. Curtain movement can be automated.

Stable Ventilation Openings

Figures 6.22, 6.23, and 6.24 provide recommendations for the minimum acceptable cold weather openings and warm weather options. Greater openings at the eaves, except for the coldest days, are desirable to assure good air quality within the stable during cold and cool weather. If sufficient ridge vent is not provided, then double the eave vent opening sizes. Center-aisle (Fig. 6.22) and single-aisle (Fig. 6.23) stables are easy to properly ventilate.

The recommended ventilation openings for a double-aisle stable, with four rows of horse stalls across width (Fig. 6.24), attempt to overcome the shortcomings of this building design. The central

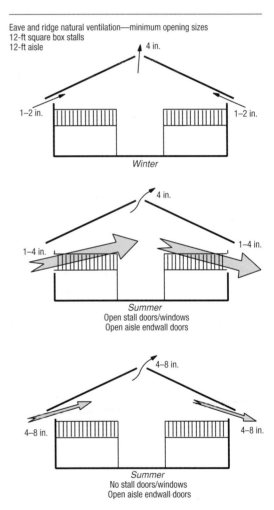

Figure 6.22. Recommended ridge and eave openings for center-aisle stable with stalls on both sides.

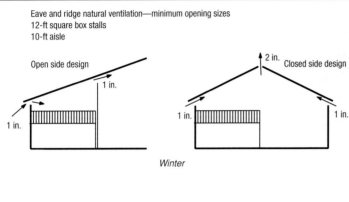

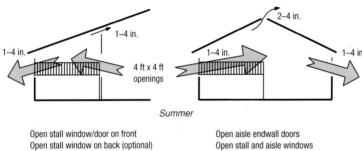

Figure 6.23. Recommended ridge and eave openings for single aisle stable with stalls facing an outside work aisle.

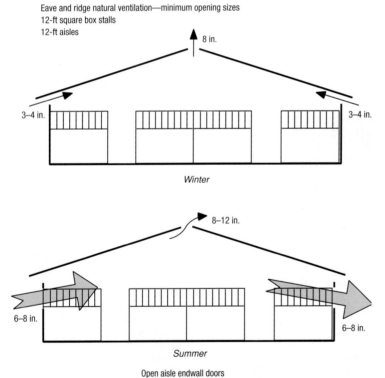

Figure 6.24. Recommended ridge and eave openings for double-aisle stable with four rows of horse stalls across width. The central stalls in the four-row layout will get almost no fresh air because they are not near a fresh air opening.

stalls in the four-row layout will get almost no fresh air, because they are not near a fresh air opening. Ventilation in these central stalls will be particularly compromised if stall walls are solid without grillwork on the top portion. With solid stall walls and a ceiling over the central stalls (for storage), there will be no fresh air movement into those stalls. This double-aisle layout is not recommended when horses will be kept inside more time than turned out. Daily stall cleanout will be important to keep ammonia and odors from accumulating in the central stalls. It is particularly important that this building design contain an open interior (and no ceiling and open grillwork on stall walls) so that fresh air can move freely (Fig. 6.25). Similar improper airflow is seen in stables that share a common sidewall with indoor riding arenas. The horses near the arena sidewall will have no access to fresh air unless openings are provided on that side of the stable.

Avoid Restrictions to Airflow

The permanently open sidewall eave openings should be constructed to be as open as possible.

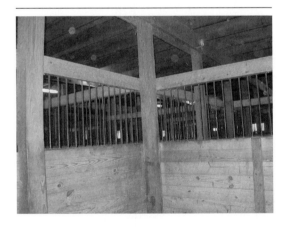

Figure 6.25. A double-aisle stable, which has four rows of stalls across the interior, has opened up the middle two rows of stalls with grillwork at the top of the stall walls and a relatively high ceiling. Fortunately, horses are turned out most of the time. Allowance for air distribution throughout the middle portion of this stable design is particularly important because these stalls do not have direct access to fresh air as the outer stalls along the sidewalls.

Ideally, they are left completely open. Do *not* cover with residential window insect screening or metal soffit treatments. Both these coverings severely restrict desirable airflow and will soon clog with dust and chaff, eventually eliminating almost all airflow (Table 6.3). Metal-sided buildings are commonly finished with metal fascia and soffit, so tell your builder that you need the ventilation air exchange at the eaves and leave off the soffit metal. The perforated metal soffit was designed for residential and commercial attic ventilation applications where the need is about one third of even the minimum airflow for horse stables. Residential soffit has very tiny holes to exclude insect entry, but it will clog with dirt and dust within months if installed in a horse stable. In addition, attics are almost dust free compared with horse stables. To discourage bird entry at the eaves, wire mesh squares of approximately ¾ to 1 inch may be installed. Since birds will enter the facility through larger openings such as doors and windows, wire mesh on the eaves is not necessary. Similar logic applies to fly entry.

Ridge Vent

Ridge opening area should match the eave opening area with a minimum of 1 square foot of opening per horse. The same recommendation for the eaves (providing at least 1 inch of continuous slot opening per 10 feet of building width) applies to the ridge opening. If no ridge opening is provided, then supply double the minimum recommended eave opening (supply 2 inches of continuous eave opening per 10 feet of stable width if no ridge vent is used). Similar to cautions raised about eave openings, be sure to avoid residential and commercial ridge vent assemblies that are overly restrictive to air movement. Insect screens restrict airflow. Remember, you are ventilating a barn and not a house attic—not only is more air exchange needed, but also the stable dust will clog small screen openings. Ridge vent assemblies from natural ventilation equipment manufacturers that specialize in agricultural buildings will offer relatively unrestricted airflow with protection from precipitation. Figure 6.26 shows several commercially available ridge vent assemblies. Some are useful in horse stable ventilation, while others restrict natural ventilation airflow. Several

Table 6.3. Open Area and Effective Area for Ventilation through Eave Inlet Treatments

Open Area (%)	Diagram	Description	To Provide 1 ft² of Opening	Effective Area
100		Simple opening	1 ft²	Recommended. Full area allows airflow.
87–94		Opening covered with 1-in. square wire mesh or poly bird netting with ¾ × 1⅛ in. openings	1 to 1.1 ft²	Recommended. Slight but acceptable restriction to air moving through mesh.
80–84		Opening covered with 2 × 2 mesh hardware cloth with ½-in. openings	1¼ to 1½ ft²	Potential for chaff, insects, and freezing condensate to clog the openings.
66		Residential insect screening 18 × 16 mesh per in.² with 0.05-in. holes	1½ to 2 ft²	Not recommended. Too restrictive to airflow and small holes will clog with dust.
43		Undereave louver or slot-vented soffit with ⅛th to 5/16th-in. slots	2½ to 3 ft²	Restrictive to airflow and often includes an insect screen, which will clog with dust.
4–6		Soffit vented with ⅛th-inch punched holes	16 to 25 ft²	Not recommended. Designed for house attic insect exclusion. Provides almost no airflow and will clog with dust within months.

Note: Some soffit coverings are so restrictive to airflow that greatly increased soffit area is needed to provide 1 sq. ft. of inlet area per stall. Tight screenings and small holes will clog with dust within months of installation, providing almost no airflow through opening.

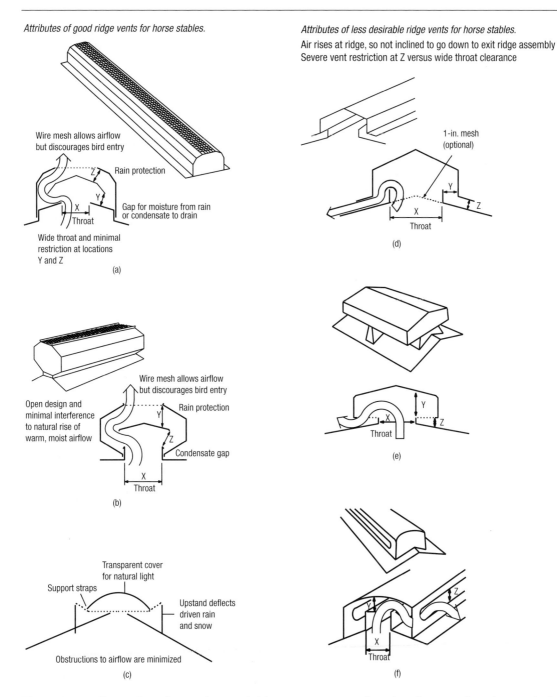

Attributes of good ridge vents for horse stables.

Wire mesh allows airflow but discourages bird entry

Rain protection

Z

Y

X

Throat

Gap for moisture from rain or condensate to drain

Wide throat and minimal restriction at locations Y and Z

(a)

Open design and minimal interference to natural rise of warm, moist airflow

Wire mesh allows airflow but discourages bird entry

Rain protection

Y

Z

Condensate gap

X

Throat

(b)

Transparent cover for natural light

Support straps

Upstand deflects driven rain and snow

Obstructions to airflow are minimized

(c)

Attributes of less desirable ridge vents for horse stables.
Air rises at ridge, so not inclined to go down to exit ridge assembly
Severe vent restriction at Z versus wide throat clearance

1-in. mesh (optional)

Y

X

Z

Throat

(d)

Y

X

Z

Throat

(e)

Z

Y

X

Throat

(f)

Figure 6.26. Examples of manufactured ridge vent construction showing opening sizes and airflow path. The narrowest part of the airflow path, at location Z, will influence air movement. Agricultural ridge vent assemblies (6.26a, b, and c) may be used in horse stables. Some commercial or industrial building ridge vent assemblies may be used on horse stables (6.26d, e, and f), although they are moderately disruptive to natural ventilation air movement. Residential ridge vents are not recommended (and not shown here) since they do not provide enough opening for horse stable ventilation and are prone to condensation, freezing the opening shut.

ridge vent designs incorporate transparent or translucent materials to allow natural light entry into the stable.

The actual ridge opening is measured at the most restrictive part of the ridge vent assembly. Manufacturers often supply the throat opening where the bottom of the ridge vent attaches to the building interior, but the key measurement for air movement is where the airflow path is narrowest. This narrowest restriction is shown at location "Z" of the vent assemblies of Figure 6.26. Some of these designs, particularly (d) and (e), prevent warm, moist air from naturally flowing upward and out of the building ridge vent when no wind is blowing. Warm, moist air flows up and is not inclined to move downward to get out of the ridge vent assembly. This air trapped in the ridge vent will not only

block ventilation but may condense, leading to dripping or freezing during cold weather. The simplest and most effective ridge vent is an unprotected opening at the ridge (Fig. 6.27). The building trusses or rafters are protected from precipitation and the stable interior is managed so that occasional rain entry is tolerated. Figure 6.27d shows a ridge opening with vertical upstand boards on each side of the opening that increase air movement through the ridge opening.

The ridge vent can be a continuous opening or a series of intermittent vent assemblies spaced uniformly along the structure. During winter, a portion of the vents can be closed to provide only the recommended permanent opening area, while all the vents are opened during warmer weather when more air exchange is needed.

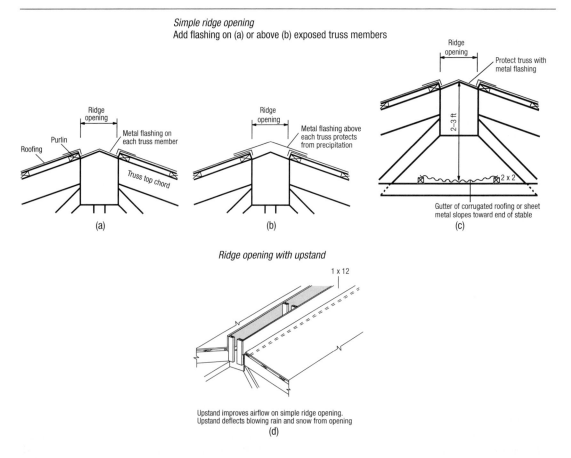

Figure 6.27. The simplest and most effective ridge opening is an unprotected opening. Four design options are shown. From *Natural Ventilating Systems for Livestock Housing.* MWPS-33. MidWest Plan Service, Ames, Iowa. 1989.

Ridge Opening Options

The ridge vent does not have to be a continuous opening, although this offers the most benefit in uniform air quality within the stable. Cupolas are a popular architectural feature in many stables, and they can be used as a ridge opening (Fig. 6.28). Measure the open area at the most restrictive construction of the cupola, which is often at the louvers. A cupola may have a 3-foot square opening into the stable area that offers 9 square feet of ventilation opening, but make sure that the louvers above this opening also have at least 9 square feet of effective open area. Louvers commonly block 50% of the open area they are protecting. Be aware that some cupolas are purely decorative and have no way for stable air to move through them. For visual balance of the cupola with the stable size, provide about 1 inch of cupola width for every foot of roof length. Most cupolas are square in width at the opening to the stable and tall rather than wide. For example, a 48-inch-square by 80-inch-tall cupola will look properly proportioned on top of a 30- to 36-foot-wide by 40- to 60-foot-long stable (Fig. 6.29).

In stables with a ceiling, chimneys are a popular construction for moving air from the stable area and exhausting it at the roof peak (Fig. 6.30). The vertical duct of the chimney travels through the roof or

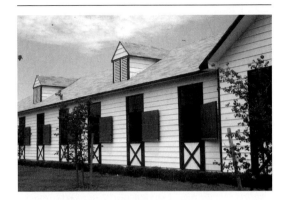

Figure 6.29. This stable offers ridge ventilation via louvered horizontal "cupolas" on the roof design. Mild weather fresh air is admitted to each stall via Dutch doors with top portion open, as shown. When the bottom portion is likewise opened, a full-screen mesh door prevents the horse from exiting while allowing entry of plenty of fresh air. Glass plastic panels above each door admit light year round.

upper story of the stable (attic or hay mow). When chimneys run through an attic or mow, insulate the chimney walls to R-10 to discourage condensation as the relatively warm stable air is ducted through the cold areas. The chimney exit must extend at

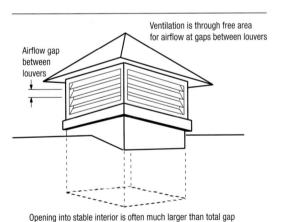

Figure 6.28. Cupolas are a popular horse stable design feature and can provide ridge ventilation if sufficient louvered openings are provided. Ridge vent assemblies that are made for livestock building ventilation are a good option for unrestricted airflow.

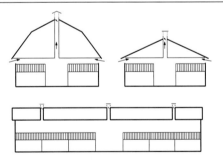

Figure 6.30. Chimneys are useful as the high opening on stables with ceilings. Provide chimney opening equivalent to $\frac{1}{2}$% to 1% of stable floor area with a minimum 2-ft square chimney size for one-story buildings and minimum 4-ft square for two-story buildings. A damper, controlled via cable from below, is useful in cold climates. The damper with 90% closure is located near the top of the chimney to keep the shaft charged with warm air for more controlled airflow.

least 1 foot above the building peak (i.e., stable air is not discharged into the attic or mow).

Condensation and Insulation

Condensation occurs when moisture is released from air as it cools in contact with a cold surface. Insulation is used to keep potentially cold surfaces near the interior building temperature, reducing condensation. Unheated barns need R-5 insulation at the roof to discourage condensation on roof steel, even under well-ventilated stable conditions. Condensation not only leads to annoying dripping but also shortens the life of metal and wood roof materials. Shingle roofs over plywood construction provide an insulation level near R-2. A 1-inch thickness of polystyrene provides R-5 insulation value and is resistant to moisture absorption. Polystyrene also has good vapor barrier properties, although each rigid board joint needs to be sealed against moisture movement.

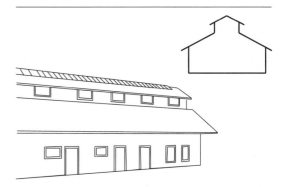

Figure 6.31. Monitor roof design offers high openings via soffit vent and/or windows that open near the roof peak.

Sizing of the cupola and chimney opening is the same as for continuous ridge vent (at least 1 square foot of opening per horse housed) with additional chimney requirements for proper airflow being no smaller than 2 feet by 2 feet for one-story buildings and 4 feet by 4 feet for two-story buildings. On a long stable, it is better to provide more than one cupola or chimney at approximately 50-foot intervals. Avoid screening cupolas or chimney openings other than to discourage bird entry (approximately 1-inch square wire mesh).

A monitor roof (Fig. 6.31) offers high openings at windows that open near the peak. Vent area can also be provided along the soffit at the eaves of the monitor section. Light from the windows along the monitor roof is another benefit of this roof design.

The Breathable Wall

An additional way to allow fresh air exchange in a stable is the breathable wall concept. With barn board siding there are thin cracks between the boards that allow a bit of air movement at each juncture. This is known as a breathable wall. Battens added to the boards will reduce this effect, as will tongue-and-groove siding. Modern construction with large 4-foot by 8-foot (and larger) panels have

eliminated the breathable wall via eliminating the cracks (large panel construction requires eave and ridge vent to replace the crack openings). Taking a look at an older barn, much of its informal ventilation was through the airy nature of the breathable wall provided by the barn siding. The air coming in the cracks is nicely uniform throughout the structure and by being such a tiny air jet, is quickly dissipated, thereby not becoming drafty.

Comfortable and uniform fresh air conditions can be maintained within the stable, even under windy conditions. Some stables are still built with this deliberate breathable wall concept. Siding boards may be butted tightly against each other and still leave a very narrow gap, or in moderate climates the vertical barn boards are spaced ¼ to 1 inch from each other. Rough-cut green lumber may be attached as siding. Once dry, gaps will provide diffuse ventilation. From the stable exterior, the breathable wall siding looks solid and well constructed. From the stable interior, sunlight can be seen penetrating between the boards indicating that air can enter (Fig. 6.32).

THREE DESIGN FEATURES TO IMPROVE HORSE STALL VENTILATION

Remember that the objective of ventilation is to get fresh air to the horse. Getting fresh air into the stable is the first important step for good ventilation; the next is distributing this fresh air to the stall occupants. Air distribution within the stable is improved by an open, airy interior. The horse stalls provide obstruction to getting air to where the horse

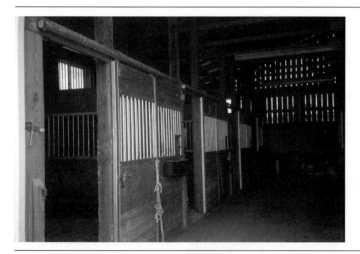

Figure 6.32. Stable interior showing airflow gaps of the breathable wall siding at end of stable aisle. This stable has other good ventilation features, including eave and ridge vents, a window that opens for each stall, open grillwork on stall partitions, and no overhead airflow obstructions.

is, but a solidly built stall is necessary for safe confinement of the horse (Fig. 6.33).

Open Stall Partitions

Ventilation air movement is greatly improved by providing openings for air to flow in and out of the stall (Fig. 6.33). Open grillwork on the top portion of front and side stall partitions is highly recommended than solid stall partitions. Open partitions provide benefits beyond the obvious improvement

in ventilation. Open partitions allow horses to see each other for companionship, which is important for this social animal. Open partitions improve management by allowing the caretaker to see horses from almost anywhere in the stable. Horses are less prone to be bored and develop bad habits in a stable with open partitions, because they can see other horses and stable activities. A horse in a stall with limited visibility of stablemates and activities is in virtual solitary confinement. See

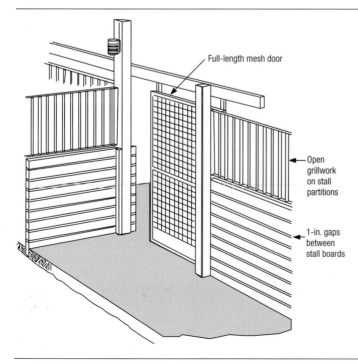

Full-length mesh door

Open grillwork on stall partitions

1-in. gaps between stall boards

Figure 6.33. Features that improve air movement into and out of the horse stall include gaps between partition boards, open grillwork on upper portions of stall partitions, and door with full-length open grillwork. Adapted from *Horse Housing and Equipment Handbook*, MWPS-15. MidWest Plan Service, Ames, Iowa. 1971.

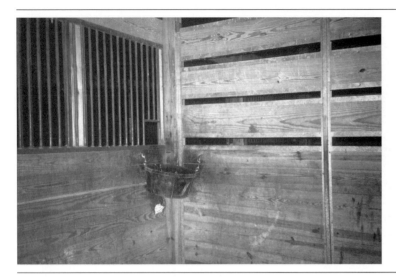

Figure 6.34. Stall wall with gaps for improved air movement within the stable when solid walls are used between stalls.

Chapter 1 for more information on the nature of horses.

Admittedly, some horses are a hazard to their neighbors. A reason to provide solid sidewall partitions is to decrease bickering between horses in adjacent stalls. One option is to provide open grillwork throughout the stable but cover the grillwork partition with a panel (i.e., plywood or spaced boards for more air movement) for unneighborly horses.

With solid sidewalls, the front stall wall becomes more important for stall ventilation. Provide openings for air movement into the stall with 1- to 2-inch gaps between boards in the solid portion of the stall wall (Fig. 6.34) and/or a full-length wire mesh stall door (Fig. 6.35) or stall front. The mesh stall door or front is particularly effective in providing air movement to the stall interior.

For isolation stalls and specialized buildings, such as veterinary practices and some high-traffic breeding facilities, solid washable partitions between stalls may be desirable. Solid walls will limit air distribution around the stable interior. Provide fresh air access in each stall and an airflow path for stale air removal. A mechanical ventilation system with fan and ducted air can be used to con-

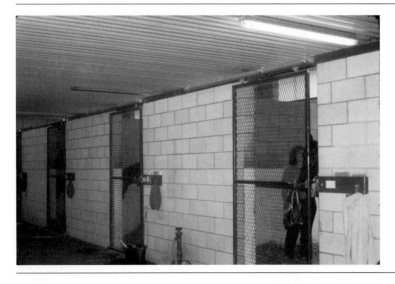

Figure 6.35. For stable designs that chose to have solid sidewalls, and in this case solid front walls, the ability to get fresh air into each stall is limited. In these cases use full mesh doors, high ceilings, windows, and eave and ridge inlets to ensure fresh air entry to each stall to provide as much internal air distribution as possible.

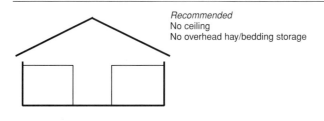

Recommended
No ceiling
No overhead hay/bedding storage

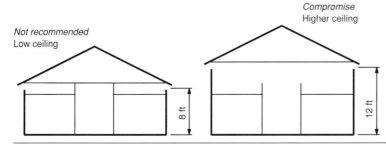

Not recommended
Low ceiling

Compromise
Higher ceiling

8 ft

12 ft

Figure 6.36. It is recommended to have no ceiling with ridge vent at roof peak. Avoid stable design with low ceilings, which inhibit airflow within the stable.

trol air exchange and to limit air mixing with the rest of the stable environment. In most applications, the natural ventilation principles using fresh air openings for each stall and ridge vent should be sufficient.

No Ceiling

When the interior has no ceiling and is open to the roof peak (and ridge opening), more air exchange and distribution can occur. If a ceiling must be used in a stable, position it at least 12 feet above the floor to allow air circulation (Fig. 6.36). Stables with ceilings, and particularly low ceilings, appear more confined and are darker than an open, airy structure (Fig. 6.37).

No Overhead Hay and Bedding Storage

To improve air quality and distribution, do not incorporate overhead hay and bedding storage in the stable. If hay and bedding must be stored overhead, construct the storage over the work aisle so that the horse stall has no ceiling and air is better circulated (Fig. 6.38). Leave at least 3 feet of clearance between the height of overhead stored items and the roofline to allow an airflow path to the ridge opening. Ridge openings above overhead hay storage

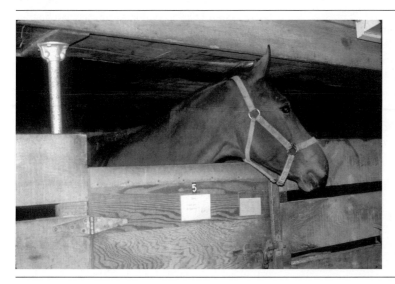

Figure 6.37. A low ceiling, as shown, is never deliberately designed into a horse stable; but with some old barn conversions, one is handicapped by original construction. Be sure to provide plenty of airflow via gaps between stall wall boards and ducted fresh air if necessary. In this case, the horses were not confined to the barn for long periods.

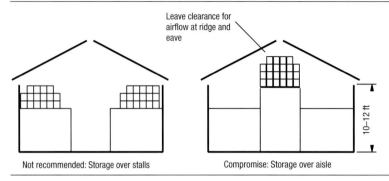

Leave clearance for airflow at ridge and eave

Not recommended: Storage over stalls

Compromise: Storage over aisle

10–12 ft

Figure 6.38. Do not store hay and bedding overhead. By eliminating overhead hay storage, the stable will have increased air movement within the stable and reduced dust and fire hazard. As a compromise, provide storage over the aisle to maximize airflow to the horse stalls.

should not allow precipitation or condensation to fall onto the forage.

The most often cited reason to eliminate overhead hay-bedding storage is for decreased dust and allergens in the stable. Managers of redesigned stables, where the hay and bedding are now stored in a separate building, provide testimony to the decreased dust irritation. Dust, chaff, and molds rain down on the stalled horses from overhead hay storage.

When the overhead hay storage is completely separated from the horse area with a full ceiling, dust and mold generation is minimized for the horses except when hay bales are being tossed down. Dust and mold can be somewhat contained in the hayloft, particularly if trapdoors to the stall hay feeders are kept closed except when in use. Recall that full ceilings need to be relatively high to allow proper natural ventilation of the horse stalls. See the "Hay and Bedding Storage" section of Chapter 13 for overhead and long-term hay storage design ideas.

Stored hay is a spontaneous combustion fire hazard when not properly cured. Adequate ventilation is needed for removal of heat generated during the curing process. Chapter 9 has more information on ways to reduce fire risk.

> ### Improve Horse Stall Ventilation
> *Unobstructed airflow and air quality are improved by the following:*
>
> 1. *Open grillwork on top of front and side stall partitions*
> 2. *No ceiling with interior open to roof peak*
>   *Compromise: High ceiling at 12 feet*
> 3. *No overhead hay-bedding storage*
>   *Compromise: No storage over horse stalls*

WHY INADEQUATE VENTILATION?

Two major factors lead to inadequate ventilation in modern stable construction. First, some stable designers are unfamiliar with how much air exchange is needed in a horse stall. Second, horse owners tend to be most comfortable in copying residential building practices. The belief that indoor housing provides a more desirable environment for horses is true only if a well-designed ventilation system is an integral part of the stable.

Very limited information has been available for horse stable builders and designers to refer to when properly designing horse stable ventilation systems. Many of these architects and builders work primarily in the residential and commercial building industry, where moisture, odor, and dust loads are much lower than in horse stables. Even when the differences in environment are appreciated, the ventilation system may fail because of a lack of understanding on how to get fresh air into each horse's stall. Fewer builders are specializing in agricultural (i.e., horse and other livestock) construction and the environment within these structures. It is better to find an experienced builder who understands horse stable design and ventilation features; but properly supplied with design ideas, inexperienced builders can tackle horse stable construction. With the low animal density of horse stabling (at about 4 pounds of horse per square foot) compared with other commercial livestock enterprises (for example, a freestall dairy at 13 pounds of cow per square foot) and with horses often being outside for a large portion of the day, the stable ventilation system can be a bit forgiving of imperfect design.

Good-intentioned horse owners are the second part of the ventilation problem. Most horses are kept in suburban settings, with few horse owners being familiar with ventilation performance and benefits. With most horses kept for recreational purposes, the effects of poor ventilation often manifest as chronic but mild respiratory conditions compared with the quickly measurable drop in performance seen in other livestock (decreased milk or meat production).

Stable designs often have a distinctly residential flair and may not be suitable for the health of the horse. Airtight buildings are for people. Horses need a more open environment and are, in fact, healthier when kept outside most of the time. Good agricultural builders regret the compromise to proper ventilation at the request of a client who wants the building completely closed tight to warm the building with horse body heat. Other builders are caught between providing proper ventilation openings and the ire of the building owner when a bit of snow or rain blows in. Better to allow a chance for a bit of precipitation to enter the stable for a few moments in a year than a whole season of the barn being too stuffy. The solution to inadequate ventilation is a familiarity with proper ventilation attributes and some experience in well-ventilated facilities to understand the benefits.

MEASURING VENTILATION RATE

Measuring a building ventilation rate seems quite simple, but in practice it is nearly impossible to estimate accurately for naturally ventilated structures, such as horse stables. When the guidelines presented in this chapter for opening sizes are followed, the stable will ventilate naturally and appropriately. The most challenging weather for naturally ventilated structures is during hot but windless days. Fortunately for horses, there is relatively low body heat accumulation in a stable that is equipped with plenty of warm weather ventilation openings. A ridge opening will let the hottest air escape out of the top of the building.

A rough estimate of ventilation rate may be made by measuring the velocity of air entering (or leaving) the stable through ventilation openings and multiplying this by the opening size. Air velocity is measured with an anemometer (Fig. 6.39), in feet per minute, and multiplied by the opening area, in square feet, to get ventilation rate in cubic feet per minute (cfm). To calculate the air changes per hour, divide the ventilation rate by the building air volume. The stable volume is the floor square footage multiplied by the average roof (or ceiling) height.

Measure the incoming ventilation air speed at several openings and at several locations on large openings, then average the velocities and multiply by the open area of airflow. With wind variations moving air into and out of the stable, the air speed (and possibly direction) at each ventilation opening is going to be frequently changing as the measurements are made. This variation of conditions is the primary difficulty in accurately estimating a natural ventilation rate.

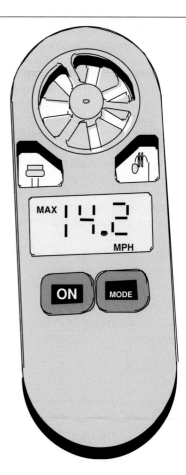

Figure 6.39. A vane anemometer measures air speed. A rough estimate of ventilation rate may be made with inlet air speed multiplied by area of ventilation opening. This instrument also measures relative humidity and temperature, so it can also be used to monitor conditions in the stable and horse stalls.

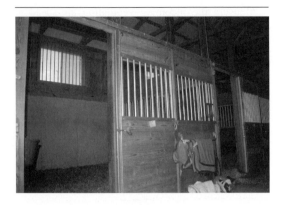

Figure 6.40. This picture is provided as an example with the recommended attributes of stable interior that will have excellent air quality. The center-aisle stable is equipped with large, 13-inch hardware-mesh covered eave inlets, and R-5 roof insulation to protect against moderate condensation below the metal-roofed structure. The stable has a covered, unobstructed 6-inch open ridge vent. Each stall has a metal-bar guarded window that can be opened in addition to endwall aisle doors (not shown). All wooden siding boards were installed to offer breathable wall diffuse ventilation. Open front and sidewall stall panels complete the design for air circulation and improved horse behavior, because confined horses can see activity and other horses.

SUMMARY

Well-ventilated stables are necessary for horse health and are the hallmark of good management.

Modern construction practices and "residential" influences have resulted in inadequate ventilation in many new stables. There is a need to demystify ventilation; the objective is simply to get fresh air to the horse. Ventilation is primarily driven by wind forces, so good ventilation is achieved by allowing wind to bring fresh air into the building while drawing out stale air. A permanent opening along both eaves that allow air entry into each stall will provide fresh air to each horse. Ridge openings are important for stale, warm, and humid air to escape. Figure 6.40 shows features that will improve fresh air exchange and distribution in horse stables. Most stables are naturally ventilated allowing wind and thermal buoyancy air movement to move fresh air into and stale air out of the stable. Mechanical ventilation using a fan-inlet system may be used for a more controlled air exchange rate when the stable or riding arena is heated.

Good ventilation is ideally designed into the original stable plans by the following:

- Providing permanent openings at eaves and ridge for winter moisture removal and summer heat relief. Breathable walls offer diffuse air entry around the stable perimeter.
- Providing windows and/or doors that open into stalls for warm weather breezes.
- Promoting interior airflow and improved air quality with open partitions and no overhead hay storage.

7
Flooring Materials and Drainage

The importance of good flooring becomes more evident as a horse spends more time in his stall. The fitness of a horse's legs and feet can be greatly affected by the type of stall flooring chosen. The most suitable floor is highly dependent on management style, while personal preferences can have a strong influence. Fortunately, there are many options for suitable floors in a horse facility. The objective of this chapter is to provide information on stall and stable flooring materials, including flooring material attributes and options for overcoming some deficiencies. Subfloor construction and drainage features are presented as these strongly influence floor integrity.

TWO MAJOR TYPES OF HORSE STABLE FLOORS

The two major categories of stable flooring materials depend on whether the material is porous or impervious to wetness (Fig. 7.1). Floor construction, from the ground up, will depend on what type of material is chosen. Porous floors will have an underlying foundation of sand and/or gravel to aid water movement down into the ground below the stable. Impervious floors may be sloped toward a drain so that urine and water can run out of the stall. Even impervious floors have a few inches of sand or fine gravel underneath for material stability and drainage of subsurface water. With either type of stall flooring, often enough bedding is used to absorb excess water and urine so actual liquid runoff is minimal except after a stall washdown.

STALL FLOOR MATERIALS

Opinions differ on which type of stall flooring material is the best, but there is one thing most owners agree upon: a good floor is important to the horse's well-being. No one type of material seems to offer all the attributes of an ideal floor. Material selection depends on which disadvantage you are willing to

work with. For example, concrete may meet most of your stall flooring criteria, but more bedding or solid rubber mats will be needed to protect the horse's legs. Table 7.1 summarizes the attributes of common flooring materials that will be described in more detail.

Characteristics of the Ideal Floor

These are ranked in importance of the horse's well-being, followed by the owner's interest:

- Easy on legs; has some "give" to decrease tendon and feet strain
- Dry
- Non-odor retentive
- Provides traction; nonslippery to encourage the horse to lie down
- Durable; stays level, resists damage from horse pawing, and has a long life
- Low maintenance
- Easy to clean
- Affordable

Stable Management for Stall Floors

Consider manure and urine management when selecting the stall flooring material. On average, a horse produces 0.5 ounces of feces and 0.3 fluid ounces of urine per pound of body weight every day. So a 1000-pound horse produces about 31 pounds of feces and 2.4 gallons of urine daily. Floors that allow urine to be absorbed and travel down through the flooring material layers can retain odors. A well-bedded stall will have less odor problem because the urine is more readily absorbed into the bedding. Impervious floors depend on slope for drainage and/or bedding to soak up urine.

Stall floors must be durable but also play an important role in the overall health of the horse. Leg soundness and fatigue are affected by the flooring material, with more forgiving floors generally being preferred to hard floors. A horse needs to lie down and get back up with confidence and without injury,

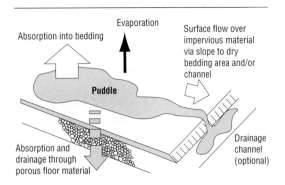

Figure 7.1. Water-flow paths within and out of a stall.

so good traction is necessary. Stall floors that retain odors can deteriorate the respiratory system of the horse. Because horses spend a great deal of time with their heads down, high ammonia concentrations at the floor level can damage the lining of the throat and lungs. A good floor can inhibit internal parasite survival in the stall environment.

Horse behavior results in uneven wetting and use of the flooring. A wet, porous material, such as soil or clay, is less capable of bearing weight. Wet material will work its way into adjacent areas through hoof action, creating holes and high spots. In addition, horses often paw near the stall door or feed bucket from impatience or boredom, or out of habit. This creates low spots. If given enough space, most horses are good housekeepers. Often, a mare will urinate and defecate in one spot in her stall, away from the resting and feeding areas. Geldings are more limited in how they use their stalls but typically defecate in one area and urinate in the center.

POROUS FLOORING MATERIALS

Figure 7.2 shows a cross section of the construction of porous floor.

Topsoil

At first this seems the most natural as it resembles pasture footing. Drainage and durability properties depend on the type of soil. Some soil types can resist drainage and result in mud or puddles, while others may become dry and dusty. Sandy topsoil will shift from use, creating uneven footing. A concrete or asphalt apron can be used at the stall door to discourage "digging."

Advantages
• Highly absorbent
• Nonslip
• Easy on legs
• Inexpensive
• Drainage varies

Table 7.1. Characteristics of Stall Floor Materials Based Solely on the Material Itself, with No Base or Drains

	Easy on Legs	Absorbs Wetness	Does Not Retain Odors	Nonslip	Durability (Stays Level)	Ease of Cleaning and Disinfecting	Low Main-tenance	Cost per 12 ft × 12 ft Stall
Topsoil	✓	✓	?	✓	β	β	β	very low
Clay	✓	?	?	✓	β	β	?	very low
Sand	✓	✓	✓	✓	β	β	β	low
Concrete	β	β	✓	?	✓	✓	✓	medium
Asphalt	β	β	✓	?	✓	✓	✓	medium
Road Base Mix	?	✓	✓	✓	?	✓	?	low
Solid Rubber Mats	✓	β	?	✓	✓	✓	?	medium-high
Grid Mats	✓	✓	✓	✓	✓	?	✓	high
Wood	✓	?	β	β	✓	✓	✓	medium
Mattress	✓	β	✓	?	✓	✓	✓	high

✓ = good to excellent; ? = highly dependent on other factors; β = poor.

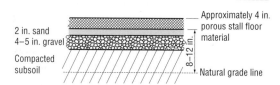

2 in. sand
4–5 in. gravel
Compacted subsoil

Approximately 4 in. porous stall floor material

8–12 in.

Natural grade line

Figure 7.2. Porous floor cross section (includes topsoil, clay, sand, road base mix, and grid mats). Porous floor will have underlying sand, gravel, or crushed stone foundation to allow urine and water to drain away from the floor and the stable.

Disadvantages
• Porosity can retain dampness and odor
• Needs to be leveled and replaced often
• Can be difficult to muck out
• May freeze hard
• Difficult to disinfect

Clay

This is traditionally the horse owner's favorite flooring. The types of clay locally available will vary. Pure clay tends to pack too tightly and become impervious to drainage. Pure-packed clay is slick when wet. It is recommended to mix clay with other soils. A mix of 1 part fine stone dust and 2 parts clay is common over a sublayer of gravel to aid drainage. Areas of frequent urination are most likely to develop dips and holes. The urine softens the clay and reduces bearing strength. As the horse steps in these areas, the clay is pushed toward the drier area, creating a pit or hole. Promote drainage by sloping the floor (1 inch per 5 feet) toward an alley channel, although maintaining an even slope is difficult. If pawing at the stall door is a problem, a concrete or asphalt apron can be a deterrent.

Advantages
• Closest to a natural tread
• Easy on legs
• Noiseless
• No dust
• Keeps hooves moist
• Highly absorbent
• Relatively warm
• Resists wear when dry and compacted

• Affords a firm footing unless wet
• Inexpensive

Disadvantages
• Can be difficult to keep clean
• Needs to be leveled and repacked each year
• Needs to be replaced every few years because of holes and pockets from constant pawing
• Remains damp longer than desirable
• May retain odors

Sand

Sand is one of the most forgiving floor materials for a horse's legs and has excellent drainage. However, pure sand does not compact and will move easily, creating tracks and pockets with repeated use. The uneven surface should be raked smooth daily. Sand can become mixed with bedding materials (especially shavings and sawdust), making cleaning difficult and creating a need for frequent replacement. If sand is used, monitor horses for signs of intestinal impaction and colic. New horses and those fed off the floor may be especially prone to ingesting the sand. Sand may have a drying effect on horse hooves, with more hoof wall cracks and splits.

Advantages
• Highly absorbent
• Soft surface
• Noiseless
• Good drainage
• Nonslip

Disadvantages
• Does not pack well
• Damp in a cold climate
• Drying effect on hooves
• Mixes with bedding, so harder to clean stall
• Must frequently replace discarded sand when stall cleaning
• Sand colic can develop when horses eat sand with dropped food or by habit

Road Base Mix

This mix is known by many names, depending on the region of the country. It has been called limestone dust, washed sand, quarry waste, and stone dust, just to name a few. Road base mix is usually decomposed granite mixed with a small amount of clay or other binding material that results in a well-graded, compactable material used for road building. The exact mix depends on the area and types of rock and binding agents available. Different grades of road mix are available, ranging from coarse, large particles to very fine. Road mixes with the fewest and smallest rocks are recommended. This material is easily compacted but can be as unforgiving to a horse's legs as concrete if compacted too much. If the floor is not compacted properly, it will be easily dredged and mixed with bedding by the digging horse. Because it is easy to level and offers some drainage through it, road base mix is often used as a subfloor for rubber mats. Road base mix flooring material should be 4 to 5 inches thick over a 6- to 8-inch base of sand or small gravel to allow drainage.

Advantages
- Packs well
- Good drainage
- Easy to level

Disadvantages
- Small rocks on surface are undesirable but can be raked up once packed
- If not compacted well enough, holes develop and material mixes with bedding

Wood

Once a common flooring in the era of horse-drawn transportation, wood is used less often in modern horse facilities because of the relatively high initial cost of hardwood boards. In addition, concrete and asphalt have become more available over this time. Wood provides a low-maintenance, level floor that aids in stall mucking. Planks should be at least 2-inch-thick hardwood (often oak) with preservative treatment. Gaps between boards allow urine drainage and should be packed with sand, road base mix, or clay (Fig. 7.3). To aid drainage, planks are placed

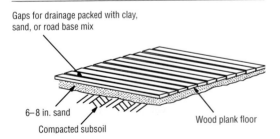

Gaps for drainage packed with clay, sand, or road base mix

6–8 in. sand

Compacted subsoil

Wood plank floor

Figure 7.3. Wood floor construction.

over a level surface of 6 to 8 inches of sand or small gravel or set into asphalt or concrete.

A wood floor helps alleviate stiffness in the muscles and joints by insulating the horse from the cold ground. It offers a softer footing than concrete or asphalt, but may become slick when wet and is difficult to disinfect because of wood's porous nature. Gaps between planks create a holding space for spilled grain, inviting insect and rodent infestation. Correct construction and adequate bedding can minimize rodent and moisture problems.

Advantages
- Easy on legs
- Warm to lie upon
- Rough wood has good traction
- Low maintenance
- Durable

Disadvantages
- Porous; difficult to clean and disinfect
- Retains odors
- Slippery when wet
- Must be checked often for signs of wear
- Prone to insect and rodent damage if constructed poorly
- High initial expense

Grid Mats

This flooring style is an open grid pattern designed to support another type of flooring material (Figs. 7.4 and 7.5). Grid mats may be manufactured from rubber or plastic (polyethylene). By design, the mat is placed over a compacted, level subfloor and topped with another flooring material such as clay, soil, or road base mix. The open spaces aid in drainage, and the matrix prevents holes and damage from pawing. Stall floor characteristics match the topping material characteristics, but the grid mat matrix decreases material movement because of wetting and hoof action.

Another option in grid stall floor design uses pressure-treated 2 × 4 lumber set on edge that span the stall width. A 1½- to 3-inch gap is left between boards, so that the lumber grid is filled and topped with a porous stall flooring material (clay, soil, road base mix). This offers similar characteristics to the manufactured grid mat product in a homemade design. Longevity of the lumber grid is expected to be less than that of rubber or plastic.

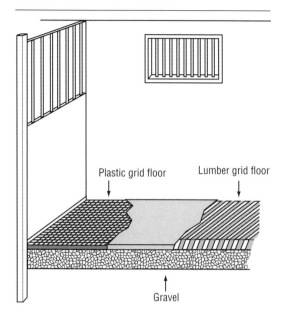

Figure 7.4. Two examples of grid floor design: one using a plastic mat and the second using lumber.

Advantages
• Durable
• Easy on legs
• Remains level
• Uses less bedding than concrete
• Low maintenance

Disadvantage
• Expensive

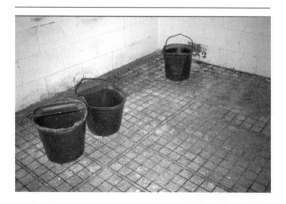

Figure 7.5. Clay material fills the space within the grid used in this floor at a veterinary facility.

IMPERVIOUS FLOORING MATERIALS

Figure 7.6 shows a cross section of impervious floor construction.

Concrete

This type of flooring has become popular because of its durability and low maintenance. It is easier to muck out and clean a concrete floor stall than most other materials. Concrete has different finishing options. Steel troweling brings fine aggregate and cement to the top, forming a glazed and slippery surface. Smoothed concrete is slick and horses are reluctant to lie down and get up. For this reason, it is not recommended for use in stalls, although it is often suitable in a feed room where its smoothness eases cleaning. Wood-float and broom-finished surfaces provide better traction; however, they tend to become smooth with wear. The brushed concrete, with its small ridges that give it the appearance of being swept with a broom, can be abrasive to lying horses without a deep bedding layer. Broomed concrete with a rough finish for traction and durability would be suitable in an aisleway.

Concrete is very durable but hard on horses standing in the stall all day. Some owners recommend that a horse be turned out at least 4 hours per day when housed on concrete flooring. Using a thick layer of bedding or solid rubber mats can minimize some of concrete's disadvantages. Provide a minimum 4-inch

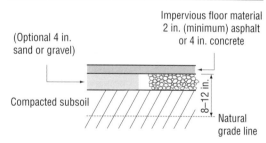

Figure 7.6. Impervious floor cross section (includes concrete, asphalt, solid rubber mats, and brick or tile aisle floor). Not all impervious stall floors are sloped to drains or channels but instead rely on deep bedding to manage urine and water removal. Impervious floors require a level, evenly compacted sublayer. Sand or fine gravel may provide structural support and underground drainage. Solid rubber mats are often laid over concrete or well-packed road base mix.

thickness for concrete floors under stalls and where vehicle use is limited. Provide 5 inches of concrete for drives and alleys with moderate vehicle traffic (such as heavy pickup trucks and manure spreaders). A well-drained sand or gravel base under the concrete is desirable, but not required.

Advantages

• Durable, long life
• Easy to clean
• Possible to disinfect
• Rodent-proof
• Difficult for the horse to damage
• Low maintenance

Disadvantages

• Hard on legs, unyielding
• May discourage normal behavior (lying down, etc.)
• Cold and damp in cold climates
• Needs more bedding or solid rubber mat
• Relatively expensive

Asphalt

An alternative to concrete, asphalt provides ease of cleaning and longevity with a bit more forgiveness to the horse's legs and feet. Asphalt is a mixture of aggregate stone and sand held together with a tar compound. Asphalt needs to be applied thickly enough to prevent cracking and chipping. A minimum 2-inch thickness is needed in stalls when installed over a solid, level subsurface. For aisles with vehicle traffic, similar to driveway use, 3 to 4 inches is recommended. Under extra heavy use, asphalt may need to be replaced in several years.

Asphalt can be installed as either a slightly porous or almost impervious floor material. Unsealed asphalt is relatively porous compared with concrete. Porosity can be improved by minimizing the amount of sand and small particles in the aggregate mixture. New asphalt floors are not smooth and provide adequate traction. However, repeated travel by horses will smooth out the floor, making it slick. Hot asphalt that has its surface raked rather than rolled will have more texture for traction. Likewise, asphalt with larger aggregate size will provide more traction.

Advantages

• Less expensive to install than concrete
• Easy to clean
• Slightly more give than concrete
• Long wearing, but not as durable as concrete
• Provides traction

Disadvantages

• Hard and cold; not as bad as concrete
• Surface irregularities can trap urine, creating sanitation problems
• May crack and chip if applied too thin
• Relatively expensive

Solid Rubber Mats

Mats are typically used over another flooring, often to cover up faults such as hardness or slipperiness. They are gaining popularity despite their expense. Mats will reduce the amount of bedding that is needed to provide cushioning, or textured models can even be used alone, which is one payback on their cost. Mats are installed on top of an even, compact surface such as 4 to 5 inches of road base mix or concrete. If the mat does not cover the entire area of the stall, then multiple mats should interlock or be anchored to the floor. Without a secure connection between mats, keeping multiple-piece stall mats in position can be difficult, as their smooth surface allows the mats to "walk" and bedding chaff in the cracks eventually pries mats up and apart. Horses can lift up areas that are not properly secured. It is often necessary to have several people move the mats because they are heavy (a 4-foot by 6-foot mat weighs about 100 pounds) and cumbersome, but they are durable and can withstand a lot of abuse. Care should be taken with horses wearing studded shoes, because the studs may damage the mat surface.

A range of mat thicknesses is available; the most common are from ½ - to ¾ inches thick. Top surfaces should be rippled or bumped to add traction, and the base of the mat should be grooved to help remove any urine that leaks through joints from the surface. Untextured mats are slippery when wet. A mat surface makes stall cleaning easy, but care must be taken with forks to prevent cutting the surface. Shop around for mats and delivery costs, because many manufacturers offer good warranties.

Advantages

• Provides good footing for breeding shed, foaling stalls, and recovery stalls
• Long life with many companies offering 10-year-plus warranties
• Easy to clean
• Easy on legs
• Low maintenance

Disadvantages

- Not as comfortable as traditional bedding
- Will move unless anchored or secured by walls or interlocking pieces
- May retain odors
- Expensive

Mattress

A mattress stall mat is a two-piece system with a secure top cover over a multicelled mattress. This technology was developed in the dairy industry, where cow comfort has been emphasized, and rugged design features were built into the mattress system. It is a highly cushioned assembly with claims of having more shock absorbance than a ¾ -inch rubber mat or 6-inch layer of wood shavings. The multicelled mattress looks like an air-filled mattress or water raft but is typically made from a durable fabric containing uniformly sized crumb rubber. Narrow cells are more durable than earlier mattress designs with one large or a few wide cells. Additional crumb rubber is added on top of the installed mattress to evenly fill the gaps between adjoining cells for a level surface. The top cover is a vulcanized rubber impregnated geotextile. A tough top cover over the mattress is necessary to decrease damage from horseshoes. The system is impervious, so it does not absorb water or urine. The top cover is securely and continuously fastened to the stall walls for placement and to prevent bedding and stall waste from getting underneath.

Advantages

- Easy to clean
- Reduced bedding, because only for urine and not softness
- Durable
- Easy on legs
- Low maintenance

Disadvantages

- Expensive
- Horseshoes may damage

SPECIALTY FLOORS AROUND THE BARN

Aisleways

Alley floors can be of the same material as the stalls, but this area has more diverse uses and often has different requirements for the floor. Horses are not housed on the aisle floor, but this area sees just as much abuse as the stall floor. See Table 7.2 for characteristics of different flooring materials.

Alley floors should be:

- Dry
- Durable
- Easy to sweep clean
- Nonslip and skidproof
- Fire resistant

Common alley floor materials are the same as the stall floors. Compare material properties listed for stall floors, with the demands of an aisle floor in

Table 7.2. Characteristics of Aisle Floor Materials Based Solely on the Material Itself, with No Base or Drains

	Stays Dry	Low Maintenance	Ease of Cleaning and Disinfecting	Nonslip	Fire Resistance	Wearability— Holds Up Well Under Heavy Use
Topsoil	β	?	β	✓	✓	?
Clay	?	?	β	?	✓	?
Sand	✓	β	β	✓	✓	?
Concrete	✓	✓	✓	?	✓	✓
Asphalt	✓	✓	✓	?	✓	✓
Road Base Mix	✓	?	✓	✓	✓	?
Solid Rubber Mats	✓	✓	✓	✓	✓	✓
Grid Mats	✓	✓	✓	✓	✓	✓
Bricks	✓	✓	?	?	✓	✓
Synthetic Bricks	✓	✓	✓	✓	✓	✓

✓ = good to excellent; **?** = highly dependent on other factors; β = poor.

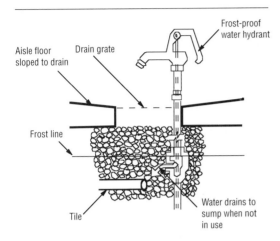

Figure 7.7. Drainage near water hydrant.

mind. Wide aisles that are used for exercising horses should have a floor of sand or a footing material suitable for use in riding arenas.

Clay is not very durable for aisleways and does not wear evenly. Concrete and asphalt are durable yet noisy and can become slippery, especially with wear. If concrete is used, use only roughened concrete. Synthetic surfaces are resilient and have good footing but are expensive. Topsoil floors vary depending on the soil type, but they can freeze and be dusty or very muddy. Soil floors may be suitable in smaller private stables where the aisle has limited traffic.

Unlike the stall floor, an alley floor should not absorb water but redirect the water elsewhere. Alley floors can be sloped toward the sides if an alley gutter is provided or toward a drain. It is recommended that drains be provided, especially under or near water hydrants (Fig. 7.7). Avoid drains in the middle of alleys heavily trafficked by horses or in areas that are commonly soiled by hay, dirt, or bedding material. Grates or drain covers can minimize clogs and should be cleaned regularly to prevent backups.

Older and more elaborate barns use bricks or tiles for the aisle floor. These floors are very attractive but are labor intensive and costly to install. Brick and tile come in a range of textures. The smoother the texture, the more slippery the surface can become, especially when wet. Bricks have also been criticized as being difficult to disinfect because of their porosity. In the past few years, rubber has been used to model the look of a traditional brick floor (Figure 7.8). This addresses some of the disadvan-

tages of the porous brick. An adequate base is essential to the longevity of the floor. Soil upheaval or improper installation may make the surface uneven to walk on. See Figure 7.6 for more details.

Feed Room

This area receives a lot of use in a horse facility. Because it is especially vulnerable to visits from rodents, a floor that facilitates the cleanup of spilled grain and dirt is recommended. A rough floor texture is not desirable in the feed room. Four-inch-thick concrete with steel trowel finish or sealed asphalt provides a long-lived, rodent-proof floor that can be easily cleaned.

Tack Room

A tack room floor is usually an impervious material if it is indeed a separate room and not a tack "area." The room can function as a lounge by adding indoor and outdoor carpeting. Concrete or asphalt has the advantage of being easy to clean and rodent proof.

Wash Area

In this area, a nonslip floor impervious to water is desirable. A drain and grate will also be needed. Some of the more resilient floors include very rough or grooved concrete, textured rubber mats over concrete, and sealed, large aggregate asphalt. The floor should slope toward a drain that is located on the side or in the back of the wash area, not in an area

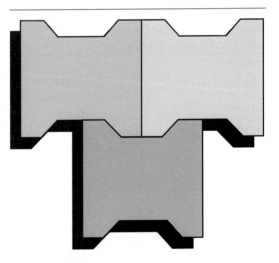

Figure 7.8. Example of a rubber paving brick configuration.

heavily trafficked by horses. Horses may be reluctant to stand on drain covers, and the drain covers themselves may become a safety hazard. Drain design should consider the need to remove clogs. Installing cleanouts and traps will add to the life of the drain.

STALL FLOOR CONSTRUCTION AND DRAINAGE

All stall floors need some way of handling fluids. Most often, bedding is used to soak up urine. Without adequate amounts of dry bedding, the extra urine will have to drain somewhere. A water-flow path provided either along the floor surface or through the floor to sublayers will allow the fluid to move away from the stable. Floor drains are not common within horse stalls because they are frequently clogged with bedding and stall waste. Many horse stall floors function well with no drainage other than careful bedding management for urine removal. When additional drainage is desired, either the floor should be sloped toward a drainage channel or porous floor layers provided that allow liquids to flow from the stall. When water is added during disinfecting or washing, then drainage becomes more important than urine management alone.

Principles of Good Stall Floor Construction

Stall floors are built from the bottom up.

- Remove vegetation, roots, stone, and topsoil, and compact the subsoil below the stable site to prevent settling and cracking of the stable and flooring. Soil with low and moderate clay content is adequate for compaction. In lieu of compaction, allow subsoil to settle for several months before construction. Avoid high-clay soils as subsoils.
- Slope the ground surface 5% away from the stable, and divert surface and groundwater away from the stable site (Fig. 7.9).

- To ensure adequate drainage for the stable when using any type of flooring, elevate the top of the stall floor at least 12 inches above the outside ground level. Often the compacted subsoil is covered with 4 to 5 inches of gravel and 2 inches of sand or pea gravel for good drainage. Then 4 inches or more of stall floor material is applied on top.
- Floors benefit from some slope to distribute urine and water spills to areas with drier bedding. A 1½ to 2% (¼ inch per foot; 1 inch per 5 feet] incline is enough to move water without causing a noticeable slope to the horse.
- For drains, shallow and safe open channeling is preferred to the complexity of an underground drainage system. See "Stall Drainage System Design" for more information. Channeled water is taken outside the stable where a rock layer of large gravel or stones that extends well beyond the stable foundation assists drainage.
- If the groundwater table is high, damp floors can be overcome by subdraining. This is a layer of drain rock laid before building the normal foundation. Severe problems require tile drainage, extra fill, and nonporous floors. See "Water from Below" for more information.

STALL DRAINAGE SYSTEM DESIGN

When improved stall drainage is desired, a safe open channel along the stall wall is recommended to catch surface wetness. Slope the stall floor toward this channel. Do not use a drain in the middle of the stall, because it will get clogged with bedding. Underground drains with inlets protected by heavy metal grates (which support horse and light vehicle traffic) may be used, but they are complex and cost more to construct and will almost surely clog with stall waste. A disadvantage of the open channel is potential odor from stall waste accumulation,

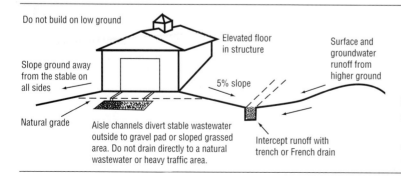

Do not build on low ground

Elevated floor in structure

Surface and groundwater runoff from higher ground

Slope ground away from the stable on all sides

5% slope

Natural grade

Aisle channels divert stable wastewater outside to gravel pad or sloped grassed area. Do not drain directly to a natural wastewater or heavy traffic area.

Intercept runoff with trench or French drain

Figure 7.9. Proper floor design considers site-related features to promote drainage from the building. Do not build on low ground.

although proper sanitation management can minimize this. Open channels can be built with gradually sloping sides to reduce injury for horses and people stepping into them, or they may be filled with large gravel. A heavy, open grill or solid grate may be placed over the channel in areas of horse and vehicle traffic, such as at doorways. An enhanced drainage system may not be desirable if freezing will occur in the barn.

Sloped floors offer drainage advantage, particularly after a stall washdown. Slope of about 1 inch per 5 feet is effective. Avoid noticeable sloping floors because this can strain tendons when horses are standing in the stalls. Stall runoff is easily hosed away with a sloping floor. Three options for floor slope and drainage system are provided in Figure 7.10.

- The stall floor can be sloped toward a channel outside the front of the stall in the working aisle. This single-slope floor is relatively easy to construct. Provision for water to escape from the stall into the aisle channel is needed along the bottom of the front stall wall. Keep any gap to less than 2 inches to minimize hoof entrapment.
- The stall floor could be sloped toward one corner where a cutout in the wall allows fluid access to the channel or drain. One drain channel can serve two stalls. Construction of the double-slope floor is a bit more complex than the single-slope floor. This design offers advantage for collection of stall wastewater for an underground drainage system.
- The stall floor may be sloped to the exterior wall of the stall where a sloping gutter drain is provided along the inside of that wall. Provide a small trench 2 inches wide extending from the top stall flooring material down to the gravel subfloor layer to collect runoff. Fill the trench with small stone or large gravel to enhance water movement.

Water from Below

Fine soils, such as clay, draw water by capillary action from a water table, resulting in saturated soil conditions under the building. A high water table causes similar problems. Saturated soil has less weight-bearing strength than dry soil. Freezing of this water can result in frost action such as heaving and odd settlement of the floor and building foundation. To prevent frost damage:

- Lower the water table with well-drained subsoil or perimeter tile drains with suitable outlets.
- Provide granular fill, which has low capillary conductivity, under the flooring to break the water's upward travel. Large gravel or crushed rock, with the fines screened out, is desirable. In the worst case, subsoil will need to be excavated to the maximum frost penetration depth and replaced with the gravel.
- Raise the building floor to move away from the water table. Any building floor should be at least 12 inches above the surrounding grade, but it may be higher if water damage is anticipated.

SUMMARY

Many options are available for suitable flooring materials in horse stables. Selection will most often depend on what characteristics are important to the stable manager and local availability of materials. Stall floors become very important to leg and foot fitness when a horse spends a lot of time confined to a stall. Proper floor materials can aid stable cleaning and manure removal. The floor is more than the top surface on which the horse stands. A properly constructed floor has layers of materials that provide suitable support, drainage, and structural integrity for the top surface layer.

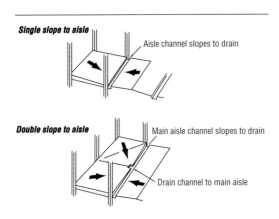

Single slope to aisle

Aisle channel slopes to drain

Double slope to aisle

Main aisle channel slopes to drain

Drain channel to main aisle

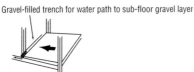

Single slope to back wall gravel-filled trench

Gravel-filled trench for water path to sub-floor gravel layer

Figure 7.10. Three types of stable floor slope and drain (exaggerated slope shown).

8
Manure Management

Manure handling is a necessary evil of stable management, with horse owners naturally preferring to ride rather than clean stalls. Making sure that stall cleaning and other manure handling chores are done efficiently can lead to more time spent with the horse. It is important to recognize that horses produce a large amount of manure that quickly accumulates! About 12 tons of manure and soiled bedding will be removed annually from each horse stall (housing a full-time occupant). Careful consideration of how this material is moved and stored is needed for efficient manure management. Getting the manure out of a stall is only the beginning. A complete manure management system involves collection, storage (temporary or long-term), and disposal or utilization. This chapter provides information to stable managers on horse manure characteristics and options for its movement and storage. Associated issues such as odor control, fly breeding, and environmental impact are addressed in relation to horse facilities.

Manure management practices within horse facilities deserve careful attention. Because most horses are kept in suburban or rural residential settings, it is essential for horse owners to be good neighbors. Often, suburban horse facilities have limited or no acreage for disposal of manure and soiled bedding. Several alternatives for handling manure include land disposal, stockpiling for future handling, removal from stable site, and composting. Some stables have developed markets to distribute or sell the stall waste. Whether in a suburban or rural setting, proper manure management is based on simple principles that will virtually eliminate environmental pollution impacts and nuisances such as odor and flies.

STALL WASTE PRODUCTION AND CHARACTERISTICS

Manure includes both the solid and liquid portions of waste. Horse manure is about 60% solids and 40% urine. On average, a horse produces 0.5 ounces of feces and 0.3 fluid ounces of urine per pound of body weight every day. A 1000-pound horse produces about 30 to 36 pounds of feces and 1.9 to 2.4 gallons of urine daily, which totals around 50 pounds of total raw waste per day (Fig. 8.1 and Table 8.1).

Soiled bedding removed with the manure during stall cleaning may account for another 8 to 15 pounds per day of waste. The volume of soiled bedding removed equals almost twice the volume of manure removed, but it varies widely depending on management practices (Fig. 8.2). So for each stall, about 60 to 70 pounds of total waste material is removed daily. This results in about 12 tons of waste a year per stall with 9 tons being manure from a 1000-pound horse (Fig. 8.3).

The density of horse manure is about 62 pounds per cubic feet. Therefore, 51 pounds of manure would occupy about 0.82 cubic feet. The soiled stall bedding removed with this manure would be about twice this volume, so the total volume of stall waste removed per day per 1000-pound horse may be estimated as 2.4 cubic feet. To put all these numbers in perspective, annual stall waste from one horse would fill its 12-foot by 12-foot stall about 6 feet deep (assumes no settling). Plan now for handling this material!

Barn chores include a daily cleanout of manure and soiled bedding, leading to a steady stream of waste to handle. There are several common stall-bedding materials, and each has different characteristics in handling, field application, suitability to composting, and acceptance for sales. Availability and cost of bedding materials in the stable area will probably have the greatest influence on bedding selection. (See Tables 8.2 and 8.3.)

The manure management needs of pastured horses are different from those of stabled horses. The field-deposited manure is beneficial because it serves as a

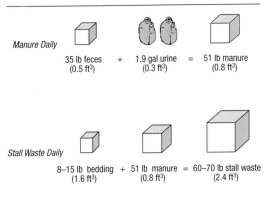

Manure Daily

35 lb feces   +   1.9 gal urine   =   51 lb manure
(0.5 ft³)   (0.3 ft³)   (0.8 ft³)

Stall Waste Daily

8–15 lb bedding + 51 lb manure = 60–70 lb stall waste
(1.6 ft³)   (0.8 ft³)   (2.4 ft³)

Figure 8.1. Daily manure and stall waste production from a typical 1000-pound horse.

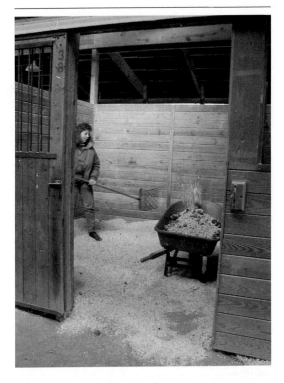

Figure 8.2. Most stable stall cleaning is still done by hand, but automation can be used to move large quantities of manure from the stable to storage.

fertilizer. Substantial amounts of manure can accumulate where horses congregate around gates, waterers, favorite shade areas, feeders, and shelters. These areas should be cleaned weekly for better pasture management and parasite control and to diminish fly breeding. Manure collected from paddocks and pastures may be added to the stall waste stockpile.

Horse manure has been considered a valuable resource rather than a "waste." Fertilizer value of 8½ tons of manure produced annually by a 1000-pound horse is about 102 pounds of nitrogen, 43 pounds of P_2O_5 (phosphorus pentoxide

Table 8.1. Estimated Weights and Volumes of Typical As-excreted Horse Manure (Urine and Feces Combined)

	Total Manure		Feces	Total Solids
Activity Level[a,b]	(lb/day)	(ft³/day)	(lb/day)	(lb/day)
Sedentary	51	0.82	35	7.6
Light exercise	46	0.74	30	6.9
Moderate exercise	48	0.77	32	7.2
Intense exercise	52	0.83	36	7.8

Note: Use these values only for planning purposes. Values will vary for individual situations because of genetics, dietary options, and variations in feed nutrient concentration, animal performance, and individual farm management.

[a]Values for 1000-lb horse; urine 16 lb/day for all activity levels; 85% moisture content w.b.; density 62 lb/ft³.

[b]Values apply to horses 18 months of age or older that are not pregnant or lactating. Production values for horses from 850 to 1350 pounds can be roughly estimated by linearly interpolating the table values. "Sedentary" activity level would apply to horses not receiving any imposed exercise; "light" activity level would include horses ridden at low intensities for a few hours per week, such as pleasure riding; "moderate" activity level would include horses used for showing, lower level combined training, and ranch work, and "intense" activity level would include race training, polo, and upper level combined training.

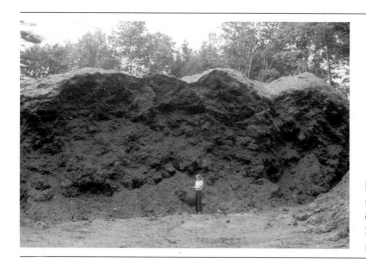

Figure 8.3. Racetracks and large stabling complexes need dedicated manure storage areas. Shown is a pile of finished compost from racetrack facility.

[phosphate] = 43.7% P), and 77 pounds of K_2O (potash = 83% K). The nutrient content of horse manure can also be represented as 12 pounds per ton of N, 5 pounds per ton of P_2O_5, and 9 pounds per ton of K_2O (nutrient values for any manure vary widely, so these are only guidelines). Traditionally, nitrate-nitrogen is the component that presents the most pollution potential, because it moves freely in the soil. Most of horse manure's nitrogen is contained in the urine.

These values are an average for horse manure (urine and feces). With the large amount of bedding material mixed with manure in typical stall waste, the fertilizer nutrient value would vary. A summary of published nutrient values is presented in Table 8.5 in the "Direct Disposal" section.

Table 8.2. Approximate Water Absorption of Dry Bedding Materials (Typically 10% Moisture)

Material	Pound Water Absorbed per Pound Bedding
Wheat straw	2.2
Hay-chopped mature	3.0
Tanning bark	4.0
Fine bark	2.5
Pine chips	3.0
Pine sawdust	2.5
Pine shavings	2.0
Hardwood chips, shavings, sawdust[a]	1.5
Corn shredded stover	2.5
Corn ground cobs	2.1

Source: Livestock Waste Facilities Handbook, MWPS-18.

Note: Not recommended for horse stall bedding: flax straw, oat straw, black cherry, and walnut wood products. The horse may eat oat straw.

[a]Walnut shavings cause founder, so all hardwood shavings are often avoided as horse stall bedding on the chance that some walnut shavings would be mixed in.

Table 8.3. Hay and Bedding Material Density

Form	Material	Density (lb/ft³)
Loose	Alfalfa	4
	Nonlegume hay	4
	Straw	2–3
	Shavings	9
	Sawdust	7–12
	Sand	105
Baled	Alfalfa	8
	Nonlegume hay	7
	Straw	5
	Wood shavings	20
Chopped	Alfalfa	6
	Nonlegume hay	6
	Straw	7

Source: Livestock Waste Facilities Handbook, MWPS-18.

ENVIRONMENTAL IMPACT

Minimizing Nuisances

For a suburban setting, one potential problem includes overcoming misconceptions about the nuisance and pollution potential of horse facilities. Most people enjoy horses; yet neighbors can be more concerned that horses are manure-generating, fly and odor machines. A horse facility operating with a large number of horses on limited acreage can intensify nuisance problems not noticed at small stables. Generally in the northeast, 2 to 3 acres of good pasture per horse is needed for summer feeding purposes; up to 5 acres per horse during times of slower grass growth. More horses per acre are common and successfully managed with supplemental feeding. Fortunately, careful management and attention to detail can overcome potential problems of intensive horse operations.

Pests commonly associated with animal agriculture are flies and small rodents, such as mice and rats. Flies and odors are the most common complaints, but proper manure management can virtually eliminate farm pests and odors. Figure 8.4 shows some simple, yet important, site-planning features to minimize nuisances associated with manure management.

INSECTS

It is always easier and more effective to prevent fly breeding than it is to control adult flies. Eliminating the habitat required by the larvae to hatch and grow significantly reduces fly populations. Because flies deposit eggs in the top few inches of moist manure, minimizing moist manure surface area is one reduction strategy. Eggs can hatch in as little as seven days under optimal temperature and moisture conditions. The fly breeding season starts when spring temperatures get above 65°F and ends at the first killing frost in the fall. Under ideal breeding conditions, it has been calculated that one fly can produce 300 million offspring in about 60 days! Few flies will develop if manure is removed from the stable site or made undesirable for fly breeding within a maximum seven-day cycle.

Keep manure as dry as possible, below 50% moisture, to make it less desirable for egg deposition. Spread manure out in thin layers during field application or field dragging, or keep out precipitation by roofing or tarping the permanent holding area and covering any dumpsters or temporary manure storage. Cleaning up decaying organic material is essential to fly control. Filth flies lay eggs in any decaying organic matter, including spilled feed, manure left in stall corners, grass clippings, and manure piles. Store small amounts of manure in containers with tight-fitting lids. Cleaning up spilled grain will not only suppress filth fly populations but also reduce feed sources for mice and rats. Further information is available in *Pest Management Recommendation for Horses* (see the "Additional Resources" section).

RODENTS

Clean out trash, dumps, piles of old lumber or manure, and garbage where rats and mice hide. Keep weeds trimmed around buildings to reduce hiding places. Stacked feedbags create ideal passageways in which rodents can eat, hide, and breed. Store feed in rodent-proof bins, preferably metal or lined with metal or wire mesh. A 30-gallon trash can will hold a 100-pound sack of feed. Feed from these containers rather than from an open bag, and clean up any spills immediately. Areas under feed bins, bunks, and buckets are excellent feeding grounds for rodents. Concrete floors and foundations deter rodent entry, as do metal shields on doors and screens over small openings. Young mice can squeeze through an opening as small as ¼ inch. Overfed pet cats are not usually good mousers but a barn cat can deter rodents. Poison bait is not often safe around horse facilities because of the presence of pets and children; however, secure bait boxes are effective.

ODOR

Nuisance odor from the horses themselves is generally minimal. Offensive odors can be generated from manure. If manure is allowed to decompose without enough oxygen, it will be anaerobic (without oxygen) and will usually produce offensive odors. Aerobic (with oxygen) decomposition, such as composting, does not produce such odors because the microbes decomposing the waste use the nutrients and produce odor-free compounds (water vapor and carbon dioxide, for example) as a by-product. Anticipate some odor from the manure storage area because fresh manure is added daily. Place the area downwind of the stable facility and residential areas to minimize odor problems.

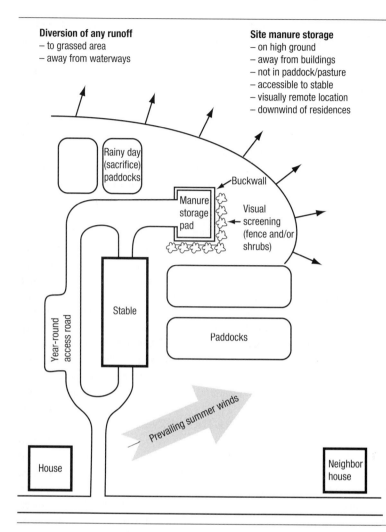

Diversion of any runoff
– to grassed area
– away from waterways

Site manure storage
– on high ground
– away from buildings
– not in paddock/pasture
– accessible to stable
– visually remote location
– downwind of residences

Rainy day (sacrifice) paddocks

Buckwall

Manure storage pad

Visual screening (fence and/or shrubs)

Stable

Year-round access road

Paddocks

Prevailing summer winds

House

Neighbor house

Figure 8.4. Farm plan showing manure management for minimizing nuisances.

Summer breezes are the main concern if winter and summer prevailing wind directions are not the same. Neighbors will be less tolerant during warm weather because they are outdoors more often and have open house windows.

AESTHETICS

Another nuisance associated with waste management can be the visual aspect of large manure storage piles. Keep the storage site screened from view with vegetation, fencing, and/or by location in a remote area. A well-designed and managed stall waste facility can be reasonably contained and not offensive visually. Screening the storage site is worthwhile because "out of sight is out of mind," if the storage is otherwise well managed.

Preventing Water Pollution

MANURE PILE RUNOFF

Any on-site manure storage should not contribute to ground or surface water pollution. Leachate is the brownish liquid that has "leached" from the solid pile contents and drains off a waste pile bottom. Not all piles will have leachate; in fact, proper management can avoid leachate formation. Stall waste is typically very dry with little leachate. When water or pure manure, such as from paddock or arena cleanup, is added, some leachate may form. A covered storage area will have much less leachate than one exposed to precipitation. Prevent any pile leachate from contaminating groundwater or nearby waterways by capturing or diverting it. A concrete pad with sidewalls is necessary to contain leachate from very large, uncovered piles. Leachate drainage to a treatment system such as a grassed infiltration area (see "Vegetated Filter Area" sidebar) is necessary to prevent runoff to geologically and socially sensitive areas. Another potential source of water pollution is from field-applied manure that is subject to surface run-off conditions or is deposited near waterways. Apply stall manure so runoff is minimized; guidelines are provided in the "Direct Disposal" section.

STALL FLOORING

The type of stall flooring may determine the potential for groundwater pollution from the stable. Concrete, most asphalt, and well-packed clay floors are considered impermeable to water flow. However, with any stall flooring material, there is so much bedding used in horse stalls that urine and any liquid from the manure are soaked up by bedding. Therefore, free urine in contact with the flooring material is minimized compared with other livestock housing. Drains are not necessary in horse stall floors, except under circumstances noted later in this chapter.

Floors in wash stalls should have impermeable and durable floors such as concrete or asphalt. Drains are recommended for wastewater removal to an approved discharge area (see "Vegetated Filter Area" sidebar). Some stalls are frequently washed down and disinfected, such as foaling stalls or hospital stalls. When large amounts of water are used, impervious floors and drains are necessary.

Drains located in the stall should be outfitted with a removable cover and located to one side of the stall to prevent discomfort when the horse lies down in the center of the stall. The floor should slope slightly (1 inch per 5 feet is adequate) toward the drain. An alternative is to slope the stall floor toward the front stall door where a shallow, narrow gutter (about 1 inch deep by 4 to 12 inch wide) is positioned along the front stall wall in the aisle floor. This gutter would then slope along the aisle toward drains. Chapter 7 contains more information on drainage.

The floor in an open-sided shelter usually consisting of the native material found on the building site. Pastured horses do not spend much time in the shelter unless encouraged to do so by feeding or fencing. Groundwater pollution is minimal because little manure is deposited in the shed. If horses are fed or confined in this facility, then a more durable floor may be desirable along with a plan to collect and dispose of the accumulated manure. Packed limestone screenings work very well in open sheds by providing good drainage and ease of cleaning.

RAINY-DAY PADDOCKS

Many farm managers have rainy-day paddocks that are exercise lots with no pasture grass. They are used for turnout during inclement weather when horse traffic on grass pastures would tear the turf into a muddy mess. Ungrassed paddocks also work well for horses kept on limited acreage or when pastures are reseeded, fertilized, or rested as part of rotational grazing program. Some managers use outdoor riding arenas for turnout paddocks. Locate exercise paddocks on high ground with provision for cleaning the area of manure and decreasing runoff potential (Fig. 8.4). A stone dust footing works well by decreasing mud, aiding drainage, and providing a surface to collect manure. The rainy-day paddock should be surrounded by well-established sod so that any runoff is captured and diverted from adjoining buildings and pastures. Fence sensitive areas around streams and natural waterways to alleviate further water pollution.

MANURE HANDLING

Efficient Movement

When handling large quantities of bulky material, straight-line movement through wide doors is the most efficient. Avoid stable designs that necessitate turns and tight passages for travel from the stall to manure deposition area. Hand labor is most common in horse stall cleaning. To increase worker efficiency, provide plenty of stall light, minimize lifting, and make the temporary manure stockpile area easily accessible from all areas of the stable (Fig. 8.5).

In most stables, stalls are cleaned daily and manure is temporarily stockpiled in an accessible area near the barn (Fig. 8.6). To avoid additional handling, workers can temporarily stockpile manure in a vehicle, such as a manure dumpster or spreader. Once the stall cleaning chores are finished or the temporary storage is filled, the stockpile is moved to the long-term storage location or removed from the stable site. Manure from heavily used turnout paddocks and riding arenas will add to the manure storage, so plan a route for fairly easy movement of manure between these sites. Chapter 4 presents considerations in locating short- and long-term manure storage.

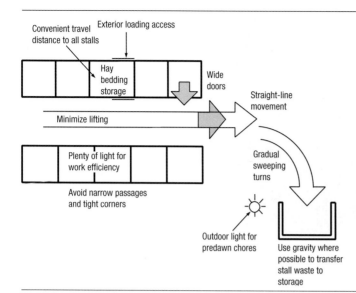

Figure 8.5. Efficient handling of large quantities of bulky material includes straight-line movement through wide doors to a convenient stockpile area.

Mechanization

Mechanization can replace some hand labor of stall cleaning. A common adaptation is a motorized vehicle pulling a cart through the working aisle of the stable. The engine exhaust and the repositioning of the cart can detract from its ultimate usefulness and become a health hazard if the stable is inadequately ventilated. The cart can efficiently transport material to areas more remote from the stable. A front-end loader and/or manure spreader can similarly be used to move stall waste outside the stable and to storage or disposal sites. For large operations, straw-based stall waste can be tossed into the work aisle then picked up with round baler equipment for movement and storage (Fig. 8.7).

A mechanized alternative is the barn cleaner, which automatically moves the waste from the stall area to the temporary stockpile area. A barn cleaner is a scraper that operates in a narrow gutter (about 16 inches wide) and has closely spaced flights on a chain drive (Figs. 8.8 and 8.9). It is designed to handle wastes with high solids content typical of horse stall waste. The gutter cleaner can be located under the floor at the back of the stall or along the side of an aisle servicing the stalls (Fig. 8.10). The primary advantage is that minimal worker effort is required

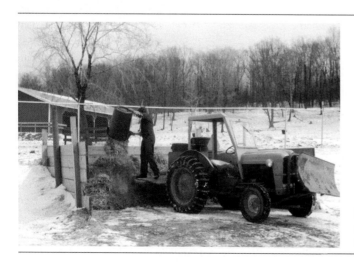

Figure 8.6. Use gravity where possible to make easier transfer of stall waste into the storage.

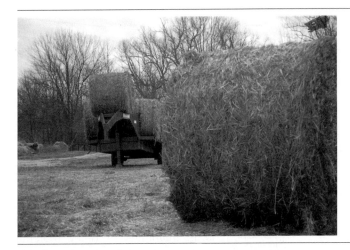

Figure 8.7. A round baler was used to pick up straw-based stall waste thrown into the central stable aisle. Waste is stored in round bale format until delivered to off-site composting processor.

to move stall waste into the gutter: no lifting, no moving carts, and no travel to the temporary stockpile area. The disadvantages are the initial cost, complex installation, and maintenance of the gutter system. Stall gutters must be covered and bedded over when horses are in the stall. With aisle gutters, horses get used to stepping around them even if gutters are left uncovered. Safety may become an issue if normally covered aisle gutters are left open.

MANURE STORAGE

The stall waste will have to be stored somewhere whether temporarily or long term. Keep stored manure in a fly-tight area during the warm months, or manage to prevent fly breeding and protect from rainfall and surface runoff. A well-built storage pad or container aids in waste handling and minimizes pollution potential from the pile. The pad can be as informal as a level, well-packed surface with a wood

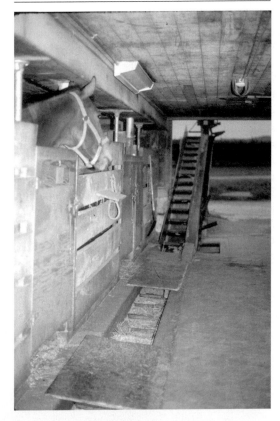

Figure 8.9. Some converted traditional dairy barns will have an operating manure gutter cleaner that can be converted for horse stall waste transport.

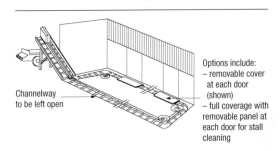

Channelway to be left open

Options include:
– removable cover at each door (shown)
– full coverage with removable panel at each door for stall cleaning

Figure 8.8. Automated barn cleaner. Adapted from *Livestock Waste Facilities Handbook.*

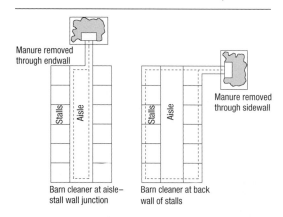

Figure 8.10. Options for automatic barn cleaner gutter and stockpile placements.

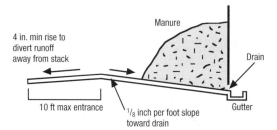

Figure 8.12. Manure pad slope and drainage. Drain and gutter are recommended in all cases, especially if the manure stack will not be protected from rainfall. Leachate (effluent) must be directed to a storage tank and/or suitable method of disposal. Reproduced with permission from *Livestock Waste Facilities Handbook*, MWPS-18.

or masonry backstop (Figs. 8.11, 8.12, and 8.13) or can be a covered structure with impermeable flooring. If topography permits, a below-grade storage container is a less-objectionable structure because it keeps the manure contained to a small area, is out of view, can be covered, and is easily filled using gravity to dump waste into it (Fig. 8.14). One side should be at ground level for emptying. Long-term manure storages are often more substantial structures than short-term storages. Large quantities of manure require a storage designed with wide door(s), a high roof, and strong construction to allow cleanout with power equipment. Construction features are shown in Figure 8.15. Additional details of large manure storages are available in the *Livestock Waste Facilities Handbook* (see Additional Resources). Manure for commercial pickup can be stored in a container or dumpster. With any large or small manure storage, a

tarp or other cover is recommended to minimize leachate production from rainfall.

Construction of the Manure Storage

Size the storage for about 180 days of long-term storage in cold climates. This provides winter storage when fields are not accessible and for summer when crops may be present. An estimated waste production of 2.4 cubic feet per day per horse would require 432 cubic feet of storage for each stalled horse. Base sizing figures on estimates that reflect the specific stable's management. It is better to have a slightly larger storage facility than one that is too small. Whether constructing a simple manure pad or more formal storage structure, some common practices will minimize labor and make nuisance control easier.

Slope entrance ramps upward with a minimum 10:1 slope (Fig. 8.12) to keep out surface water. Provide a rough-surfaced, load-out ramp at least 40 feet wide if commercial-sized agricultural machinery will be used to load and unload the storage. A smaller width of 20 feet is acceptable for smaller farm and garden tractors, leaving enough room to maneuver the tractor during unloading. Angle grooves across the ramp to drain rainwater. Install a 4-inch-thick concrete floor and ramp over 6 inches of coarse gravel or crushed rock (up to 1½-inch aggregate size). Two inches of sand can replace gravel as fill under the concrete when placed over undisturbed or compacted soil. Smaller or private stables can suffice with well-packed stone dust.

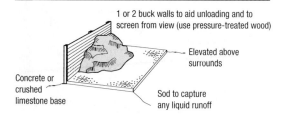

Figure 8.11. Simple manure stockpile pad with backstop, which is suitable for a small stable. Use a tarp or other cover to minimize leachate production from precipitation.

Bucking walls (backstop) are recommended to aid in unloading; options are provided in Figure 8.13.

If liquids such as unabsorbed urine, snowmelt, and rain are to be stored, slope the floor toward a

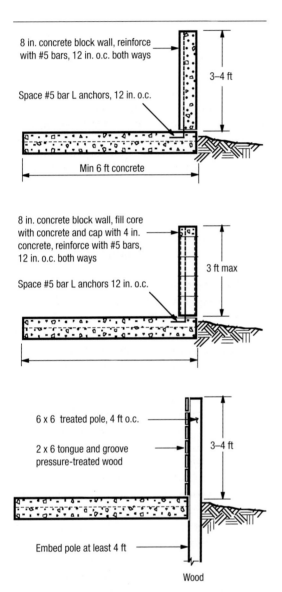

Figure 8.13. Bucking wall options.
Note: These drawings are general representations and are not meant as construction drawings. A site-specific design is recommended in all cases. If soil backfill is to be placed behind the wall, a more economical wall may be possible. Adapted from *Livestock Waste Facilities Handbook*, MWPS-18.

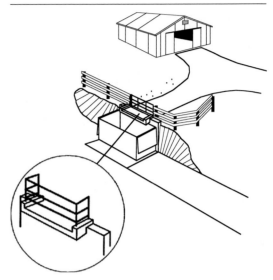

Figure 8.14. Manure storage container uses topography and gravity for ease of waste-handling chores. Two options are shown for manure drop-off protection.

closed end. The floor may be sloped to one or both sides, with openings on the low side to a gutter or surface drain (Fig. 8.16). Unabsorbed liquids may be diverted to a gently sloped, grassed area that acts as a vegetated filter (Fig. 8.17). Additional problems of handling separated liquids may make use of roofs or extra bedding a better solution. A large, unroofed storage (such as those serving multiple stables at a track) may need floor drains connected to underground corrosion-resistant 8-inch pipes to carry away liquids. Provide removable grills for

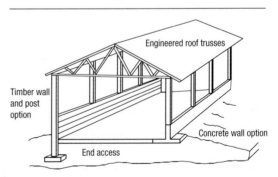

Figure 8.15. Features of large, roofed, solid-manure storage.

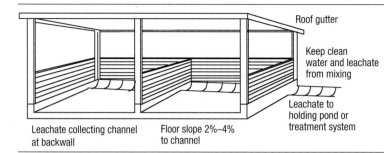

Figure 8.16. Covered storage with leachate collection for wet materials.

Roof gutter

Keep clean water and leachate from mixing

Leachate to holding pond or treatment system

Leachate collecting channel at backwall

Floor slope 2%–4% to channel

periodic cleaning, or start the stack with 6 inches of absorbent material such as wood or bark chips to absorb some liquids and permit drainage.

Siting the Manure Storage

The waste stockpile areas must be accessible to trucks or tractors in all weather conditions. A location on high ground will usually provide firm soil well above groundwater, forming a suitable base for the storage facility and access road. Keep manure away from building materials, as corrosive chemicals in the manure can damage them. Do not store manure where runoff or floodwater will cause nutrients to enter nearby waterways. Table 8.4 lists distances to separate the manure storage from sensitive areas such as nearby water sources or residences. Do not store manure in paddocks because of increased parasite exposure for the horses. Locate storages downwind from both the farm and neighbors' residences. Consider the aesthetics of the storage placement so that it can be screened from view (Fig. 8.4). Use natural or artificial screening such as a hedgerow or fence to improve the aesthetics and help contain any odors. Remember that for many perceived nuisances, out of sight can be out of mind for neighbors. Provide for easy filling of the storage with a tractor-mounted manure loader or scraper elevator stacker unit. Unload waste with a tractor-mounted bucket.

Good drainage at any manure storage site is absolutely necessary. The site may be graded to divert surface runoff without creating erosion. Poor drainage results in saturated conditions leading to muddy access and pools of dirty water. Divert any surface drainage water and runoff from nearby roofs away from the pile area. *On-Farm Composting Handbook*, NRAES-54, has details of surface water diversion and site grading. Many stables and indoor riding arenas do not have gutters and downspouts, causing substantial runoff from these buildings. A gutter and downspout system will collect and divert water away from the building foundation and bypass the manure storage. Tarps or a roof over the manure storage can minimize rainwater entry if leachate containment becomes a problem. Do not allow polluted runoff to pool because mosquitoes and flies will breed in the moist area.

Management of the Stored Manure

With proper management, flies and odors from manure storage can be minimal. The major deterrent to fly breeding in horse operations is to keep the manure as dry as possible. Other wet organic material sites also need to be removed. Remove manure from the farm at least every seven days during fly breeding season, or operate a properly managed composting facility.

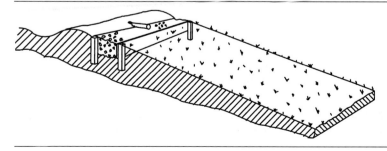

Figure 8.17. Grassed filter area for treating manure storage leachate. Use a site-specific design of the vegetated filter based on leachate production and site characteristics.

Table 8.4. Minimum Separation Distances Commonly Recommended for Composting and Manure Handling Activities

Sensitive area	Minimum separation distance (feet)
Property line	50–100
Residence or place of business	200–500
Private well or other potable water source	100–200
Wetlands or surface water (streams, pond, lakes)	100–200
Subsurface drainage pipe or drainage ditch discharging to a natural water course	25
Water table (seasonal high)	2–5
Bedrock	2–5

Source: On-Farm Composing Handbook, NRAES-54.

Add new stall waste to the pile as a large block of material to minimize fresh manure surface exposure. This reduces the area of odor volatilization and access to moist manure for fly breeding. Avoid dumping new material on top of a pile where it spreads out and falls away down the sides creating a large, fresh, and wet manure surface area promoting flies and odor. Flies lay eggs in the top 2 inches of moist manure.

Naturally occurring fly predators, tiny nonstinging wasps and parasites, are beneficial to the manure storage. Avoid indiscriminate use of larvicides and other pesticides that kill predator wasps and parasites. Depending on the species, wasps have 10- to 28-day egg and larva stages. Wasps are active during fly season (some are killed by cold temperatures), and their activity depends on manure conditions, with dry manure being the best. Wet manure decreases wasp effectiveness.

When cleaning out the storage, leave a 4-inch *dry* pad of manure over the bottom of the storage area to provide a stock of fly parasites and predators. Manure removal can be staggered to leave one section per week to supply fly predators and parasites. Remove a winter's stockpile of manure during cold weather (<65°F) before fly breeding begins.

Vegetated Filter Area

A grassed, gently sloped area may be used as a filter and infiltration area for wastewater (Fig. 8.17). Wastewater is piped to the filter area and spread evenly across the top portion of the filter. As it flows through the soil profile and down the slight slope, biological activity and adsorption in the soil matrix removes waste materials. Most biological activity occurs in the topsoil layer where aerobic (using oxygen) activity provides for odor-free treatment. Obviously, not all soils are equally suitable, as some provide rapid infiltration for limited treatment while others are rather impermeable and provide surface run-off. Frozen soil will not act as a proper filter. Get professional help from your Natural Resources Conservation Service or County Conservation District, for example, for proper filter sizing and design.

Vegetated filter area is a relatively low-cost farm wastewater treatment system. These areas can be variable in cost, approaching that of a septic system. In size, one rule of thumb is to provide about 10 square feet of vegetated filter for each gallon of wastewater being handled. The spreading device at the head of the filter strip is important for establishing even flow to minimize short-circuiting wastewater through the area. A settling tank before the filter strip will be needed if manure solids are allowed into the wastewater.

These filter areas need to be well vegetated before they are put to use. Keep animals off the filter strip, as the frequent wet soil conditions lead to destruction of the sod cover by horse grazing and exercise. If the storage facility will hold the manure from more than a few horses, the volume and strength of the leachate may be too great to send directly to a vegetated filter. In that case, the liquid should be collected in a tank and be dosed to the vegetated filter every three or more days, or be irrigated on pasture. In any case, a site-specific design is recommended.

MANURE DISPOSAL

Direct Disposal

Direct disposal involves the on-farm use of the stall waste via field application. Proper field application demands equipment such as a tractor and spreader so that the manure is applied in a thin

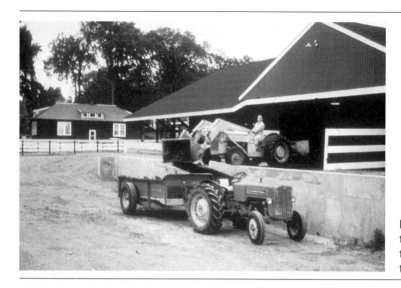

Figure 8.18. Stall waste transfer from stable collection vehicle to field application machinery.

layer over the soil (Fig. 8.18). The thin layer is essential for drying the manure to discourage fly breeding and also spreads the nutrients for more optimal plant use. Weekly spreading in the summer will disrupt fly breeding and egg development cycles. To minimize pollution from runoff, do not spread manure on frozen ground or near waterways. It may not be possible to spread manure each week, year round, in which case the manure must be stockpiled. In cold climates, figure on 180 days of stockpile storage space. Manure application may be limited to preplanting and postharvest dates for cultivated fields. Fields may not be accessible because of heavy snow accumulation or soil that is too wet to support equipment traffic.

Spreading manure in thin layers has been thought to reduce parasite numbers by desiccating the eggs. This does hold true under dry and extreme cold or hot conditions. Under the moist conditions encountered in the northeastern United States, the practice of spreading manure in thin layers on pasture is being questioned (as far as parasite control is concerned; the other nutrient, aesthetic, and fly egg desiccation characteristics remain). Recent evidence suggests that spreading thin layers of manure on pastures can enhance grazing horses' parasite exposure by spreading viable parasites over a larger area. The recommendation is to leave the manure piles in clumps and pick them up for disposal outside the pasture area.

Field application is based on fertilizer needs of the crop or pasture grass through soil sampling (Fig. 8.19). The approximate fertilizer value of

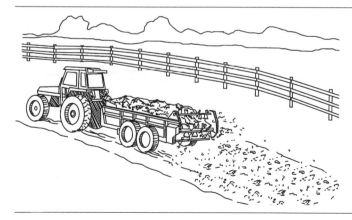

Figure 8.19. Proper application with a tractor and spreader provides a thin layer of stable waste over the soil to improve manure drying and fertilizer application along with decreased fly breeding. Adapted from *On-Farm Composting Handbook*, NRAES-54.

manure from bedded horse stalls (46% dry matter) is 4 pounds per ton ammonium-N, 14 pounds per ton total N, 4 pounds per ton P_2O_5 (phosphate), and 14 pounds per ton K_2O (potash). Fertilizer value of manure at 20% moisture without bedding is approximately 12-5-9 pounds per ton (N-P_2O_5-K_2O). Horse manure nutrient values surveyed from published literature are presented in Table 8.5. Nutrient values vary widely, so use these values as guidelines and have the manure analyzed if more specific data are needed. The amount of organic nitrogen mineralized (released to crops) during the first cropping season after application of horse manure is about 0.20. Organic nitrogen must be released through mineralization before plants can use it. About 20% of the organic nitrogen from horse manure is available to the pasture grass the year of application.

Table 8.5. Equations from Which Nitrogen, Phosphorus, and Potassium Daily Excretion Can Be Estimated

Nitrogen Excretion (mg/kg BW)
Sedentary horses:
$$N_{out} = 55.4 + 0.586 \times N_{in} \qquad (R^2 = 0.76)$$
Exercised horses:
$$N_{out} = 42.9 + 0.492 \times N_{in} \qquad (R^2 = 0.94)$$
Phosphorus Excretion (mg/kg BW)
Sedentary or exercised horses:
$$P_{out} = 4.56 + 0.793 \times P_{in} \qquad (R^2 = 0.85)$$
Potassium Excretion (mg/kg BW)
Sedentary or exercised horses:
$$K_{out} = 19.4 + 0.673 \times K_{in} \qquad (R^2 = 0.62)$$

Note: The equations were developed from dozens of published studies that documented daily intake and excretion of these three nutrients. For nitrogen, different equations should be used to estimate excretion by working and nonworking horses. For phosphorus and potassium, the same equation may be used because there were no significant differences between sedentary and exercised horses. Calculated values apply to mature body weights of (850 to 1350 pounds) nonpregnant and nonlactating horses.

Notations: N_{in}, nitrogen intake (mg/kg BW); N_{out}, nitrogen excretion; P_{in}, phosphorus intake (mg/kg BW); P_{out}, phosphorus excretion; K_{in}, potassium intake (mg/kg BW); K_{out}, potassium excretion; BW, body weight (kg)

Organic nitrogen released during subsequent seasons is usually about 50% (second year), 25% (third year), and 13% (fourth year) of the first-year mineralization.

Contract Disposal

Another manure disposal option is to contract with a hauler who will remove the waste from the stable facility. The waste can be used in a commercial composting operation or for other functions where the waste disposal is the responsibility of the hauler. Dumpsters are positioned at the stable for temporary stall waste storage (no trash or garbage); a full dumpster is replaced with an empty one. Dumpsters should be sized so that the contents are emptied at least weekly during the fly breeding season. Place the dumpster in a convenient location where barn waste can be dumped into it and trucks can access and empty the dumpster during all weather (Fig. 8.14). A concrete tank or pad is useful to contain any dumpster leachate.

A less formal "contract" disposal is to interest neighbors in free garden organic material. The key is to locate the organic fertilizer enthusiasts. Owners of small stables have had success with newspaper ads and locating "free" bagged manure at curbside. Empty feed sacks filled with horse manure are a useful package for manure distribution.

By-product: Compost

An alternative to "disposing" of horse manure is to compost it into a by-product of the operation. Composting occurs naturally if stall waste decomposes in the presence of oxygen and is kept relatively moist, above 50% moisture content (Fig. 8.20). The

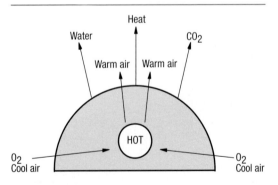

Figure 8.20. Simple process of a composting stall waste pile.

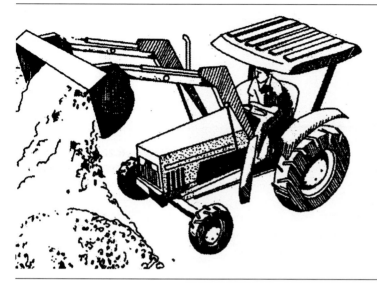

Figure 8.21. A front-end loader (pictured) or specialized compost turning equipment is used to turn compost in professionally managed composting facilities. Reproduced with permission from *On-Farm Composting Handbook*, NRAES-54.

microbes that decompose the bedding and manure occur naturally in stall waste. In fact, commercial composters and mushroom substrate preparation facilities often seek straw-bedded horse stall waste. Composting provides a material that is more readily marketable than raw stall waste. Finished compost is partially degraded manure and is more organically stable, presenting less of a pollution threat. Its finer texture, high organic matter content, and fertilizer value make it desirable as a garden soil amendment. Composting reduces the volume of waste by 40% to 70%. Horse manure, with its associated bedding, is almost perfectly suited for composting because it has appropriate levels of nitrogenous material and carbon-based bedding material. (The carbon-to-nitrogen ratio of stall waste is 20:1 to 30:1.) Stables have successfully given away, or even sold, bulk and bagged horse compost. Golf courses and nurseries provide an outlet for truckloads of compost.

Pathogens and fly eggs are killed by the high temperature of composting. Parasite eggs can be killed with a 30-minute exposure to 140°F that will occur on the inside of a properly composted pile. These temperatures are not reached on the pile exterior, which is one reason the pile is periodically mixed and turned so that exterior material is incorporated into the middle for full composting. Stall waste composts well in piles that are at least 3 feet square by 3 feet deep. Smaller piles will not retain enough heat to reach the proper composting temperature.

There is a trade-off between the complexities of composting facilities versus the amount of time to produce finished compost. For example, static pile composting, which is informally practiced at most stables, involves simply piling the stall waste and letting it "compost" for 6 months to 2 years. In contrast, with more ideal conditions and intensive management, the same stall waste could be composted in about 4 weeks. Intensive management of a composting operation entails daily monitoring and periodic (perhaps weekly) attention to mixing the raw ingredients, forming the pile, and perhaps turning the compost (Fig. 8.21).

Compost microbes live most comfortably at certain temperatures (130–140°F) and moisture levels (50%–60%). They need oxygen (5%–15%), so waste pile aeration is necessary. The more carefully these biological factors are controlled, the more sophisticated the compost facility becomes. It takes 2 weeks to 6 months to produce finished compost under professionally managed conditions. The benefit of faster production is that less space is needed for compost processing and storage. Large, commercial compost facilities provide near-ideal conditions for composting to speed the process and minimize space. Aerated bunkers in buildings may be used at large compost finishing facilities where a uniform product is ground and bagged for sale (Figs. 8.22, 8.23, and 8.24) A good and thorough guide to on-farm composting is available (see Additional Resources).

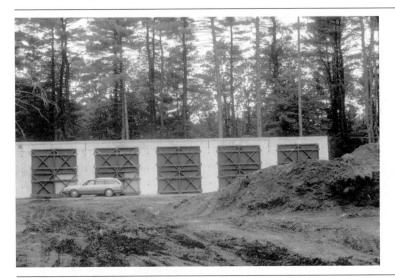

Figure 8.22. Composting facility where bunker rooms contain horse stall waste subjected to forced aeration to speed process versus static pile composting. Finished compost is stockpiled in the foreground.

Intensive composting will be another daily operation at the stable. This responsibility may not be of interest to all stable managers. The sale or disposal of the compost must also be considered. Marketing and potential liability becomes important if off-farm disposal is desired. Having a ready outlet for compost will make the facility and time investment more worthwhile. With limited hauling, a centralized cooperative facility could be managed for several farms, with more effective process labor and marketing of compost being additional benefits.

OTHER STABLE WASTES

Waste management is not confined to horse stall waste at a large facility. Keep trash separate from manure and soiled bedding for disposal. Recyclable materials are also kept separate for collection. Medical waste (e.g., syringes) usually has special disposal requirements. Fertilizers and pesticides and their containers sometimes have disposal restrictions. Human waste from a bathroom requires a septic system or connection to municipal sewer. Gray water, such as shower and sink water, may also go to the septic or sewer unless it is needed for groundskeeping or other uses where high-quality water is not necessary. A grassed filter area may be used to treat wastewater from the stable's horse wash stalls, tack area, laundry, showers, and feed room.

Drainage and surface runoff from pavement, building roofs, unvegetated paddocks, and exercise

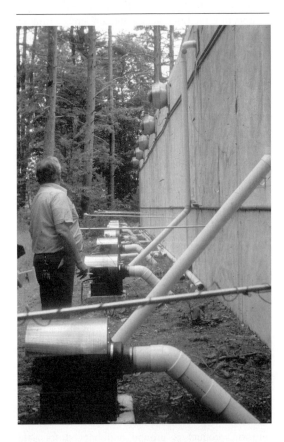

Figure 8.23. Fan, temperature instrumentation, and air distribution piping behind aerated bunker composting facility.

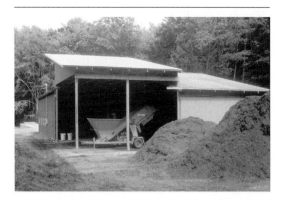

Figure 8.24. Further processing of composted stall waste is often needed prior to sale to provide uniform material. Shredding and sieving are typical processes before being bagged, and even for many bulk sales.

areas need to be managed. This is especially important for areas where manure is allowed to accumulate between rainfall or thawing events. Run off should not enter natural waterways, where it could increase nutrient level of the water or contribute to increased erosion. Pick up excess manure from paddocks and exercise areas and add to manure handling system.

KEEPING IT LEGAL

Among state and federal agencies, there are various regulations for protecting environmental quality that are aimed at manure management. Often, categories of livestock (including horse) operations are defined that relate to their potential to cause environmental harm. When stable facilities and manure storage structures are properly designed, constructed, and managed, the manure is an important and environmentally safe source of nutrients and organic matter. Proper land application of manure will not cause water quality problems (Fig. 8.25). The intent of regulations is to ensure that economically practical techniques are used in all aspects of manure handling. In some states, all farms are required to properly handle manure in accordance with water quality laws, but formal nutrient (manure) management plans are generally not required of all farms.

Many states have enacted nutrient management legislation aimed at higher density livestock farms to address water quality concerns. The law defines the regulated community as animal production facilities having more than a target threshold of animal equivalent units (aeu) per acre. An animal equivalent unit is 1000 pounds of animal, or about one horse or four market-weight hogs, and so forth. Although most horse facilities would be smaller in total animal equivalent units than the currently targeted Concentrated Animal Operations (CAO), stable owners should be aware of the regulatory emphasis being placed on environmental stewardship. Regulations originally targeted 1000-aeu facilities, but smaller farms, many of which are horse facilities, are now in the regulated community. Be aware that

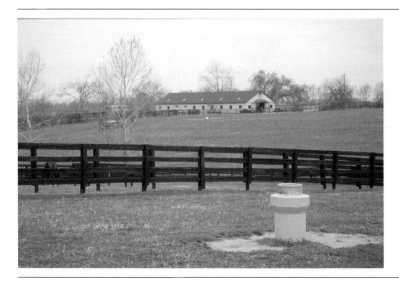

Figure 8.25. Stall waste is part of a pasture fertilization management plan if enough acreage is available to properly apply the manure.

many suburban horse farms are considered higher *density* livestock farms according to some nutrient management guidelines, because they have more than two animal equivalent units per acre.

Environmental information related to water quality and manure management is usually available from a state's department that regulates and enforces environmental protection. A local source of conservation-minded assistance for manure management planning and design are county Conservation District and Natural Resources Conservation Service offices. Check the phone directory blue pages under County Government and United States Government (Agriculture), respectively.

HAVE A PLAN

It is recommended that managers of large stables (10 or more horses) prepare a written manure management plan. This is a useful tool for the operator and shows that a proactive stance has been taken if

methods of manure handling are questioned. Keep it simple, but address exactly how and where manure is stored and disposed. Address leachate management and manure storage siting for reducing water pollution. Address water run-on and runoff from the stable and storage site. Even preparing a simple handwritten plan is beneficial in thinking through how to efficiently handle tons of manure and soiled bedding.

SUMMARY

Making manure management a more thoughtful and efficient chore benefits both horse owners and their neighbors. Time spent planning for proper and easy manure disposal will pay back in many more hours spent enjoying the horses through decreased time and effort in stall cleaning and manure disposal chores. Maintaining good neighbor relations through fly and odor minimization will assure the compatibility of horse stables within the neighborhood.

9
Fire Safety

Many of us know the legend of Catherine O'Leary's infamous cow accused of kicking over a lantern and starting a barn fire on the night of October 8, 1871, leveling three square miles of Chicago. A barn fire in today's world is not likely to destroy a city, although it is likely to devastate the barn. In the blink of an eye, a fire can destroy a barn structure and all its occupants while the owners stand by helplessly. Many advances in residential fire protection have been made, but protecting barns is much more difficult because of their harsh environment and housing requirements of the horses in them.

In barn fires, the old adage "an ounce of prevention is worth a pound of cure" could not be truer. Planning is the greatest asset in fire prevention (Fig. 9.1). This chapter provides an understanding of fire behavior and how fire and fire damage can be minimized or prevented through building techniques, fire detection options, and management practices.

HOW A FIRE BEHAVES

A fire occurs when a fuel source comes in contact with an ignition source. A fuel source can be any item that contains wood, plant material, plastic, paper, fabric, combustible fuel, and so forth. After contact with the ignition source (anything that would cause the fuel to burn, e.g., spark, intense heat), the fuel starts to smolder. Oxygen availability, fuel type, and physical arrangement are factors that determine the length of the smoldering process. Smoldering can vary from minutes to hours. Fires caught during this stage have the greatest chances of being controlled with minimal damage but are still extremely dangerous. Smoldering fires may also be difficult to detect and completely extinguish, especially with smoldering hay or wood shavings, when the fuel itself helps to insulate the fire and prevent water penetration. The time it takes a fire to grow and spread is again related to a number of factors, such as the fuel source, the fire temperature, and the time the fire has to burn.

Smoke and heat production increase as the fire smolders. By the end of this smoldering or "incipient" phase, enough heat has been generated to produce flames. Once flames are present, the fire is extremely dangerous and unpredictable. It grows rapidly and the heat produced becomes intense. The capabilities of fire extinguishers as a line of defense will soon be surpassed. After flame eruption it only takes a few minutes for ceiling temperatures to exceed 1800°F. As ceiling temperatures continue to rise, the building acts as a boiler and the "flash point" is soon reached. When fire has reached the flash point, often in as little as 3 to 5 minutes, the hot air temperature simultaneously ignites all combustibles within the space. At flash point, survival within the structure is unlikely, and the building contents are destroyed.

Smoke is produced in the earliest stages of fire development. The color and density of the smoke are dependent on fuel and burning conditions. Low-temperature fires produce more visible smoke particles, creating darker, thicker smoke, whereas hotter fires have smaller particles in the smoke, making it less visible. Smoke and heat are the fire's killing attributes. Smoke contains noxious gases and vapors specific to the fuel. The most common products of combustion (fire) are carbon monoxide and carbon dioxide. As the fire consumes the available oxygen in the room, it releases carbon monoxide. When inhaled, carbon monoxide combines with blood hemoglobin more readily than oxygen would, resulting in suffocation, even if an adequate supply of oxygen is available. Elevated levels of carbon monoxide and carbon dioxide increase respiration in an attempt to obtain more oxygen, resulting in the inhalation of more deadly gases. The consequences are swift, thorough incapacitation and asphyxiation. Bodily harm from smoke is increased by its intense heat. When this superheated mass of gases is inhaled, the respiratory

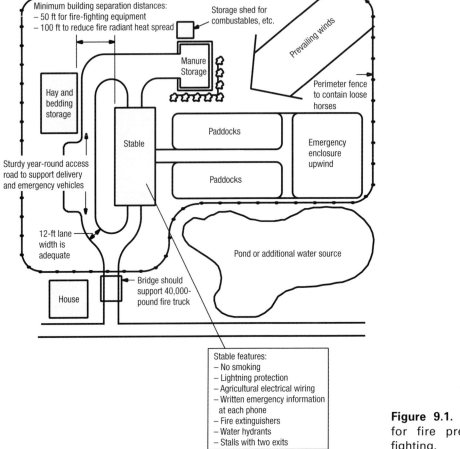

Minimum building separation distances:
– 50 ft for fire-fighting equipment
– 100 ft to reduce fire radiant heat spread

Storage shed for combustables, etc.

Prevailing winds

Manure Storage

Hay and bedding storage

Perimeter fence to contain loose horses

Stable

Paddocks

Emergency enclosure upwind

Sturdy year-round access road to support delivery and emergency vehicles

Paddocks

12-ft lane width is adequate

Pond or additional water source

Bridge should support 40,000-pound fire truck

House

Stable features:
– No smoking
– Lightning protection
– Agricultural electrical wiring
– Written emergency information
  at each phone
– Fire extinguishers
– Water hydrants
– Stalls with two exits

Figure 9.1. Site features for fire prevention and fighting.

tract will be seared. Smoke damage can occur even before flames are visible.

Once all available fuel sources have been used, the fire will "burn out." Unfortunately, this is not necessarily the end of the fire. Barns and agricultural buildings often contain large quantities of fuel sources that can be impervious to water (e.g., hay, petroleum fuels, and fertilizers). It is common for some of these fuel sources to remain unburned during the initial fire, then continue to smolder. These smoldering pockets often reignite or "rekindle" another fire, requiring another visit from the fire department.

Fire Prevention Is the Best Protection

There is no such thing as a fireproof building, especially in agricultural settings. Building design, management, and safety practices are the best way to minimize the risk of fires. It has been estimated that the root cause of 95% of preventable horse barn fires is from careless smoking, with faulty electrical systems high on the list. Fires can grow quickly and give no warning. In most cases, if you see flames, it is already too late. The damage a fire causes grows exponentially with the amount of time it has burned. Fire is extremely dangerous at any stage of growth and controlling it is best left up to the professionals.

Most barn fires occur in the winter when most forage and bedding is stored, electrical use is high, and equipment repairs and upgrades are traditionally made. Most of the components in a horse barn are highly flammable. Stall walls are frequently constructed with wood, and horses are usually standing in ample amounts of dried bedding, eating dried forages.

HAY FIRES

Hay fires are unique to the horse and agricultural industry. Baled hay can be its own fuel and ignition source. The majority of hay fires occur within 6 weeks of baling, usually caused by excessive moisture in the bale. Ideal moisture range for hay at baling is 15% to 18%. Even after grass and legume forages are harvested, plant respiration continues and generates a small amount of heat. In properly harvested forages, respiration decreases and will eventually cease during drying and curing. The heat of respiration is normal and under appropriate curing is inconsequential. However, if moisture levels are too high, the respiratory heat will provide an environment suitable for the already-present mesophilic microorganisms (that require moderately warm temperatures) to grow and multiply. As these microorganisms grow, heat is produced as a by-product of their respiration and reproduction. Once the bale interior reaches temperatures of 130 to 140°F, the environment becomes unsuitable for these organisms and most die. If microorganism activity declines, the interior bale temperature also declines. This cycle may be repeated several times, but the maximum temperature will be lower each time. Hay that has sustained these heat cycles has lost its quality as a feeding source but poses no threat as an ignition source.

Baled hay becomes a potential fire hazard when the interior bale temperature does not cool after the first heating cycle. If conditions are favorable, the heat created by the mesophilic organisms provides an environment for thermophilic, or heat-loving, microorganisms to take over. When the thermophilic microorganisms begin to multiply, their heat of respiration can raise the interior bale temperature to 170°F before they die from the heat. This is an extremely high temperature and can cause the bale to ignite if oxygen is present. The growth of microorganisms within the hay bale creates a microscopic cavernous environment, similar to a sponge. The damaged material in the bale combines readily with oxygen and, in its already-heated state, can self-ignite quickly. A burning bale of hay may be difficult to detect because the inside of the bale burns first. Hay fires are very difficult to extinguish completely. The tightly laced forages prevent water from penetrating to the core. Only a forceful blast of water can penetrate deep enough to extinguish the fire.

Hay temperature monitoring can be done to ensure that bale temperatures never reach critical levels. Under less-than-ideal field curing conditions, hay may have been baled above the recommended 15% to 18% moisture level. Check newly baled hay twice a day for heat buildup.

A temperature probe is available at most farm supply companies (i.e., Nasco, Gemplers) and stores (Agway) for $12 to $20. If bale temperatures have reached 150°F, monitor the interior bale temperature frequently, as the temperature is most likely to climb. By the time the interior bale temperature reaches 175 to 190°F, a fire is about to occur, and at 200°F, a fire has already erupted (Table 9.1).

An alternative to purchasing a temperature probe is to make one, using a metal rod $\frac{3}{8}$ to $\frac{1}{2}$ inches in diameter. Drive the rod into the hay and let it stand for at least 15 to 20 minutes before removing it. If the temperature within the bale is less than 130°F, you should be able to hold the metal comfortably in your bare hand. If the bale has reached a temperature of 160°F or greater, the rod will be too hot to hold comfortably in your bare hands. If the rod is too hot, let it cool for a few minutes and then reconfirm by taking another sample. When hot hay bales are found, summon the fire department. Be sure to tell the dispatcher that you have hot hay bales that may ignite instead of saying that you have a hay fire. This will help the fire company in planning on how to deal with your situation.

Hay Storage Recommendations

There are plenty of theories about how to stack bales in a storage or mow. It is a good idea to stack bales on their sides, with the stems of the cut hay running up and down. This allows convection ventilation of warm, moist air up and out of the bale. The greener or moister the hay, the looser it should be packed to allow cooling and curing without danger of mildew formation or combustion. Realize though that loosely packed bales are more prone to tumbling out of their stacked formation. Using pallets, or at least a layer of dry straw, under the bottom row will reduce storage losses from ground moisture. One strong recommendation to reduce fire hazard (with an added benefit of decreasing dust levels in the barn) is to store hay and bedding in a separate building from the horse stable.

Table 9.1. Determining Hay Temperatures with a Probe

Temperature	Interpretation
Below 130°F	No problem.
130–140°F	No problem yet.
	Temperature may go up or down.
	Recheck in a few hours.
150°F	Temperature will most likely continue to climb.
	Move the hay to provide air circulation and cooling.
	Monitor temperature often.
175–190°F	Fire is imminent or may be present a short distance from the probe.
	Call the fire department.
	Continue probing and monitoring the temperature.
200°F or above	Fire is present at or near the probe.
	Call the fire department.
	Inject water to cool hot spots before moving hay.
	Have a charged hose ready to control blazing when moving hay.

Note: You should use a probe and thermometer to accurately determine the temperature inside a stack of hay. Push or drive the probe into the stack, and lower the thermometer to the end of the probe on a lightweight wire. If the probe is horizontal, use a heavier wire to push the thermometer into the probe. After about 15 minutes, retrieve the thermometer and read the temperature.

SITE PLAN AND CONSTRUCTION CONSIDERATIONS

Fire Codes for Barns

In many states, horse barns and agricultural buildings do not have state-mandated fire code requirements. Some states such as New Jersey have enacted fire codes for their agricultural community, and there is some speculation that other states are not far from doing the same. Fire codes consider building materials and designate fire prevention techniques on the basis of floor area and use. Fire codes do vary among municipalities, so check the local zoning and building codebook while in the planning stages of construction.

Site Planning for Fire Fighting

Facility design plays an important role not only in fire prevention but also in fire suppression (Fig. 9.2). Design the facility for accessibility of large rescue vehicles. Be sure that all roads and bridges providing access to the property and between buildings are large enough for emergency vehicles. A 12-foot-wide lane is sufficient, and any bridges should support a 40,000-pound fire truck. Bridge requirements will vary depending on the span of the bridge. It may be a good idea to contact

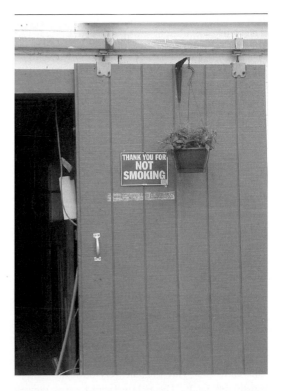

Figure 9.2. Post and enforce a no smoking policy in the stable, hay and bedding storage, and riding arenas.

your local fire chief to ensure that you meet any requirements for your lane.

An effective tool to prevent the spread of fire between buildings is to place buildings at least 50 to 100 feet away from the stable. The 100-foot distance reduces the chance of fire spreading from building to building through radiation. The 50-foot gap between buildings provides access for fire-fighting equipment. The ground around all buildings should be compacted or sturdy enough to support the weight of heavy equipment, such as a fire truck, during wet conditions. Fire hoses can deliver 250 gallons of water per minute and the ground around the building and truck will get saturated. The fire department will not risk endangering their lives or equipment at a fire scene. Having a surface that can provide access to buildings allows the fire department more options to attack the fire efficiently and safely.

Building Materials

The three rating systems for building materials are flame spread, smoke development, and fire rating. Each rating system compares how well the material in question behaves in a fire compared to a standard. The standard materials are concrete and raw wood, usually red oak. Flame spread ratings indicate how well or poorly a material will prevent flames from traveling along it. Concrete has a flame spread rating of 0; and raw wood, 100. The lower the flame spread rating, the longer it takes for flames to traverse the surface of the material.

A good or low smoke development rating indicates that the material produces less smoke as it burns. Less smoke improves visibility, decreases the quantity of noxious gases, and decreases fire progression through smoke particles and gases. Fire ratings tell important characteristics about how long (in minutes) the material contains a fire. The longer the progression of the fire is blocked, the greater chance rescue and fire suppression efforts will have at being successful. Each rating has inherent differences in controlling fires. For example, metal siding on a barn has a good flame spread rating, preventing the spread of flames, but because metal is a good conductor of heat, it has a poor fire rating and it could conduct enough heat to ignite combustible materials behind it.

Use rated fire-retardant or -resistant products, such as masonry, heavy timber, or fire-retardant treated wood whenever possible. Masonry will not burn, but it may be too costly to install, and because masonry construction is so tight, it tends to obstruct airflow around the stable interior. Heavy timber has a greater ratio of volume to surface area. The small surface area compared to the total volume prevents the wood from burning as quickly. In heavy timber construction, fire chars the wood to a depth of approximately 1 inch. The charred surface prevents the flames from accessing the wood in the center of the post, maintaining its structural integrity.

Fire-retardant treated wood decreases flame spread by 75% (flame spread rating is 25 for treated wood, 100 for untreated), and if the treatment is properly applied, it will be effective for at least 30 years. Lumber or plywood treated with fire retardant releases noncombustible gas and water vapor below normal ignition points, usually 300 to 400°C or 572 to 752°F. When the wood is exposed to flames, a hard carbon char layer forms on the surface of the wood, insulating it from further damage. Because of this insulation (charring), heavy timber and wood treated with fire retardant retains its structural integrity longer than unprotected steel during a fire.

Treated wood products may withstand the harsh, humid barn environment better than untreated products, but it depends on the ingredients used. Obtain information on wood strength and recommended fasteners from the manufacturer. The fire-retardant ingredients can be more corrosive to fasteners, especially in a high-humidity setting, characteristic of barns and indoor riding arenas. Be sure that any fire-retardant treated wood is stamped with either the Underwriter's Laboratory or Factory Mutual seal to ensure the products meet recent fire-retardant standards of the American Wood Products Association.

Some care must be taken while selecting fire-retardant lumber and plywood. The fire-retardant ingredients contain inorganic salts, such as monoammonium and diammonium phosphate, ammonium sulfate, zinc chloridem, sodium tetraborate, boric acid, and guanylurea phosphate, and may not be safe for chewers, cribbers, and foals. Most salts are water soluble and will leach out of the wood if it is frequently washed (such as a wash or foaling stall) or if the barn is continually damp because of poor drainage or inadequate ventilation. In these situations, select fire-retardant wood with low hygroscopicity. Instead of salts, low-hygroscopicity materials use impregnated water-insoluble amino resins or polymer flame-retardants grafted directly to the wood fiber. These retardants bond directly with the wood and will not wash out.

Lightning Protection Systems

All barns, regardless of age, should be outfitted with a lightning protection system, commonly referred to as "lightning rods." Lightning storms occur in every state, but most prevalently in the central and eastern United States. It is estimated that there are 40 to 80 lightning strikes per square mile each year. Lightning is a stream of pure energy, ½ to ¾ inches thick, surrounded by 4 inches of superheated air, hot enough to boil and instantaneously evaporate all the sap from a tree at the moment of impact. It looks for a path of least resistance from ground to cloud and has the potential to burn, damage, or kill anything in its path.

A properly installed and grounded lightning protection system is good insurance to minimize the chance of a horse barn catching fire from a lightning strike. The metal air terminal (rod) is the highest part of the building to intercept the lightning bolt; direct it through a heavy conducting cable, deep into the ground to be harmlessly dissipated. These systems are inexpensive to install on existing or newly constructed barns and should be periodically inspected by a qualified professional to ensure that all connections are intact and still work properly. Lightning protection systems should only be installed by a certified installer, not by an amateur. An improperly installed system cannot only fail, but increases the potential of the building to be struck by lightning. Certified installers can be found by contacting the Lightning Protection Institute (335 N. Arlingtons Heights, IL 60004, 1-800-488-6864) or the Underwriter's Laboratory (333 Pfingston Road, Northbrook, IL 60062, 1-847-272-2800).

SIMPLE SOLUTIONS TO MINIMIZE FIRE RISK

The Best Way to Prevent Fire Is to Minimize Fuel Sources

- Keep the grass mowed and the weeds down to improve the aesthetics and eliminate a frequently overlooked fuel source (dried plant materials).
- Store hay, bedding, and equipment in a separate section of the barn or, preferably, in its own building.
- Remove less frequently used combustibles from the stable. Store all combustibles properly and be sure to provide appropriate receptacles to dispose of rags soiled with combustibles.
- Keep the barn clean and free of cobwebs, chaff, and dust, which are easily combustible and make excellent fuel sources.

- An ignition source includes the obvious cigarettes and heaters to those not so obvious, such as machinery exhaust systems. Trucks driven into the hay and bedding storage area have been known to ignite materials in contact with the hot exhaust and catalytic converters. Space heaters should only be used according to the manufacturer's guidelines and should not be left unattended.
- Post and enforce a no smoking policy (Fig. 9.2). All smoking should be banned from the barn and immediate premises. If smokers do frequent the barn, provide them with a smoking area away from the barn that is equipped with a receptacle for butts and matches.

Stable Design and Management to Minimize Fire Risk

Having water hydrants (more than one) with adequate water volume and pressure located in and around the barn helps in early suppression before the fire company arrives. An alternative is having enough hose available to reach all areas in the barn. In all facilities, hydrants need to be frost free. If heat tapes are used (but their use is discouraged), be sure to read, understand, and follow all manufacturer warnings and directions. An improperly installed heat tape is a fire hazard.

Locating additional water sources around the barn will save valuable time for firefighters (Fig. 9.3). Water sources include ponds, swimming pools, cisterns, and manure lagoons. The major reason for fire suppression problems in rural communities is the lack of water supply. Any potential water source

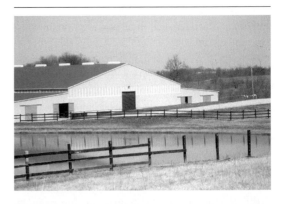

Figure 9.3. Having nearby water adds to the aesthetics of a farm site and serves as a fire-fighting water source.

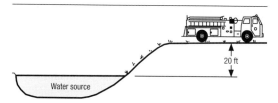

Figure 9.4. Maximum elevation difference between water source and fire truck. From *Fire Control in Livestock Buildings*, NRAES 39.

must be no lower than 20 feet below the pump truck elevation (Fig. 9.4). Most large agricultural enterprises develop a pond into the farmstead plan for fire suppression. The farm pond often provides recreational and aesthetic functions as well.

Do not overlook the importance of proper electrical wiring. Old, damaged, or improperly connected wires are a fire hazard, especially in a dusty environment. All wiring should be housed in a conduit and have an UF-B rating. The plastic used in residential wire insulators is often "sweet" and invites rodents to chew the wires, exposing them to each other. Conduit can be metal, but because of the humidity in barn environments, PVC is preferred. Chapter 10 contains details of electrical wiring and water service to horse facilities.

Overloaded circuits or outlets are another recipe for disaster. Inspect and clean electrical panels, wiring, and fixtures frequently. Use dust-tight electric switch and receptacle fixtures. Lighting fixtures and fans should be designed for agricultural use (Fig. 9.5), which is a harsher environment than in residential applications, and have appropriate dust- and moisture-resistant covers. Use products approved by the Underwriter's Laboratory, keep all electric appliances in good repair, and unplug them when not in use. Electricity to the barn may be turned off at night. Locate master switches near entrances so that light is available for rescue and fire suppression efforts.

Be sure that a charged and mounted fire extinguisher is easily accessible every 50 feet in the barn (Fig. 9.6). The most versatile type of extinguisher is

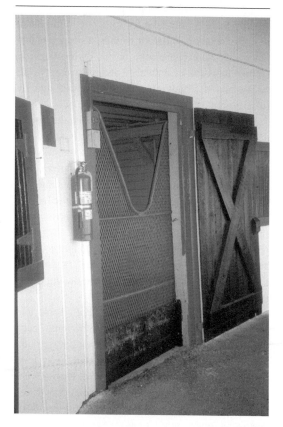

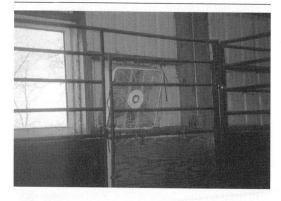

Figure 9.5. A fan designed for residential use, such as the "box" fan shown, has potential for motor to overheat because it does not have a fully enclosed motor and is not designed to remain cool under high dust accumulation. Agricultural grade fans are recommended for use in horse stables whether they are used for circulating air over individual horses in a stall or for exhaust of stale air.

Figure 9.6. Maintain fire extinguishers every 50 feet in large stabling facilities near areas of potential fire such as stalls, hay and bedding storage, and places where equipment or appliances are used. Different types of extinguishers will be needed depending on fire fuel.

the ABC type (Fig. 9.7) that extinguishes the broadest range of fire. Extinguishers are not universal. Using a water-type extinguisher can spread fires fueled by flammable liquids, such as gasoline, or become a safety hazard in electrical fires. An ABC type is recommended for locations that may experience different types of fires.

Try to design stalls with two exits for the horse to use in an escape route. An adequate number of exits are needed so that the fire will not block the only exit(s). Provide easy entrances and exits from all stalls and rooms. Have exits open into an enclosed area so that horses escaping the stable will not have access to nearby roads and traffic or destroy neighbor's property. Be sure to keep all exits clear. A fire door is not an effective exit if it is blocked. Have halters and lead ropes available for each horse.

Swinging stall doors should open out of the stall. Frantic horses will catch a hip on half-open doors. Also, if there is only time for someone to run down the alley opening stall door latches, a horse pushing out on the door can escape on his own. Likewise, sliding doors can be unlatched and pushed open. All latches and fastenings on doors should work quickly to save time.

Post evacuation plans and practice fire drills with all persons and horses in the barn. Post by the phone all emergency numbers, written directions, a list of any chemicals stored on the premises, and any other important information that emergency operators will need. Providing a map of the facility to emergency services will greatly enhance reaction time once Fire/Emergency Medical Services (EMS) is on site. This map should indicate where animals are housed, water sources that can be used to help extinguish a fire, and the location and quantity of commonly stored chemicals.

By practicing evacuation drills, both horse and handler can prepare for emergency situations. Teach the horses to walk out with their eyes covered and accustom horses to firefighter turnout gear, loud noises that simulate sirens, and smoke. If horses are reluctant to walk blindfolded during the drills, chances are that they will be even more reluctant during an emergency situation. Some fire companies are willing to meet with you to train both you and the firefighters. Most firefighters are volunteers who may have little to no horse experience, making handling a frightened horse not only difficult and dangerous, but also potentially lethal.

MORE EXTENSIVE FIRE PROTECTION

The best barn fire prevention systems incorporate building design, early warning devices, and fire suppression mechanisms. Building design for fire prevention changes the environment to minimize the spread of heat and flames and provides multiple options for escape. Barn design should increase the time it takes a fire to reach the flash point by modifying ceiling height or room volume, building materials, and building contents.

Horse Stall on Fire

Protecting a horse stall is not the same as protecting a home. The horse is standing in dry bedding material that is very flammable. Straw reaches a burning temperature of 3008F in 1 to 5 minutes and develops as much heat at the same rate as gasoline. All that is required to start this fire is a spark or match. It takes 2 to 3 minutes for a straw fire to burn an area 10 feet in diameter. Compare this to the size of a common horse box stall that is 10- to 12-feet square. After a fire starts in a stall and spreads to only 4 feet in diameter, most horses are injured. By a 6-foot diameter, its lungs are seared. With an 8-foot diameter fire, the horse will start to suffocate. By 10 feet, the horse is dead. All of this occurs in 2 to 3 minutes. If the horse is to survive unharmed, he must be removed from the stall within 30 seconds. A quick rescue is key, but fire prevention is more important.

Compartmentalization

Although not a common practice in horse barns, one way to slow a fire's spread is to compartmentalize the structure. Compartmentalization divides the stable into "rooms" not longer than 150 feet with fire-resistant barriers such as walls, doors, or fire curtains. This prevents the spread of fire within the building and allows more time for fire suppression. A true firewall must be completely sealed in a fire and should provide at least 1 hour of fire protection (Fig. 9.8). Any doors in the wall need to be fire rated and self-closing, and any openings for wiring or pipes need to be sealed. In a stable with a frame-constructed roof, the wall itself needs to extend at least 18 inches above the roof; the higher the wall extends, the longer the fire protection. Fire curtains (Fig. 9.9) or fire barriers are walls that divide up the open

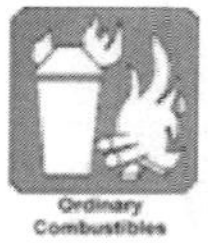

Symbol	Description	Description	Symbol
A Ordinary Combustibles	Class A extinguishers will put out fires in ordinary combustibles, such as wood and paper. The numerical rating for this class of fire extinguisher refers to the amount of water the fire extinguisher holds and the amount of fire it will extinguish.	Water extinguishers contain water and compressed gas and should only be used on Class A (ordinary combustibles) fires.	Ordinary Combustibles
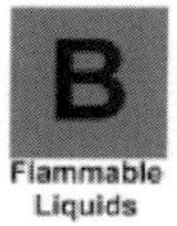 **B** Flammable Liquids	Class B extinguishers should be used on fires involving flammable liquids, such as grease, gasoline, oil, etc. The numerical rating for this class of fire extinguisher states the approximate number of square feet of a flammable liquid fire that a nonexpert person can expect to extinguish.	Carbon dioxide (CO_2) extinguishers are most effective on Class B and C (liquids and electrical) fires. Because the gas disperses quickly, these extinguishers are only effective from 3 to 8 feet. The carbon dioxide is stored as a compressed liquid in the extinguisher. As it expands, it cools the surrounding air.	Flammable Liquids
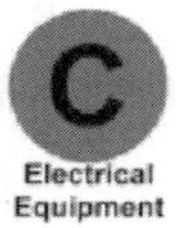 **C** Electrical Equipment	Class C extinguishers are suitable for use on electrically energized fires. This class of fire extinguishers does not have a numerical rating. The presence of the letter "C" indicates that the extinguishing agent is nonconductive.	Halon* extinguishers contain a gas that interrupts the chemical reaction that takes place when fuels burn. These types of extinguishers are often used to protect valuable electrical equipment because they leave no residue to clean up. Halon extinguishers have a limited range, usually 4 to 6 feet. *carcinogenic and damages ozone	Electrical Equipment
A Ordinary Combustibles **B** Flammable Liquids	Many extinguishers available today can be used on different types of fires and will be labeled with more than one designator, e.g., A-B, B-C, or A-B-C.	Dry chemical extinguishers are usually rated for multipurpose use. They contain an extinguishing agent and use a compressed, nonflammable gas as a propellant.	

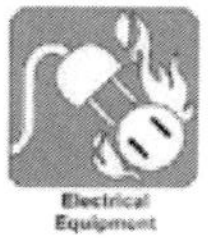

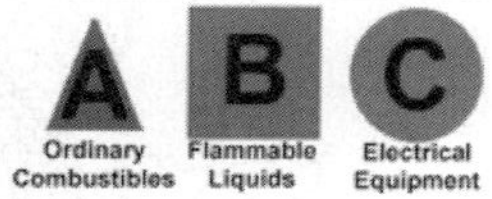

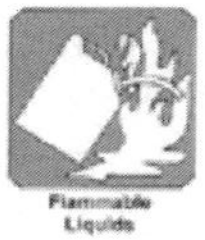

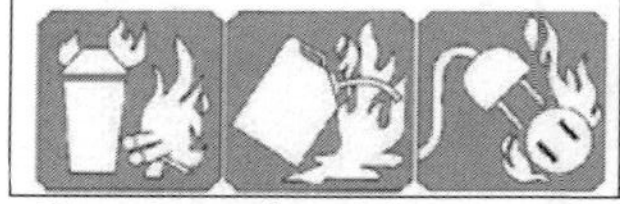

Class D extinguishers are designed for use on flammable metals and are often specific for the type of metal in question. There is no picture designator for Class D extinguishers. These extinguishers generally have no rating, nor are they given a multipurpose rating for use on other types of fires.

Figure 9.7. Fire extinguisher types and codes. Adapted from Hanford Fire Department Web site information.

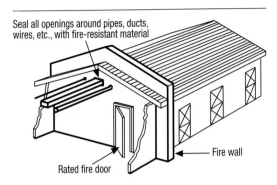

Seal all openings around pipes, ducts, wires, etc., with fire-resistant material

Fire wall

Rated fire door

Figure 9.8. Fire wall to prevent or delay the spread of fire. From *Fire Control in Livestock Buildings*, NRAES-39.

space in the roof trusses and prevent the spread of heat and smoke through the attic space. This prevents the truss area from becoming a natural tunnel for heat and flame travel. Building design determines the size of the fire curtain; the taller the fire curtain, the greater the effectiveness.

Compartmentalization is not as simple as just adding a wall. Preventing the exchange and redirection of superheated air and flame is the operating principle of a firewall or curtain. Although if not properly installed, it disrupts the everyday air patterns needed for proper ventilation in the stable. An option more common at horse facilities is to "compartmentalize" by having entirely separate

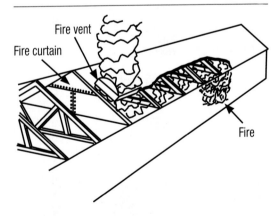

Fire vent

Fire curtain

Fire

Figure 9.9. Fire curtain to delay and limit the horizontal spread of heat, smoke, and flame. From *Fire Control in Livestock Buildings*, NRAES-39.

structures rather than dividing up one extra large building. This is one reason why many racetracks have several modest-sized stables rather than one huge stable.

Fire Ventilation

Proper ventilation will also improve survival by removing gases from occupied areas, directing flow of air currents and fire spread, and providing for the release of unburned gases before ignition. Roof vents are an effective way to ventilate a barn during a fire. Recommendations for vent spacing and sizes are set by the National Fire Protection Association on the basis of building material types and area to be vented. The most important factor to determine the space needed between vents is the rate at which burning material gives off heat. Horse barn fires burn with moderate-to-high heat production. Stables should have 1 square foot of ceiling vent space for every 100 square feet of floor area. Buildings with hay storage need 1 square foot for every 30 to 50 square feet of floor area. Options include a continuous slot opening along the ridge; roof vent monitors with louvers or thin glass that are opened by the superheated air; and unit vents that are designed to melt, collapse, or spring open at predetermined temperatures. Each of these vents increases gas removal during the fire. Vents on heat-triggered fuses (usually set to open at 212°F) may not open unless a hot, free-burning fire produces smoke temperatures high enough to activate fuses. This may mean that the fire has had time to progress, depending on its origin. Do not assume that just because vents are installed, the environment within a burning barn is livable. A smoldering fire can produce enough toxic smoke to be an immediate threat to human and animal life.

Fire Detection Devices and Principles

Early warning devices can be an effective tool in fire detection, but few are suitable for barn use. In some situations, the main goal is to save the animals housed in the barn; but in other situations, minimizing property damage is the priority. Many early detection and fire suppression systems are available, but most were developed for residential use. This severely limits their practicality in horse or livestock facilities, because they tend to be dustier, more humid, and colder than residential environments. It is best to seek advice and recommendations from fire engineers or fire protection professionals familiar with the unique needs and situations found in horse facilities. If you have trouble locating fire protection professionals, contact your fire department and ask for referrals.

Early warning devices were developed to mimic human senses. There are three basic types of fire detection devices: smoke, thermal (heat), and flame detectors. Smoke detectors mimic the human sense of smell. An ionization detector charges the air within the detector, so that it will carry an electric current, and any resistance to the electrical current will set off an alarm. Smoke particles and dust will interrupt the air's ability to conduct electrical current. An ionization detector is more responsive to a flaming fire than a smoldering one. For earlier smoke detection, a photoelectric smoke detector is recommended. Within a chamber in the smoke detector is a light-sensitive photocell. Smoke particles and dust will act like miniature mirrors, scattering a light beam and directing it toward the photocell. Once the amount of light detected by the photocell reaches a predetermined point, the alarm is activated.

Smoke detectors are the best line of defense for early warning of fires (Fig. 9.10). They identify the fire while it is in the smoldering or early flame stages. Smoke detectors are not as reliable in the dusty and humid environment of horse barns. Airborne dust and dander or humidity may trigger

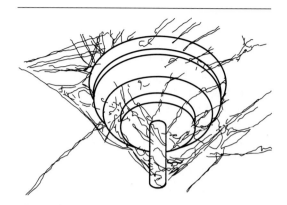

Figure 9.11. Keep all detectors free of cobwebs and dust. From *Fire Control in Livestock Buildings*, NRAES-39.

false alarms (Fig. 9.11). In more controlled environments, such as a residential-style lounge or office, a smoke detector is better suited.

Thermal detectors, developed in the mid-1800s, are the oldest type of automatic detection device. They are inexpensive to install and easy to maintain. The most common thermal detectors are fixed temperature devices, set to operate when temperatures reach a predetermined level, usually 135 to 165°F. Another class of thermal detectors, called rate-of-rise detectors, activates an alarm when the temperature climbs at an abnormally fast rate. Both fixed temperature and rate-of-rise detectors are spot detectors and activate sooner with a closer proximity to the heat source.

A third type of thermal detector, the fixed temperature line detector, does not require the sensor to be as close to the heat source for activation. Two wires are run between detectors. Alarms are activated when the insulators, designed to degrade at a specific temperature, are damaged. The benefit of this fixed temperature line sensor is that floor area coverage can be increased at a lower cost. Thermal detectors are highly reliable and are not as affected by a dusty, moist environment. However, their adequacy in a horse barn is debatable because they require the fire to be in the later stages of progression before the sensor recognizes it and signals the alarm. The longer a fire has to develop, the greater damage it can cause and the more difficult it is to control, especially in a barn. This is why they are usually not permitted as the sole detection device in life safety applications, such as in residential use.

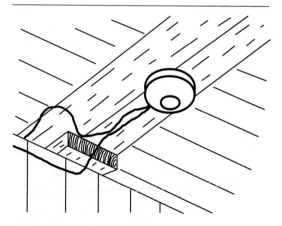

Figure 9.10. Many fire detection devices, such as this smoke detector, were developed for residential use, which severely limits their application to dusty, humid barn environments. From *Fire Control in Livestock Buildings*, NRAES-39.

The most reliable and expensive early warning detection device is the flame detector. These sensors imitate human sight and are most commonly used in aircraft maintenance facilities, refineries, and mines. As with other spot detectors, flame detectors must be "looking" directly at the fire source. Flames are classified by short wavelengths of electromagnetic radiation flickering in the range of 5 to 30 cycles per second. When the device senses these conditions, it is preset to monitor the source for a few seconds, before sounding the alarm. By recognizing the flame's wavelength, cycle, and consistency, flame detectors differentiate between hot objects and actual fires, minimizing false alarms. The farther the flame is from the sensor, the larger it must be before the sensor will respond to it. Flame detectors are highly reliable early detection devices, especially for hot burning fires that are not likely to give off smoke, such as alcohol or methane fires.

Early warning systems can add valuable time to rescue efforts, if someone is available to hear them. One way to ensure that someone is alerted when a fire is detected is through a telephone dialer. A telephone dialer provides 24-hour alarm monitoring. The dialer can be connected to a professional monitoring service, family, neighbors, or directly to the fire department. It may be best to alert someone near the premises first to prevent calling the fire department for any false alarms. However, best judgment should prevail, and if the nearest neighbor is too far away, contacting the 911 operator may be a better alternative. A phone dialer will need its own line to ensure the availability of a phone connection after a fire has been detected.

Automatic Fire Suppression

Sprinkler systems are an effective tool for controlling fires but are not common in rural horse barns. Most sprinkler systems open to apply water to a fire when a sensing element in the individual sprinkler head comes in contact with intense heat. Only the sprinkler heads that come in contact with the fire's heat react, minimizing the water needed to extinguish the fire. A sprinkler system usually suppresses a fire with as few as two sprinkler heads and is very effective at controlling fires before they get out of hand. However, for a sprinkler system to be effective, an adequate water supply needs to be available at all times to provide enough gallons and sufficient pressure to extinguish the fire. It is often difficult for

rural horse farms to meet this criterion. On average, one sprinkler head will deliver 25 gallons of water per minute to extinguish the blaze. As more sprinklers are activated, more water must be available to maintain pressure in the line (47 gallons and 72 gallons per minute for activation of the second and third sprinklers, respectively.) If water availability is a problem, a tank can be installed. This is an extremely expensive addition that will need regular service checks and maintenance.

If the facility's water supply is sufficient, several options are available for sprinkler systems (Fig. 9.12). A sprinkler system that holds water all the time is called a wet-pipe system. These are the most inexpensive systems to install and require the least amount of maintenance. However, in climates where the barn temperature is too low to prevent freezing, the wet-pipe system will not work.

In freezing environments, a dry-pipe system is employed. The supply lines are pressurized with air or nitrogen gas to hold a valve closed, preventing water from entering the system. In a fire, the sprinklers are activated, releasing the pressure and opening the valve. If the pressure is released through damage to the supply line, the valve is also released. This poses problems if the valve release is not found and temperatures are low enough for freezing to occur. Dry-pipe systems are more limited in design. The reliance on pressure to close a valve creates strict requirements on the overall size and locations of the sprinkler heads and supply lines. The increased system complexity requires more components, has more opportunity for fail-

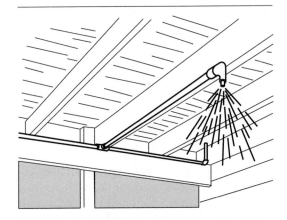

Figure 9.12. Sprinkler installed in barn. From *Fire Control in Livestock Buildings*, NRAES-39.

ure, and increases the costs of installation and maintenance.

A pre-action system was designed to eliminate the danger of accidental valve release on the dry-pipe system. A pre-action system uses an electronically operated valve to prevent water from prematurely entering the pipes. In order for the valves to be opened, an independent flame, heat, or smoke detection device must identify a fire or potential fire. Once a fire is detected, the valve is released and the water is available to the sprinkler heads. The sprinklers open when triggered by heat, not by the valve detection device. As with an increasingly complex system, installation and maintenance costs increase along with the potential for malfunction.

One promising technology for areas with limited water supplies is the water mist. This system was originally designed for controlling severe fires on ships and oil-drilling platforms, where excessive water use could make the vessel capsize. Currently, these systems are standard on marine vessels and have a proven record of extinguishing maritime fires. Their applications in buildings have been recognized and used in Europe. Water mist systems are highly pressurized, ranging from 100 to 1000 pounds per square inch and produce finer droplets 50 to 200 micrometers in diameter (sprinklers deliver 600- to 1000-micrometer droplets). These smaller droplets are exceptionally efficient at cooling and fire control with 10% to 25% less water than a sprinkler system. Because of its limited availability, this technology is significantly more expensive than sprinkler systems. Currently, insurance companies do not recognize water mist systems as a fire suppression system and will not give rate incentives for them. Recognition of and advancements in this technology should bring it closer to affordable horse farm applications.

WHAT TO DO IF YOU HAVE A FIRE

1. Remain Calm

The most important thing to do is remain calm. The situation may be perilous, but panic is only going to make it worse. Panic can create situations that endanger lives. Take a deep breath, stop, and plan.

2. Survey the Scene

This is the most important and most often forgotten step. *If the area is not safe, get out!!!* Botched acts of heroism will only jeopardize lives and the structure. Look and see what the fire is near. A smoldering pile of hay is not nearly as deadly as one smoldering near bags of fertilizer. Take a quick inventory of available resources. Are there other people present? Use their skills in the most efficient manner possible. Remember that because of their behavior patterns, horses are the most difficult domestic livestock species to evacuate from a burning barn. Always send the most qualified person to do the task. Persons who are not qualified to do the task are more of a liability than assistance. A person who is unfamiliar with operating a fire extinguisher may spread the fire. Someone unfamiliar with the behavior of a panicked horse puts others, himself or herself, and the horse in greater danger. If the area is unsafe to enter, do not put yourself or anyone else at risk. Be alert for potential hidden dangers. Firefighters cannot concentrate on saving the horses until they have rescued the people.

> *Surveying the fire scene only takes a fraction of a second, but it is the single most important step to ensure everyone's safety.*

Investigating a smoldering haystack or mow is especially dangerous. If smoke is seen or smelled in hay, do not attempt to move it or walk on it. Disturbing the hay may expose the smoldering sections to oxygen, causing it to flash quickly. Smoldering cavities are prone to collapse. Burned-out cavities may collapse under weight and trap a person who was attempting to stand or walk on the bale.

3. Call 911 or the Fire Department

Regardless of the size of the fire or potential fire, call the fire department. Even if the fire was contained without professional help, contact the fire department immediately and have the area inspected to ensure the fire has been completely extinguished. Firefighters are trained, certified, and experienced in fire control. It is better to catch a blaze in the earliest stages than have it get out of hand.

Be sure that whoever is calling the emergency dispatch operator is capable of giving clear and concise directions and other valuable information. Also include the county, state, and municipality if using a cell phone. The nature of the fire (barn fire, hay storage shed, etc.), how far the fire has gone (still

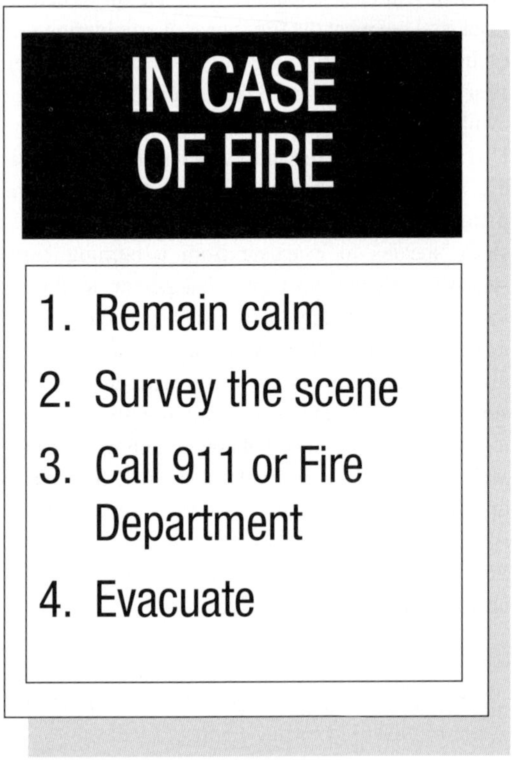

IN CASE OF FIRE

1. Remain calm
2. Survey the scene
3. Call 911 or Fire Department
4. Evacuate

Figure 9.13 Sign for survey scene.

smoldering, flames erupted, structure totally engulfed), and whether any people or animals are trapped in the structure are invaluable pieces of information for dispatching emergency crews.

4. Evacuate

If time permits, get the horses out and into a safe pasture. Once the flames have erupted, the fire will spread quickly and pose an immediate danger to life. Put horses in a secure, fenced area, as far away from the commotion as possible. During a fire, many situations are present that can distress even the most "bomb-proof" horse. Loose horses running amid the lights, sirens, and moving trucks can be hit, injure firefighters, or even run back into the burning barn. Using a pasture right next to the barn will endanger the horse(s) and inhibit fire-fighting measures.

SUMMARY

Although a serious threat because of their rapid spread and destructiveness, horse barn fires are largely preventable. Take steps to reduce the chances of fire in your facility. Fortunately, much of fire protection involves simple, common-sense prevention measures.

- Fire requires a fuel source, an ignition source, and oxygen and goes through four growth stages: incipient, smoldering, flame, and heat production.
- Baled hay can be its own fuel and ignition source if it is baled too wet. Wet hay should be monitored for heat buildup, caused by microbial respiration.
- Store hay and bedding in a separate building from the horse stable.
- Minimize fuel and ignition sources in and around the barn. Be sure to store and dispose of combustible materials properly.
- Keeping the barn neat and clean has aesthetic appeal, will minimize the risk of fire, and increase the chances of escape during a fire.
- Post and enforce a no smoking policy.
- Be sure that the facility is accessible to emergency vehicles and that the ground around the buildings is sturdy enough to support them.
- An effective tool for preventing fire spread is to separate the buildings.
- The three fire control rating systems for building materials are flame spread, smoke development, and fire rating.
- Fire-retardant -resistant products include masonry, heavy timber, and fire-retardant treated wood.
- All barns should be outfitted with a lightning protection system and inspected regularly. Only certified professionals should install and inspect the lightning protection system.
- Having multiple water hydrants around the barn will give more options for early fire suppression.
- Know where additional water sources (e.g., ponds) are located.
- Have at least one charged and mounted ABC-type fire extinguisher every 50 feet.
- Make sure that wiring and all electrical equipment is rated for agricultural use, is in working condition, and is free of dust and cobwebs, and that wiring is housed in conduit. Wires with UF-B ratings are preferable.
- Design stalls with two exits that open into a secure, enclosed area and make sure that any swinging doors do not obstruct pathways.
- Have halters and lead ropes easily accessible on stall doors.

- Post written emergency information at each phone. This information should include written directions to the facility and a list of commonly kept combustibles.
- Post and practice evacuation routes.
- A more elaborate barn fire protection system may incorporate building design, early warning devices, and fire suppression mechanisms.
- Many early detection and fire suppression systems are available, but most were developed for residential use. This severely limits their practicality in horse facilities. Barn environments tend to be dustier, more humid, and colder than residential environments, which decrease the life of the detector and may cause the sensors to indicate false alarms.
- Use sprinkler systems that have adequate water pressure. These systems can be expensive to install and maintain in freezing climates but do have a proven history of containing fires and saving lives.
- Seek advice and recommendations from fire engineers or fire protection professionals familiar with the unique needs and situations found in horse facilities.
- Check local zoning and building codebooks for fire regulations in your area.
- If you do have a barn fire, do not put yourself or someone else in danger. Think out your actions first.

10
Utilities

COLD VERSUS WARM STABLE

Early in the stable design process, a decision is made to provide either cold or warm housing for horses during winter conditions. This decision will affect utility design and fixture selection.

In cold housing, the inside air temperature will be within 5 to 15°F of outside temperatures, with natural air movements being used to create the air exchange required to maintain good air quality in the building. Cold stables are typically lightly insulated under the roof to reduce condensation. During freezing weather, the interior will have freezing temperatures. A "warm" stable will be constructed with wall, roof (or ceiling), and perimeter insulation and use a fan-and-inlet system to create the air exchange required for maintaining both good air quality and a warmer environment in the stable. Some of the warmth will come from retaining more of the animal body heat in the building, but supplemental heat will be needed to maintain conditions above freezing during below-freezing outside temperatures. Most horse stables are maintained as "cold" housing with interior temperatures very close to outside temperatures to ensure that good air quality is maintained. For human comfort, an area can be insulated and heated, which may be a location where the horse is tacked, a tack room, office, and so forth. See Chapter 12 for more details.

ELECTRICITY

Electricity will be needed in stables for lights, mechanical ventilation equipment in warm barns, and small appliances (e.g., radio, tools). Electricity may be needed for laundry, supplemental heat, and office needs. Outbuildings such as hay and bedding storage, manure storage area, and pasture shelters often benefit from electricity for lighting. Lights are used in indoor riding arenas and may be used for outdoor riding areas. Security lights are used at entrances. Electric heat applications are covered in Chapter 12. Options and selection of lighting are covered Chapter 11. Overall electrical wiring and service considerations are discussed in this chapter.

Necessary Features

A well-planned horse facility wiring system must be safe, adequate, and expandable. The first requirement, safety, is the most important and will be achieved by compliance with the National Electrical Code (NEC) and, in particular, Article 547 for agricultural building wiring compliance. The NEC is *the* guide for safe and proper installation procedures and materials. Other good detailed resources are the *Agricultural Wiring Handbook* from the National Food and Energy Council and the *Farm Buildings Wiring Handbook* from the Mid-West Plan Service (see the "Additional Resources" section). The latter book provides many practical tips for proper installation. The reference to the aforementioned electrical wiring handbooks for agricultural applications presumes that the horse facility is not used by the public or required to comply with the electric code for any other reason. Even though many farm buildings are neither required to follow NEC code nor obtain an electrical permit, it is a good idea to follow its guidelines, particularly for insurance purposes.

A safe electrical system will prevent electrical fires, shock hazards, and tripping hazards. The following are important for a safe system:

- Proper sizing of electrical wires connected to properly sized fuse or circuit breaker.
- Proper fixtures for the dust and moisture exposure that are common in horse facilities.
- Proper equipment grounding circuit—the green wires and round prong on the plugs.
- Connecting grounding wires to metal building components and fixed metal equipment.
- Compatible materials—do not connect copper and aluminum together without proper connector.
- Proper tightening of all connections.

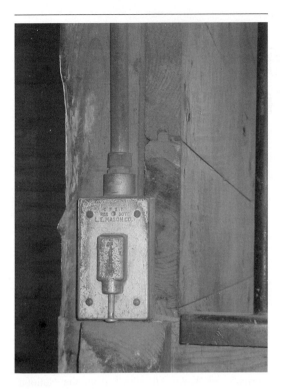

Figure 10.1. Example of a rugged, horse-proof switch located just outside stall in area accessible by the horse, as evidenced by chewing marks on wood support. Light switch is a stem that moves in and out of fixture from lower edge. Use this type or similar fixture to protect horse from electrical shock and prevent horse actuation of lights.

Electrical wiring and fixtures in stable facilities must be of more rugged construction than those used in residential construction. In the NEC code, "dry" buildings include residence, shops, and garages. "Damp" buildings include animal housing and any area that is washed periodically. "Dusty" facilities include dry hay and bedding storage areas and animal housing areas. Specialized moisture-tight and dust-tight fixtures (outlets, switches, and lamps) are required in damp and dusty areas to reduce fire-causing short circuits, heat buildup in electrical fixtures, and corrosion. Wiring and fixtures need to be protected from horse chewing or other damage when installed within horse reach, which is up to 12 foot high (Fig. 10.1). Areas where horses can reach wiring include not only the obvious stall area but also stable aisles, indoor arenas, wash stalls, and anywhere else that even a loose horse might access the wiring.

Rodents may chew exposed wiring, particularly when wires are located in areas that rodents frequent, such as along the floor and in loose insulation materials.

Protect Wiring

There are two recommended ways to protect electrical wiring from mechanical damage and resist the high moisture and dust conditions found in horse stables. One is to use underground feeder wiring. UF-B rated cable, meaning "underground feeder," is constructed for very high moisture applications (such as found underground). UF-B cable has wires that are embedded in a solid core plastic vinyl sheathing and includes a bare copper equipment grounding wire (Fig. 10.2). UF-B wiring is installed above ground in

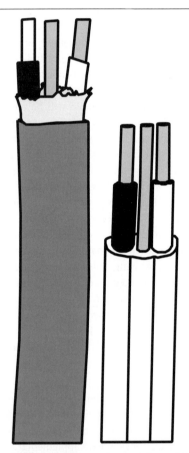

Figure 10.2. Waterproof electric cable (UF) recommended for use in damp environment such as horse facilities (on right). Note that UF wires are embedded in plastic protective cover. Typical residential electrical cable is shown on left.

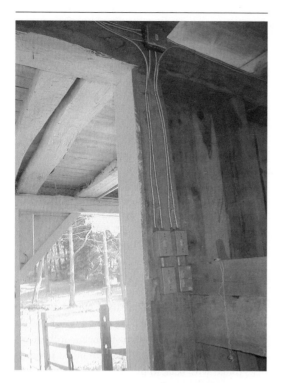

Figure 10.3. Electrical service in older barns converted to horse stabling, such as this classic bank barn formerly housing dairy cattle, need to include safe wiring. Here metal conduit and moisture-proof switches and outlets are located away from horse contact.

the stable and can be used unprotected other than in areas where horses can reach it or where it is potentially subjected to physical damage from equipment, where it should be protected by conduit. UF-B is a higher cost wire compared with residential-type wire construction. *Do not* wire with the residential-style, plastic-covered cable (type NM rating meaning "nonmetallic"). NM cable has two or three insulated conducting copper wires and a bare ground wire. Each conducting wire is sheathed in a plastic vinyl, but the entire assembly, although somewhat moisture resistant, is rated for use only in dry conditions (100% of the time) such as a home.

The second way to install electrical wiring in a damp environment is to enclose it in conduit (Fig. 10.3) appropriate for damp and dusty conditions. This option uses a less expensive wire, still choosing one that is moisture resistant, and encloses it in protective conduit. In this case, the conduit increases the cost of electrical wiring installation

but if several wires for several circuits can be encased in the conduit, this option is typically less expensive than running multiple lines of UF-B wire.

Schedule 40 PVC (polyvinyl chloride) conduit of ½- and ¾-inch diameter is the most common type used in damp buildings to protect wiring from mechanical damage. Steel conduit, such as electrical metallic tubing (EMT), will corrode in a damp environment and is not considered to be any stronger than the PVC Schedule 40. Thicker, stronger Schedule 80 PVC conduit may be used in areas that expect heavy mechanical damage potential, such as where equipment is run nearby. Plastic conduit will expand and contract with changes in temperature, and this is accounted for by installing proper expansion fittings during installation (see *Farm Buildings Wiring Handbook*, MWPS-28, for more detail). If not using UF-B cable, the conduit-enclosed wires need a type W classification (indicating moisture resistance), such as THW (submersible pump cable), THWN, RHW, THHW, or XHHW. For those inclined to use residential rated wires (type NM, which is *not* recommended practice) in the conduit, be sure to weigh the likelihood and consequences of condensation and other moisture accumulating in the conduit where it cannot escape and will saturate a wire not constructed to resist moisture. When using conduit to protect a portion of the wire from damage, seal the end after the installation is completed to keep dust and insects from entering the conduit and attached boxes.

Condensation management ends up influencing layout design and installation of electrical system. When conduit is run from a warm, heated area, such as a tack room, to a cold area, such as the horse stable, moisture in the warm air can travel within the conduit and will condense on the inside of the cold conduit. This condensation is trapped and leads to moisture level higher than residential-grade wire can resist. Condensation may run into attached electrical boxes. Avoid or minimize the number of conduits from warm to cold locations in the building. When most circuits are in the cold portion of a building, install the service panel in the cold portion. When a conduit must pass through a wall from a warm room to the cold stable, use putty (duct sealer) to seal the inside of the conduit on the warm side of the wall.

Service Panel

A service panel distributes the electrical energy to several circuits, provides a means to shut off electricity, and protects against excessive current flow in each wire. The panel size is expressed in amperes. Typical sizes range from 60 to 200 amperes. Properly sized fuse or circuit breakers protect the service panel and each circuit extending from the service panel.

The service panel may be fed from an existing service panel, a central metering point, or a separate, metered electric service. Small, privately owned stables may be able to use a subpanel fed from the residential electrical power. First, the residential panel has to have the capacity to support the subpanel to the stable. Feed the subpanel with wire properly sized for the current and wire length to maintain adequate voltage at the stable. Connect it to a properly sized fuse or circuit breaker. Secondly, if the stable is located far from the house, it may be best to have a separate stable electrical service panel to avoid the high cost of large wire that is required to limit the voltage loss between house and stable. When buildings are spread around a central location, a central meter location with feeders to an electrical panel in each building is possible. Large stables and public facilities will need their own electrical panel service, either with a separate meter or served from a central meter. Whether the stable has its own panel or a subpanel, small buildings with up to two branch circuits (pasture shelter, hay and bedding storage) may be supplied via 30-ampere switches and circuit breakers.

A typical recommendation is to locate a farm building's service panel in a mechanical room, a human-occupied office, or tack room where dust and moisture is reduced compared with the main stabling area. Also, consider placing the stable's electrical service panel either outside or in a location near an exterior doorway for emergency shutdown, but not in an animal-occupied area (Fig. 10.4). An outside disconnect switch by the service entrance can also be used to provide emergency shutdown. A rain-tight or weather-tight NEMA-4X (this is a dust- and moisture-tight design specification) designated plastic cabinet service box will be needed in a dusty or damp environment. For safety, maintain 3 feet of cleared space in front of and above the service panel, and do not run any water lines above the panel.

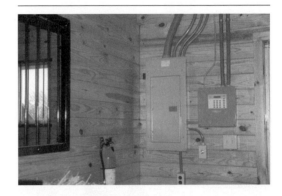

Figure 10.4. Electrical service panel located in unheated storage area on endwall of stable with easy access from outside door. Note handy fire extinguisher.

The electrical service must be grounded at the main panel via long copper rods buried in damp ground (*Farm Buildings Wiring Handbook*, MWPS-28, provides details). A subpanel needs to be likewise grounded independently or grounded via copper ground wire back to the main panel. Each piece of conductive, metallic equipment in the stable will have an equipment-grounding conductor back to the panel box grounding block. The electrical grounding system is separate from the lightning ground.

The electrical system must be expandable. Size the electric service panel for at least 50% more than the currently anticipated load, with a minimum size in any major building being 60 amperes with three-wire, 120- and 240-volt service. Branch circuits, of 15 to 20 amperes, provide electricity to sets of lights, convenience outlets, and motors (up to ½ horsepower) that are not particularly sensitive to voltage drop. Each branch is protected by a properly sized fuse or circuit breaker. Individual circuits are provided to devices with larger electrical loads, such as motors larger than ½ horsepower and heaters over 1000 watt, or loads that require continuous service, such as a water system or freezer. The rating of the receptacles and switches must match or be higher than circuit amperage.

Conducting Wires

Acceptable conducting wire sizes are based on the length of run, the ampacity (maximum expected current in amperes), and circuit protection device (circuit breaker or fuse) rating. For circuits with a 15-ampere circuit protection device, the minimum conductor size is #14. For a 20-ampere circuit protection device, the minimum conductor size is #12. Limiting voltage drop is important in sizing the conductor. To protect equipment, especially motors, the voltage drop should be limited to 5% or 6 volts for a 120-volt line. The voltage drop is dependent on the resistance of the conductor. For UF wire on a 120-volt circuit, the maximum lengths for a 5% drop include the following: #14 wire at 15 amperes for 60 feet; #12 wire at 15 amperes for 100 feet; and #12 wire at 20 amperes for 75 feet. Because the allowable length is inversely proportional to current, longer runs are possible when the known load is less. For example, a lighting circuit with twelve 100-watt light bulbs will have a known current of 10 amperes. The 5% voltage drop for a #14 wire at 10 amperes is 90 feet. The 5% voltage drop for a #12 wire at 10 amperes is 150 feet.

The selection of 15- or 20-ampere branch circuits is based on the expected loads and potential cost impacts. For small buildings with small loads, 15-ampere circuits with #14 wire can be used up to 60 feet, with maximum current flow. When a circuit will not have 100% current flow, a #14 wire up to 75 feet may be used, especially with lighting circuits. Above 75 feet, a #12 wire should be used with either a 15- or 20-ampere circuit protection device.

Wiring System

The wiring system will be adequate when it provides electrical service throughout the horse facility with enough outlets of the proper size and type and in convenient locations. Provide at least two electrical circuits in each major building. Expandability is highly important, because it is much cheaper to overestimate the initial system than it is to replace or rewire as the system becomes overloaded. This is particularly true for wires in protective conduit or in concealed locations. Before wiring a building, have a detailed plan that shows location and type of lights, convenience outlets, motors, switches, and junction boxes. Indicate those portions of wiring that will need to be protected from horse damage if all wiring is not to be installed in conduit. Include expandability in the detailed plan.

For damp and/or dusty buildings, such as stables and indoor riding arenas, every wire splice, switch, and receptacle is enclosed in a noncorrosive, dust- and water-tight, molded plastic PVC box. Gasketed covers are required to seal all junction boxes, and receptacles need spring-loaded and gasketed covers (Fig. 10.5).

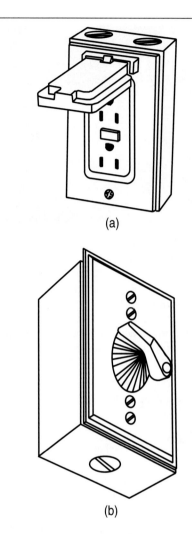

(a)

(b)

Figure 10.5. Dust- and moisture-resistant switch and convenience outlet receptacles recommended for use in damp and dusty environments, such as horse facilities.

Gasketed and spring-loaded receptacle covers for damp environments are commonly available in hardware supply stores and may be used where precipitation and wash water will not directly contact the receptacle. A ground-fault interruption (GFI or GFCI) circuit breaker and receptacle should be used to protect humans and animals from dangerous shock by cutting the circuit almost immediately upon detecting a ground-fault (current is escaping to ground somewhere in the circuit). A breakdown of the insulation or wires usually causes a ground fault. GFIs are recommended in wet areas such as bathroom facilities, wash areas, or anywhere floors may be wet or wires are run

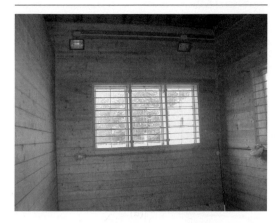

Figure 10.6. Overhead lights in wash stall and veterinary care area are located at back of stall and in similar position at front opening. Electrical wiring is protected in PVC conduit with moisture-proof fixtures on lights, junction box, and convenience outlet. Note protective bars on windows, which admit plenty of natural light, and rugged wood wall construction.

Table 10.1. Horse Stable Water Use Estimates

Purpose	Water Use
Horse drinking	12 gallons/day/horse
Riding arena footing dust control[a]	0.05–0.50 gallons/ft^2
	Total Water Use (gallons/use)
Bathroom or wash sink	1–2
Toilet flush	4–7
Shower	25–60
Automatic clothes washer	30–50
Equipment washing (horse trailer, tractor, etc.)	30
Horse bath[b]	25–60
Floor wash with hose[c]	10–20
Manured-floor wash with hose[c]	40–75

Note: Because horse facility water use is virtually undocumented, footnotes explain where estimates were drawn from similar water use purposes in other agricultural enterprises.

[a]Riding arena footing water use was estimated from similar conditions used in greenhouse crop watering to achieve good soaking of entire soil profile, which provided the high-end estimate. The low-end estimate may be used for topping off already damp footing and was established from limited horse facility data.

[b]Horse bath water use was estimated as being similar to a human shower. Although a larger body is being washed, there is an intermittent, and therefore shorter, time of water flow.

[c]Floor washing water use was estimated from dairy milkhouse and milking parlor washwater use, respectively, for typical hose-cleanable concrete floors (tack or feed room, work aisle) and floor with manure present (horse stall or wash stall).

underground (Fig. 10.6). GFIs are required within 6 feet of sinks and for outdoor circuits.

WATER

Water is a necessity in the horse stable. Water will be needed for drinking by horses and people and for stable, equipment, and horse cleaning. An outdoor water source may be needed for paddocks and turnout shelters and other auxiliary buildings. Additional water may be used in a laundry and bathroom and for dust control of the riding arena surface. In smaller private stables it may not be the case, but in larger or commercial stables it is recommended that a human drinking water supply be provided along with at least a sink for light washing. Firefighting water supply may be a nearby pond or public hydrant. The water system must provide adequate quantities of water to the desired locations, provide the proper equipment, protect the water supply from contamination, and be protected from freezing.

Drinking Water

An adequate supply of drinking (potable) water is necessary in a horse facility. The best sources will be a deep well or public water supply, with additional sources being springs and shallow wells.

Drinking water for each horse will be about 12 gallons per day. Actual water consumption will depend

on temperature, horse activity level, and diet, with more water consumed during warm weather, with high activity level, and for increased dry matter consumption. Other water demand may be estimated from Table 10.1, but water use and waste varies widely among water users. The minimum water flow rate for a small- to moderate-sized horse farmstead is 8 gallons per minute (gpm), but 10 gpm is more desirable. Large commercial facilities will have to conduct a more careful estimate to determine the larger flow rate needed. When the supply flow rate is low, a storage tank can supply the larger short-term flow rates.

Horse facilities have great variety in distribution of water within the facility. Some managers will provide horse drinking water in each stall and every outdoor paddock, which is generally recommended for horse well-being, while other managers maintain well-kept horses with limited but frequent access to group watering tanks.

Options for supplying water to each horse stall and for outside paddocks are automated waterers or hand-carried buckets (more discussion about pros and cons is in Chapter 5). Hand carrying buckets for long distances can become burdensome even with only one or two horses. Water in a garden hose will freeze in northern climates, so it is difficult to supply the horses with adequate water at all times with hoses and hand-carried buckets. Buckets may be used with nearby frost-proof water taps (Figs. 10.7 and 10.8). Use frost-proof hydrants with an integral antisiphon protection. Do not install an antisiphon to the hydrant hose bib. Installing such a devise will

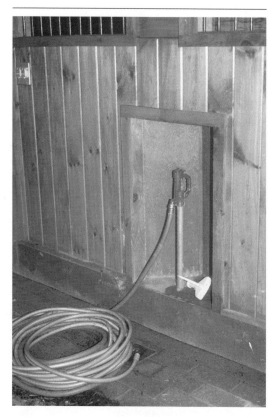

Figure 10.8. Self-draining water hydrant recessed into stable aisle wall for additional safety from horse impact.

prevent the hydrant from properly draining. Provide a place where unused water from a horse bucket can be conveniently discarded to an all-weather drain, and where water buckets can be rinsed and scrubbed and refilled with fresh water. A semiautomated system using buckets employs an overhead water line with manually activated valves at each bucket to deliver water as needed to each stall. Add pipe insulation and wrap with heat tape in freezing climates (Fig. 10.9).

Automatic watering units in stalls and outside have gained considerable acceptance with the use of durable materials that are easily cleaned; some offer water use monitoring. Choose a waterer design that is very easy to clean as this will be a frequent chore even in inclement weather. To prevent pollution of water supply, the design will need an anti-backsiphoning device or provide the water supply to the drinking bowl with an air gap between water inlet and maximum water level to prevent backsiphoning. Indoor

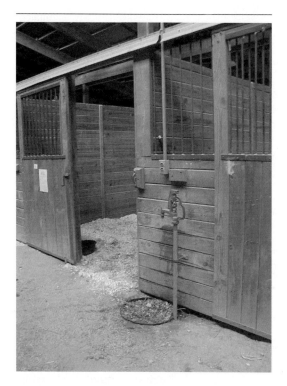

Figure 10.7. Frost-proof, self-draining water hydrant in unheated stable secured to nearby wall with overflow drainage area.

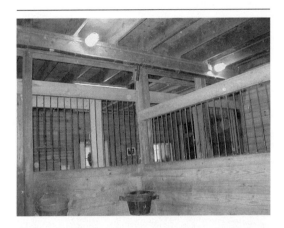

Figure 10.9. Water delivered in overhead pipeline with pull cord for dispensing water to individual buckets in each stall. Pull cord is accessible from work aisle. Water line is wrapped with electric heat tape covered with foam pipe insulation in freezing climate. Note electrical wiring protected in PVC conduit with sealed junction box. Incandescent stall lights are positioned at the front of each stall in a protective, sealed fixture. Aisle lights are fluorescent.

units are secured to a stall wall. Outdoor paddock automatic waterers are often secured to a small-diameter concrete pad with an all-weather surface surrounding (see "Outside Water Needs" section). Each outdoor waterer should have its own water supply shutoff valve.

Whether installed indoors or outside, automatic waterers have features to prevent freezing, such as an insulated mounting column that is constructed down to below the local frost line and/or heated bowls and water supply pipes (Fig. 10.10). A large-diameter pipe extends 18 to 24 inches below the local frost line to protect the water supply line. A larger diameter pipe (12-inch diameter or greater) is used in cold climates than in warmer climates (6-inch diameter may suffice) to provide more air space insulating value to the water pipe. Automatic water tanks can generally remain ice-free if at least one tank of water is consumed every 4 to 6 hours (small individual bowls will freeze more quickly). In very cold climates or when water flow will be too infrequent to prevent the water from freezing, insulation will be needed inside the ground pipe. With

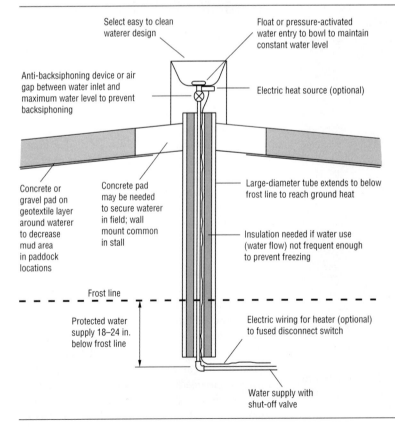

Figure 10.10. Cutaway view of automatic waterer insulated column and heated bowl showing design and installation features relating to freeze protection for plumbing.

infrequent water use, additional freeze protection will be needed near the water bowl via electric heat. Electric wiring is grounded and connects to a fused disconnect switch.

Outside Water Needs

Water will be needed outdoors for horse watering and equipment cleaning. At the minimum, an antisiphoning, frost-proof hydrant should be provided in a location that can service paddock water needs and any cleaning chores. Automatic outdoor waterers can be located nearer the center of a paddock rather than near the fenceline, but it still needs to be checked daily for water use and cleanliness; so put it in a convenient, mud-free location (Fig. 10.11). These units provide access to ground heat and perhaps supplemental heat to keep from freezing the water (see "Drinking Water" section for more detail). A durable pad or footing around a permanent location for the watering of horses will minimize mud and potholes in the area.

Outside livestock water tanks should be located to minimize freezing problems and surrounding mud. Placing the tank on a 10- to 20-foot diameter (or equivalent) concrete or hard-packed fine-gravel pad will reduce mud and frozen muck around the watering site. Slope the surface away from the tank. The all-weather surface will improve access for horses to drink and for humans to clean in this high-traffic area. Direct sunshine will reduce water tank frost and freeze-up, as will a location protected from cold winter winds. Thermostatically controlled heaters may be used. For electric and water utility access, outdoor water tanks are usually placed near

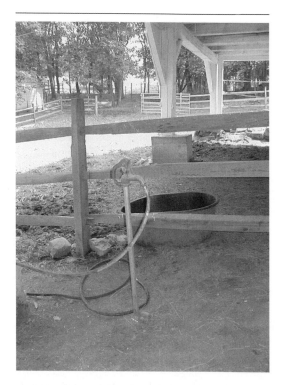

Figure 10.12. Outdoor horse watering tank with nearby frost-proof hydrant for convenient filling year round.

a paddock fenceline. When located near a human entry gate (not necessarily a horse gate), they can be quickly checked and maintained. A nearby frost-proof hydrant is convenient for filling the tank (Fig. 10.12). Use a hose cut to length and secured to reach just over the edge of the tank for water additions. When the hydrant is turned off, it can siphon the water back out of the tank if a hose is left below the water line.

Water Distribution

An underground pipe is needed to distribute water from its source to the barn. A 1-inch diameter pipe as long as 1000 feet can supply water for about 10 horses (drinking water and modest, other water uses). Below-frost water lines are also needed to conveniently supply outdoor water tanks or hydrants. Including a wire in the trench with plastic pipe will make finding the pipe at a later time easier. Placing a plastic tape in the trench about 2 feet above the pipe will warn people digging in the area of the pipe.

Water freezing in pipes is dependent on several factors. With no snow cover, soil freezes deeper

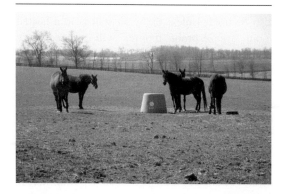

Figure 10.11. Outdoor automatic watering system in pasture.

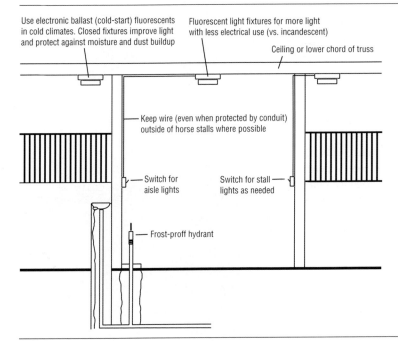

Use electronic ballast (cold-start) fluorescents in cold climates. Closed fixtures improve light and protect against moisture and dust buildup

Fluorescent light fixtures for more light with less electrical use (vs. incandescent)

Ceiling or lower chord of truss

Keep wire (even when protected by conduit) outside of horse stalls where possible

Switch for aisle lights

Switch for stall lights as needed

Frost-proff hydrant

Figure 10.13. Cross section of central-aisle stable showing plumbing for stall automatic waterer and frost-free hydrant in aisle. Also shown is electric wiring to waterer and switches for lights in aisle and stalls.

than an area protected with a blanket of snow. A pipe with running water is less likely to freeze than a pipe with standing water, because even cold groundwater is warmer than surrounding frozen soil. Outdoors and in unheated stables, installing the pipes below the frost line (frost depth) for your area is the best way to avoid frozen pipes (Fig. 10.13). Bury water lines deeper in areas where snow will be removed, such as under a road.

The other demon of freezing weather is frost heaving that raises rocks, foundations, and fence posts. Frost heaving depends on soil being saturated and cyclical freeze-thaw cycles. Drainage at the base of foundations and under arenas will inhibit frost heaving. Insulation along the exterior of the foundation of a heated building will increase temperature of the interior and the soil contained within the foundation boundaries.

Horse Wash Stall

Horse washing is one use of water that is included in many stables, particularly where show and competitive horses are kept. A dedicated wash stall is most common, but a simple area may be designated and outfitted with water and drainage to handle horse bathing. The water use and discharge in the wash stall will be equivalent to a bathroom.

While the drainage water will have substantial hair and manure addition, it may still be considered simple "gray water." The drainage system must be able to handle the hair and manure. An easily cleanable trap can catch most hair and manure before they lodge in piping. Provide cleanouts for the drain pipes to make removing clogs easier. Connect the drain to a properly designed and approved disposal system, where regulations require.

Both hot and cold water will be needed in the wash stall. A mixing faucet with hose bib will provide tempered water to a hose for washing. Separate hot and cold faucets with a "Y" hose connector can also be used. Unless the wash stall is in a heated room, freeze-proof fixtures will be necessary (Fig. 10.14). Supply the freeze-proof fixtures from a heated room. In freezing weather, be sure to remove the hose after use so that the faucets drain properly, or they will freeze. A small water heater in the heated room may eliminate long hot water lines or when the wash stall is the only place using heated water. Within the horse wash stall, either recess the faucets to be flush with the wall or shield them with a horse-strong rail if they protrude to protect horses from injury and plumbing from breakage. (Lighting and heating options for the wash stall area are covered in Chapters 11 and 12, respectively.)

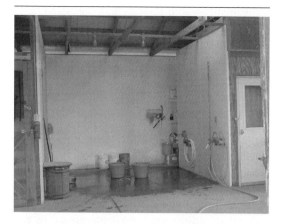

Figure 10.14. Horse wash stall water needs include hot and cold water supply and drain system for washwater and potentially a limited amount of manure waste. Area often doubles as drinking water bucket wash station and for other stable-cleaning chores.

Riding Arena Water Use

One of the most variable uses of water will be for dust control of riding arena surface material. Not all owners, but most, will use water to suppress dust in both outdoor and indoor arenas. Water is used during portions of the year when evaporation depletes the footing moisture, such as during warmer weather. Watering will need to be deep penetrating, like watering a crop soil profile. Most of the time, frequent arena footing maintenance will mean that just the topmost layer is wetted while the underlying layers remain damp. Arena footing materials that do not hold water, such as sand, will require more volume and frequent water to maintain a footing with traction than footing materials that have more organic material that can hold moisture, such as wood products. Table 10.1 shows the range of water use for differing conditions. Chapter 17 provides more information about arena footing materials, including their water and dust suppression needs.

Cleaning Water

Stable cleanup chores will require a source of water in the stable aisle. In most barns the aisle water source will be via an antisiphoning, frost-proof hydrant (Figs. 10.7 and 10.13). Horse stalls may be cleaned and disinfected in some facilities. There will likely be periodic cleaning of the floors of the aisle, tack room, feed room, and other areas.

Hot and cold water will be needed for cleaning tack and for feed mixing and equipment cleanup. Water buckets need periodic scrubbing. Provide at least one hot water faucet in the stable for these small cleaning chores (Fig. 10.14) unless these activities are performed elsewhere (such as in an adjacent home).

Lavatory and Laundry Facilities

Public and larger stables will need to include bathroom facilities for both employees and visitors. A bathroom facility can be as simple as toilet and sink, but showering facilities may be desirable. An alternative is a contract for portable toilet. Portable toilets can and should be brought in for public events because most stables will not have enough bathrooms, nor perhaps enough water supply and/or septic capacity, to handle the additional waste load generated by many visitors.

A washer and dryer may be incorporated into stables and is dedicated to horse laundry such as wraps, light blankets, and saddle pads. An adjacent laundry sink is useful for rinsing out extremely dirty items before putting them into the washer.

Lavatory and laundry rooms will need supplemental heat in cold climates to prevent freezing of the water supply. Consider durable construction materials that will survive the moist and dusty conditions found in stables. In an unheated stable, sheet rock will mildew with high winter humidity and is relatively easily damaged compared with wood and fiberglass reinforced plastic (FRP) clad hardboard materials.

Clearly, the addition of a toilet necessitates that a sewage disposal option be added to the facility (public sewer hookup or septic tank system). Nonsewage wastewater, called "gray water," may be handled without the use of a septic system. Gray water would include various washwater flows such as from a sink, shower, and laundry that are lower in organics and pollutants than the toilet sewage wastewater. Washwater can be directed to a vegetative filter (local regulations permitting) or into a tank for spray irrigation on surrounding cropland or pasture. These washwater disposal options need to be designed to handle the expected water loads and maintained for effective water distribution. In the long run, installation of a septic system, even if just for gray water disposal, may be the best option in all but the smallest horse farms.

GAS SERVICE AND SOLID FUELS

Natural and Propane Gas

Gas is an efficient source of heat for a unit heater, hot water tank, and radiant heater. Natural gas may be available on-site via underground pipeline for facilities that have distribution nearby. This is most likely for suburban and urban facilities or rural locations that happen to be close to distribution pipelines. Anywhere else, propane can be substituted for natural gas, with a slight gas burner modification that is available on most heating appliances. A contract is arranged with a local propane gas utility for storage tank installation and gas supply service. In either case, the utility company will be able to install or otherwise advise on proper equipment and hookup.

Wood and Coal Fuel

For heating needs, wood and coal may be used for energy. These burners are not commonly used in horse facilities because the heating needs are relatively low compared with other livestock and residential use, but they are a suitable energy source.

TELEPHONE AND OTHER ACCESS

Access to a telephone is a convenience in a private stable. It can often be an extension of the residential line so it rings in both home and barn. The phone is often located in the feed or tack area. Adding an extra bell in the stable area will allow you to hear when the phone is ringing while you are in the stables. When the distances are short, a cordless house phone may provide adequate coverage.

Telephone service for a commercial or public facility becomes a necessity within the stable, usually with its own dedicated number(s). An office or lounge is an obvious place for telephone service for business transactions. Also consider phone(s) in the horse-occupied areas of the stable and indoor riding arena for convenience in not having to leave an animal unattended while on the phone. The abundance of cell phone and cordless phone use has decreased the need for hard-wired phone access in multiple locations around the facility. A public facility may want a pay phone (or other dedicated phone) for customer and visitor convenience and in order to protect use of the business phone.

Additional phone lines may be needed for dedicated facsimile and dial-up Internet access for horse business-related services. Cable networks may be accessed for TV or high-speed, dedicated Internet.

11
Lighting

A high-quality work environment provides proper lighting to improve worker efficiency, safety, and comfort. Good lighting takes some of the drudgery out of the many human-labor chores associated with horse housing. Good stable light quality can have a positive influence on worker comfort. Quality of light refers to reduced glare, shadow control, and reduction in sharp differences between objects and their background. Light quality also considers the light's "color." Lighting may be used for photoperiod control of horse reproductive activities. Horses can sleep in light or dark conditions.

Lighting levels are provided to meet the requirements of different purposes or tasks. Levels range from low required to walk safely through an area to high for detailed observation and visual work. Proper lighting provides the required light levels in the proper locations for each task. In some areas, a low general light level is adequate; for example, hay storage. Other areas require a medium light level to efficiently do the work; for example, an office. A high light level is required where detailed tasks are being performed such as a vet area. A general medium light level with the ability to have a focused high light level on the critical areas can save installation and operating costs over providing a high light level for the entire space. In the case of indoor riding arenas and grooming and wash stall areas, we want to reduce or eliminate shadows as part of the lighting system design.

The amount of illumination needed in horse facilities varies from 3 footcandles in hay and bedding storage areas to 50 footcandles in an office or tack room. Up to 100 footcandles is supplied as task lighting where precise work is done, such as an office desk, veterinary care area, or shop workbench. A footcandle is a measure of light output. The English system uses footcandle (fc) per square foot and the metric system uses lumen (lm) per square meter, or lux (1 fc = 10.76 lux).

The performance of the lighting system is critical to the performance of the building. Both natural and artificial lighting is used to illuminate stable and riding arena activities. Design either system to meet the lighting needs of the specific spaces. With natural lighting the design issues are the size, location, and protection of openings for light entrance. For electrical lights, the design issues include the light uniformity, type of bulb, energy efficiency, light color, the bulb fixture and reflector, mounting height, spacing, and switch location.

NATURAL LIGHT

Natural lighting systems allow sunlight to enter the stable or arena through glazed or unglazed openings. The design includes the number, size and locations of openings, covers for each opening, and protection from horses. Covers for each opening include glass and translucent plastic panels or translucent curtain materials.

Typically, each stall should have a window. Support areas should have windows such as in the tack room, feed room, office, and lounge. During warm weather, stable doors, stall exterior doors, and movable panels provide ventilation air exchange and additional light. Design the natural lighting system to provide an acceptable light level during cold weather when large solid doors and panels are closed. Light-colored interior surfaces reflect light better than dark colors. Keep in mind that a building at night will be darker than outside (with stars and moon light) if no light-emitting openings are provided. Windows and sliding panels are positioned intermittently along the sidewalls and endwalls, while translucent panels are often installed along the whole length of the wall near the top of the wall (Fig. 11.1). Endwall doors and stall exterior doors can incorporate windows for light entry even when closed.

Direct sunlight provides a high light level but has the disadvantages of also providing glare, high

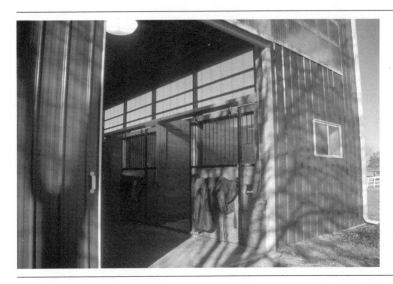

Figure 11.1. Light entry in a stable combines natural light, shown here via windows and translucent siding panels, and electric light, via HID light fixtures in this photo.

variability of light level, and heat. Reflected sunlight is more diffuse with reduced glare. Overhangs and other shading devices can stop direct sunlight entry (Figs. 11.2 and 11.3) through windows and panels. Sunlight entry and subsequent heat buildup is a problem during warm and hot weather. An overhang may be designed to shade windows from summer sun angles while allowing winter sun, at a lower sun angle, to enter the building (Fig. 11.4). An east-west orientation of the building's long axis is better for natural lighting (and natural ventilation) than a north-south orientation. Translucent panels offer uniform diffuse light when installed on the top portion of sidewalls. They may be protected from direct sunlight entry with an overhang.

For adequate natural light, a minimum of 1 square foot window per 30 square feet barn floor area is needed. One 2-foot by 3-foot stall window provides enough light for a 12-foot by 12-foot box stall with a 10-foot alley. It is best to install windows that open so they can also serve a ventilation function. Protect glass from horses with strong

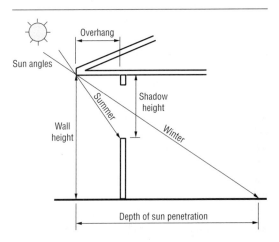

Figure 11.3. Natural light entering the building can be naturally controlled with properly designed overhangs that work with the seasonal sun angles to allow light entry during winter for warming and shade against light entry during hot weather when the extra solar heating is undesirable. From *Structures and Environment Handbook*, MWPS-1.

Figure 11.2. Example overhang that shades stall door openings against summer sunlight and heat entry. Adapted from *Structures and Environment Handbook*, MWPS-1.

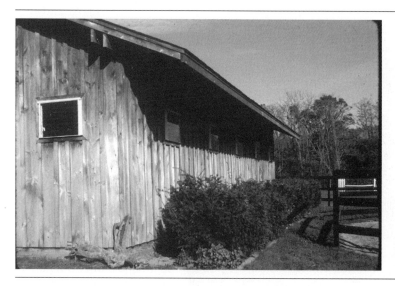

Figure 11.4. Stable windows shaded from excessive sunlight entry and glare during warm weather.

grillwork of bars or wire mesh similar to those used on stall partitions. Window height varies, but the sill should be at least 5 feet (up to 7 feet) off the stall floor. This will keep windows high enough to decrease the danger of being kicked, yet low enough so that horses can look outside. Indoor riding arenas also benefit from natural light entry through translucent siding or movable panels (Fig. 11.5).

Roof Translucent Panels

Translucent panels located in the roof cause water leakage and heat problems and are not recommended. In addition, light patterns thrown on the floor from roof translucent panels are particularly troublesome in riding arenas as they are spread throughout the arena interior and seem to have a confusing influence on horses. Horses may avoid large, dark-shadowed areas and jump sharply lit patches of the floor. Water leakage occurs because translucent panels do not have the same temperature expansion and contraction properties as the roofing materials around them, so that disparate material movements cause gaps to form even around the best-installed and -caulked panels. Finally, there is no way to block direct sunlight penetration through roof translucent panels, such as with an eave overhang.

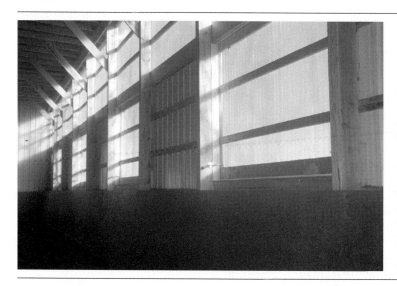

Figure 11.5. Translucent panels used in indoor riding arena for light entry. This arena has two sides surrounded by stabling that results in a limited area for natural light entry compared with a free-standing arena. A good solution was the addition of the extra translucent panels along one sidewall. These panels slide open for fresh air entry.

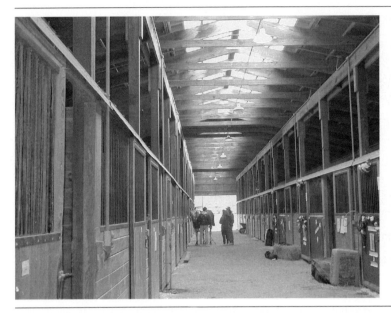

Figure 11.6. Although not generally recommended because of challenges of maintaining a leak-free construction and uncontrollable solar heat gain, roof translucent panels offer a naturally bright interior to this four-stall-wide fairground stable.

Translucent roof panels are an attractive alternative for natural lighting where the solar heat entry is welcome, for example in a building only used during cold weather, and where water leaks are tolerable (Fig. 11.6). Stables and indoor arenas in northern climates can benefit from the additional natural light without so much concern for summer overheating. Particularly for riding arenas, choose translucent panels that diffuse light entry to reduce the contrast between sunlit and shaded areas of the arena floor. Skylights, of residential design, offer light entry through the roof area with better seal against water entry than offered by translucent panels. Skylights may be installed in shingled or tiled roof construction. Some agricultural ridge vent assemblies provide translucent materials for natural light entry.

ELECTRIC LIGHT

Design of a good electric lighting system involves many factors, including light levels, light color, acceptable variability of light levels, lamp type, energy use, mounting height, light reflector, and ambient temperature. A small stable may only require one type of light such as an incandescent bulb in a dust- and moisture-proof fixture. In a large complex, a design using the light appropriate for each specific area will provide a better and more economical lighting system.

Lighting applications range from stall lights and arena lights that are typically used in cold environ-ments to tack room and office lighting where higher illumination levels are desirable and the environment may be warmer with lower ceilings. Recommended illumination levels for specific tasks are given in Table 11.1. For clarity in this lighting discussion, the words "lamp" and "bulb" are used to indicate the light bulb only, while "luminaire" and "light fixture" indicate the combination of ballast, ballast housing, reflector, and lamp.

Table 11.1. Recommended Illumination Levels for Various Tasks in Horse Facilities

Visual Task	Footcandles on Task
Prepare feed	10–20
Read charts and records	30
Haymow	3–9
Ladders and stairs	20
Feeding, inspection, cleaning	20
Veterinarian and farrier inspection area	50–100
General shop lighting, machinery repair	30–100
Riding area	20–30
Stalls—housing only	7–10
Horse handling, in-stall or work aisle	20
Office, bookkeeping	50–70
Restroom	30

Table 11.2. Light Source Considerations in Horse Facilities

| | Considerations for Lighting Applications | | | |
Light Source	Color Rendition Index (CRI)[a]	Tolerant of Frequent On-Off Cycles	Temperature Sensitive	Typical Overhead Mounting Height[b] (ft)
Incandescent	90–100	Yes	No	8–12
Quartz-Halogen	100	Yes	No	8–12
Fluorescent	70–95 [compact 80–90]	Yes Frequent on-off shortens bulb life	Yes Need cold-start ballast	8–12
Metal Halide HID	60–80[c]	No Leave on for at least 3 hr	No	12–20
High-Pressure Sodium HID[d]	20–80	No Leave on for at least 3 hr	No	12–20

[a]CRI defines the color, or degree of whiteness, of a light source. CRI > 80 is recommended where high-quality light is needed.

[b]Overhead mounting height for horse facilities has an 8-ft minimum clearance in areas with horse access. Incandescent, quartz-halogen, and fluorescent lights may be mounted at human ceiling level in areas without horse access. High-intensity discharge (HID) lights are mounted relatively high to evenly distribute light and heat from lamps.

[c]Higher CRI metal halide is available at increased cost.

[d]Low-pressure sodium HID has CRI of 0 and should not be used in indoor lighting applications.

Table 11.2 summarizes typical light source considerations such as mounting height and on-off cycles.

Artificial lights are classified according to the type of bulb used in the light fixture: incandescent, quartz-halogen; fluorescent; and high-intensity discharge (HID) are common options. The type of lamp affects the energy use and light color. Table 11.3 provides examples of the energy efficiency, bulb, and typical bulb-ballast sizes with some advantages and disadvantages of each type of light source. Realize that energy efficiency of a light fixture can vary up to 25% among different brands of the same lamp. Also included are some pros and cons used in deciding which lamp type is suitable for the various applications in horse facilities. Table 11.4 provides typical applications of lighting types in horse facilities.

Types of Lamps Useful in Horse Facilities

INCANDESCENT

Incandescent bulbs operate by using electricity to heat a tungsten metal filament in the bulb that "incandesces" and releases visible light. Incandescent bulbs have a low initial cost but are the most expensive to operate for the same level of light. Incandescent lamps have by far the shortest life and are the least energy efficient of the lamps discussed here. A 100-watt incandescent bulb only radiates 10% of its electric energy input as light; over 70% is radiated as heat in the infrared spectrum. Light output decreases to 80 to 90% of its initial value as it reaches it rated life. Incandescent light color is usually yellowish white, but lamps with different color outputs are available.

Incandescent bulbs are the best lamps for applications where lights are turned on and off frequently or where dimming is desired. They are commonly available and operate well under most temperature conditions. They can be used in low-ceiling rooms and are convenient for task lighting in an otherwise lower illumination room. Incandescent fixtures in the horse-occupied area need to be protected from physical damage and from high moisture and dust in the environment (Fig. 11.7). Incandescent bulbs get

Table 11.3. Light Source Wattage, Lifespan, Energy Efficiency, and Some Advantages and Disadvantages[a]

Light Source	Typical Wattage (W)	Initial Lumens	Ballast Watts (W)	Total Watts (W)	Average Life (hr)	Efficiency[b] (lumens/W)	Advantages	Disadvantages
Incandescent	40	400			460 to	12	• Commonly available • Inexpensive	• Short bulb life
	100	1600			1000	17		
	200	3400				20		
Quartz-Halogen	75	1400			2000–6000	15–38	• Bright white light	• Very hot bulb when on so keep away from flammable items • Oils from fingers and moisture will shorten bulb life • Efficiency low compared to other bulbs
	250	5000						
Fluorescent cool white	32	3200	8	48	20,000	66	• High energy efficiency • Bright, white light • Commonly available	• Light output decays drastically over time • Bulbs temperature sensitive, so need cold-start ballast for cold weather (<50°F)
	75	6300	16	91	12,000	69		
Metal Halide HID	175	13,000	40	215	10,000	60	• Bright, white light very close to daylight • High energy efficiency • Long lamp life	• Ballast hums slightly • High initial cost • All HID lights take minutes to warm up for full light
	250	20,000	45	295	10,000	68		
	400	40,000	55	455	15,000	88		
	1000	110,000	80	1080	11,000	102		
High-Pressure Sodium HID	150	15,000	38	188	24,000	80	• Highest energy efficiency • Longest lamp life	• All HID lights unsuitable for frequent on-off cycles • Unnatural yellowish glow to light
	250	28,000	50	300	24,000	93		
	400	50,000	55	455	24,000	110		
	1000	140,000	145	1145	24,000	122		

HID, high-intensity discharge; W, watts.

[a]These values are examples to illustrate typical lamp and luminaire performance. Use actual manufacturer values for final lighting system design.

[b]Efficiency includes ballast for fluorescent and HID luminaires.

Table 11.4. Typical Applications of Light Sources in Horse Facilities

Light Source	Tack, Feed, Lounge, Areas	Hay and Bedding Storage	Indoor Riding Arena and Stable Aisles with High Ceilings	Stalls and Stable Aisles with Low Ceilings	Outdoor Convenience and Security
			Typical Applications in Horse Facilities		
Incandescent	Yes	Yes, in sealed fixture	No, except as quick "walk-through" lights	Yes	Yes
Quartz-Halogen	Yes	No, hot bulb is fire hazard	No, except as quick "walk-through" lights	No, hot bulb is fire hazard	Yes
Fluorescent	Yes	Yes	Yes, but many lamps needed	Yes	No
Metal Halide HID	Slow startup a disadvantage Need high mounting height		Excellent use[a]	Not enough overhead clearance	Yes
High-Pressure Sodium HID	Slow startup a disadvantage Need high mounting height		Excellent use[a]	Not enough overhead clearance	Excellent use

[a]Provide incandescent lights in HID-lit area for quick on-off for checking or walk-through.

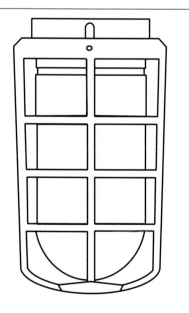

Figure 11.7 Incandescent bulb protected by rugged glass enclosure and cage for use in horse stable.

hot and should be placed in porcelain sockets when 100 watt or larger.

A quartz-halogen bulb is a type of incandescent bulb that has the tungsten metal filament in a halogen gas–sealed quartz bulb (Fig. 11.8). Halogen bulbs are slightly more energy efficient and have longer life than incandescent bulbs. A more noticeable advantage is that quartz-halogen bulbs produce a whiter light than incandescent, which is helpful where good color recognition is important. During lamp operation the halogen gas combines with tungsten molecules that have evaporated off the filament. The tungsten is redeposited on the filament rather than on the quartz bulb interior, so there is almost no bulb darkening with age as in an incandescent bulb. This halogen regenerative process requires high-temperature operation that also produces the brighter, higher color temperature light. The quartz bulb walls are necessary to withstand this high temperature but suffer from sensitivity to oil and dirt from human skin, which causes premature lamp failure.

While the lamp temperature increases with wattage, all quartz-halogen lamps, even low-wattage

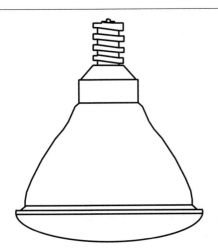

Figure 11.8. Quartz-halogen bulbs are a variation of incandescent that provide a whiter light but have very hot bulbs that are unsuitable for use near flammable materials (hay and bedding storage) or in dusty areas (feed room). Sealed floodlight models are excellent for use in areas where high-quality light is needed.

ones, operate at very hot temperatures; so *do not* use them near hay or bedding or in high-dust areas. All quartz-halogen lamps operate at high internal pressure and may unexpectedly shatter resulting in hot, flying fragments of glass or metal. Choose lamps that have the light bulb completely sealed against dust and moisture, similar in construction to a car headlight. Sealed lamps contain the bulb fragments, minimize shatter risk, and decrease ultraviolet (UV) radiation. Halogen lamps are recommended in the human-occupied areas of the stable where task lighting at high illumination or good color rendition is needed. They are also suitable for outdoor security lights. They are very effective when used as accent or display lighting or where full-range dimming is desired.

FLUORESCENT

The fluorescent bulb has a phosphor coating on the inside that glows when excited by electrical energy. Fluorescent lamps need a starter and ballast for proper current control through the lamp during operation. The ballast applies a voltage across the lamp until an "arc" forms and current begins to flow between the coils. Once operating, the ballast continues to control the coil and regulates the lamp current and power.

Fluorescent fixtures and bulbs cost more than incandescent but produce three to four times more light for the same electrical use. Fluorescent lights produce little heat or infrared light. In their more traditional tubular form, fluorescent lamps provide a relatively glare-free light due to their low surface brightness and a more uniform light distribution, because they are a linear light source rather than the point source of incandescent or quartz-halogen.

Fluorescent lamp light level decreases dramatically with age, but these lamps do last 12,000 hours or longer. Fluorescents lamp life is highly dependent on the number of burning hours per start; continuous burning can double the lamp life. This problem has been reduced with new electronic rapid-start and instant-start ballasts providing about 16,000 on-off cycles. For example, 16,000 starts at 15-minute intervals translate into a 4000-hour lamp life while with a 3-hour interval provide 15,000-hour lamp life.

The standard fluorescent bulb is commonly available as 4- or 8-foot lengths. It is housed in a fixture of the same length that contains the ballast (Fig. 11.9). Compact fluorescents are smaller, linear or globular designs that have a ballast built into the "bulb" and will fit in typical incandescent fixture.

Fluorescent fixtures are successfully used in indoor applications where ceiling height is relatively low (7 to 12 feet) and where good color rendition is desired. At heights above 10 feet, the illumination

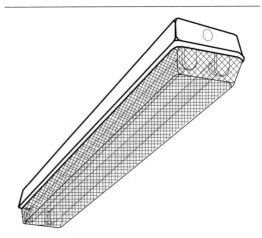

Figure 11.9. Fluorescent fixture with bulbs enclosed in sealed, gasketed enclosure that is moisture and dust tight. Electric start ballasts will provide cold-start capabilities (under 50°F) for unheated stables and arenas.

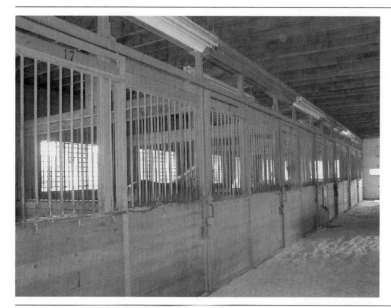

Figure 11.10. Fluorescent fixtures used in aisle and stalls of stable for energy-efficient lighting in cold climate. Locate light fixtures to side of aisle and front of stall to minimizes shadows on aisle work and horses, respectively. Fixture location is staggered in aisle and stall to provide more uniform light to both locations.

effectiveness of fluorescent fixtures is greatly reduced compared to HID fixtures. Standard white fluorescent provides the highest light output per energy of input but is not the best for color-matching tasks. Deluxe whites are about 25% less efficient than the standard, but they produce light nearest to daylight. Deluxe warm white produces light close in color to an incandescent lamp. Design and construction of the 32-watt T8 style lamps are about 40% more efficient than the older standard 40-watt T12 fluorescent style. The T8 or T12 designation refers to the tube diameter in increments of $\frac{1}{8}$ inch. T8 is 1-inch diameter and T12 is $1\frac{1}{2}$-inch diameter.

One of the reasons that fluorescent fixtures are used mainly indoors is that they have been sensitive to low temperatures and high humidity (Fig. 11.10). At lower temperatures the internal mercury vapor pressure is lower; thus there is less mercury available to start the lamp. Standard indoor fluorescent fixtures with magnetic ballasts operate well down to about 50°F and with moderate relative humidity (RH). Above 65% RH they become difficult to start because of the high humidity altering the electrostatic charge on the outside of the fluorescent tube. Fortunately, changes in ballast design have greatly improved cold-weather applications of fluorescent lamps.

Use electronic ballasts for fluorescent applications in horse facilities. With electronic "quick-start" or "cold-start" ballasts, fluorescents can be started down to –20°F. The light output is lower because the mercury is not emitting the optimum amount of UV light for the phosphor to convert to visible light. The ambient temperature of the lamp determines the light output. In cold applications, use enclosed fixtures (as shown in Fig. 11.9), which provide an 18°F rise in lamp temperature over ambient temperature. This means that at freezing temperature (32°F), an open fixture's relative light output is 50% (relative to an open fixture's 100% light output at 77°F) compared with a closed fixture (lamp at 50°F) that will provide 80% light output.

HIGH-INTENSITY DISCHARGE

High-intensity discharge (HID) lamps resemble incandescent in outward appearance yet operate more like a fluorescent using the electronic discharge principle. All HID lamps produce large quantities of light, have long lives, and are highly energy efficient. The operating pressure of HID lamps is high, so that the radiation generated by the electronic discharge is shifted from UV to visible light, thus greatly increasing the light output and efficiency. HID lamps contain mercury, halides, or sodium in the inner tube, which partially characterizes the light-emitting properties of the lamp. Metal halide and high-pressure sodium (HPS) HID lamps have virtually replaced mercury vapor, one of the original HID technologies, for use in horse facilities. They have longer life and maintain the light output better throughout the lamp's useful life.

Low-pressure sodium is a very energy efficient lamp best used for outdoor lighting. Low-pressure sodium lamps cast a very yellow light that is not acceptable for any indoor application.

HID fixtures are composed of the lamp bulb and a current-limiting ballast, which is specific to the type of bulb used (although a few luminaries are designed to switch between HPS or metal halide). The ballast will prevent an increasing current from harming the lamp as the lamp heat increases and its resistance drops during start-up. There can be a noticeable hum from the fixture as the ballast ages and when first turned on.

HID lamps are best utilized when mounted at least 12 feet high for light distribution. The luminaire itself is a large fixture with "high-bay" (about 30-inch luminaire height), "low-bay" (as small as 20-inch height) (Figs. 11.11 and 11.12), and wall pack models. The main difference between low- and high-bay HID is the wattage. Low-bay luminaries are typically lower wattage, 35 to 150 watts (some models up to 400 watt), and are mounted 10 to 16 feet high, while the high-bay luminaires are typically above 400 watts and mounted a minimum of

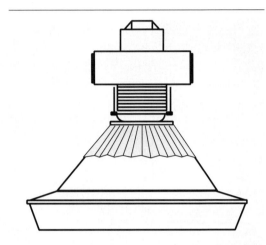

Figure 11.12. A low-bay HID model is simply a lower wattage and shorter profile fixture that can be mounted at lower heights than high-bay models.

16 feet high. At the higher wattage, and hence higher illumination, the high-bay models need to be mounted high to uniformly distribute their wide and bright light pattern. Wall packs are designed for mounting on the wall.

The reflective shield around the HID lamp is an important component of the luminaire design. Reflector shape will dictate whether a more circular or square light pattern is produced and the width (diameter) of this light pattern. Well-designed HID luminaire will have computer-designed, field-adjustable reflector mounts that allow for adjustment of the light distribution pattern to provide light in corners, for example, or to even out light patterns within an area. Manufacturers provide photometrics that show light output directly below the luminaire and to various angles from the fixture. This information is very useful in designing uniform lighting patterns at a specific illumination level. For horse facilities, use HID luminaires that are sealed against moisture and dust entry with a sealed refractor (Fig. 11.13).

Choose energy-efficient luminaires because, in the long run, electricity cost savings will far exceed original luminaire price. For example, with 3000 hours per year of use (about 8 hours per day) and an electricity price of $0.05, each 400-watt HID luminaire (455 total watts with ballast) will cost about $68 per year to operate. Over 10 years, this electrical operating cost far exceeds the original purchase price of the luminaire.

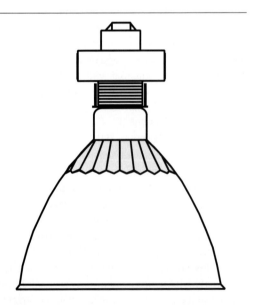

Figure 11.11. High-intensity discharge (HID) lamp in high-bay model. All types of HID lamps are highly energy efficient and provide light to a wide area. They are mounted high to take advantage of their large light output and have very long bulb life.

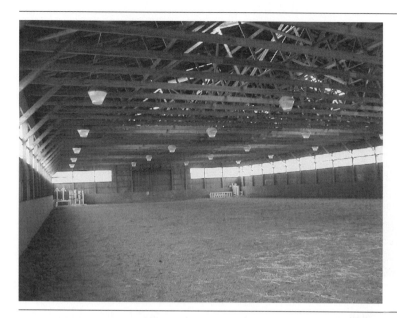

Figure 11.13. Indoor riding arena outfitted with four rows of sealed HID lamps in addition to natural lighting from translucent panels along the top of all walls.

HID luminaires operate well in cold temperatures (down to $-20°F$ for metal halide and $-40°F$ for HPS) and so have application in both warm and cold buildings and outdoors. HID lamps require several minutes to start and reach full light level; this can range from 3 to 15 minutes. Because of start-up delay and the reduction in lamp life with on-off cycles, they are not suitable for on-off cycles of less than 3 hours. In many applications a few incandescent lights are installed in areas with HID lights. The incandescent lights are used when short on times are expected such as while walking through one to another area for a quick general check of the space. The HID lights are used for longer light periods.

Metal halide light color is close to daylight and should be used when color appearance is important. High-pressure sodium has a slight yellow cast but is at least 20% more energy efficient with almost double the bulb life of metal halide. HID lights have a very low light decay over time and enjoy a long life that reduces bulb-changing maintenance in hard-to-reach locations (a humming ballast may have to be replaced more often than the bulb).

LIGHT QUALITY

Regardless of the source, light quality is determined by glare, color of the light, and uniformity of the coverage. Some places that may need high-quality light in addition to high illumination level are an office or shop workspace, the feed and tack room, a veterinary and farrier care area, and an indoor arena used for shows. High-quality light generally improves worker comfort and makes chores easier (Fig. 11.14).

Glare

Light delivery that prevents glare is needed. Glare is reduced by shielding the bulb, shading windows, placing lights above eye level, and using nonglossy, matte finish interior surfaces. The use of reflective surroundings improves the light energy efficiency (Fig. 11.15). Light-colored ceilings, walls, and floors will aid light scattering, while dark colors absorb the light. Where practical, ceilings should reflect 80% of the light striking them (white paint is common). Walls with 40 to 60% reflectance and floors at least 20% reflective are recommended. For example, white cement is about 50% reflective.

Light Color

The color, or degree of whiteness, of a light source is defined by the color rendition index (CRI). CRI values for the common light sources are included in Table 11.2. A CRI of 80 or more is recommended for areas where high light quality is needed. All light sources can be chosen to provide a CRI of 80 with the exception of low-pressure

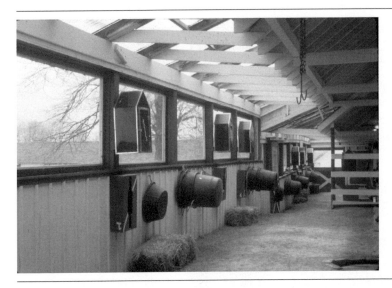

Figure 11.14. Conversion of this stable from open shed row design to an enclosed work aisle included provision for plenty of light for bright working conditions. Solar gain through roof plexiglass panels is welcome during cool weather but would be a liability on hot days.

sodium lamps that have a yellow glow and are only suitable for outdoor general lighting applications. Additional information about light color is in the "Incandescent," "Fluorescent," and "High-Intensity Discharge" sections.

Uniformity of Light

Illumination uniformity is defined as the ratio of the maximum to minimum values of light over a work area. In locations where tasks are visually challenging, such as office work or detailed horse care, the uniformity ratio (UR) should be no higher than 1.5. A UR around 5 is suitable for tasks that do not require close observation by the worker, such as horse stalls or riding arena surface. The UR is a very simple measure; divide the maximum light reading found in the area of interest by the minimum reading. A more descriptive, yet more complicated, measure of light uniformity is the coefficient of variation (CV). Table 11.5 provides example CV for fluorescent fixtures. The CV expresses uniformity as normalized with the average of all

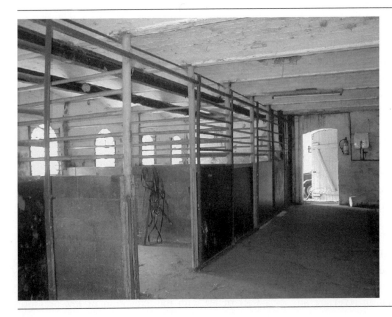

Figure 11.15. Light painted interior reflects more light than a dark interior as shown in this old yet bright whitewashed stable interior.

Table 11.5. Recommended Light Uniformity Criteria for Horse Stable Activities as Expressed by Coefficient of Variation (CV) and Ratio of Fluorescent Luminaire Mounting Spacing (s) versus Height (for up to 10-ft Mounting height)

Activity Classification	Maximum CV (%)	Spacing/Mounting Height (s/Hp) Fluorescent Lamps
Visually intensive (vet, tacking, washing, office, etc.)	25	0.85–1.0
Handling horse and equipment (stalls, aisle, private arena)	45	1.5
General lighting, low intensity	55	1.7–2.0

Hp is mounting height above work surface. Work surface height = 2 ft unless otherwise designated.

light measurements. It is defined as the standard deviation of all measurements divided by their mean value, and expressed as a percentage. Figure 11.16 shows lighting placement for working on a horse in an area where both high light level and uniformity are needed.

The uniformity of light is related to the height and spacing of luminaires in relation to their light output and distribution pattern. A ratio of the spacing between lamp fixtures to the mounting height above the "work" surface is used as one criterion in light uniformity design. This is probably the simplest method and is represented by the s/Hp ratio, where s is spacing between fixtures and Hp is lamp mounting height minus work surface height. If an obvious work height is not clear, such as workbench height of 3½ feet, then use a height of 2 feet. This 2-foot height would apply within the general stable stall area, while the "working" height of the indoor arena would be the riding surface, or floor of the building.

General guidelines for s/Hp ratios have been determined from studies in animal housing that have similar lighting and construction as horse stables and riding arenas. Provide a high level of light uniformity with an s/Hp ratio near 1.0. A spacing to mounting height ratio of 2.0 or less may be used where uniformity is not important and low cost is an objective. A guideline for horse stabling and arenas is an s/Hp ratio of no more than 1.8 for reasonable light uniformity with reasonable cost. This spacing ratio is used between fixtures within a row of lights and between rows of lights where more than one row is used, such as in indoor riding arenas. The more uniform the light needed, the more the fixtures needed, which

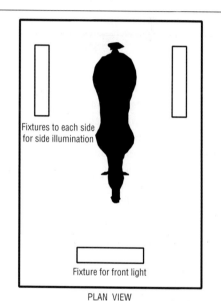

Fixtures to each side for side illumination

Fixture for front light

PLAN VIEW

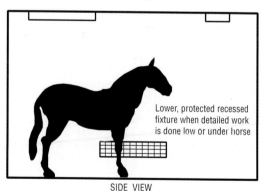

Lower, protected recessed fixture when detailed work is done low or under horse

SIDE VIEW

Figure 11.16. Example of lamp placement to achieve relatively shadow-free conditions in an area where detailed work is performed on a horse, such as in grooming, tacking, and washing areas.

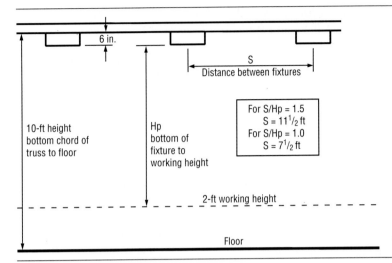

Figure 11.17. Luminaire spacing example for fluorescent lamps.

increases cost of installation and energy use. Figures 11.17 and 11.18 provide examples using common mounting heights of fluorescent and HID fixtures. Correct lamp placement is only partially explained by the s/Hp relationship. Providing uniform light depends on additional factors, such as lamp lumens and reflector design, so that s/Hp is only used as a guideline for the maximum reasonable spacing of light fixtures.

REFLECTORS

Uniformity of light in the illuminated space is more a function of the reflector than the type of lamp (for fluorescent or HID). Uniform distribution of light requires reflectors on HID fixtures. More modern HID lamp reflectors have increased the design distance between fixtures from 1.5 times the mounting height to as much as 4.5 times the mounting height while still attaining uniform light distribution. The

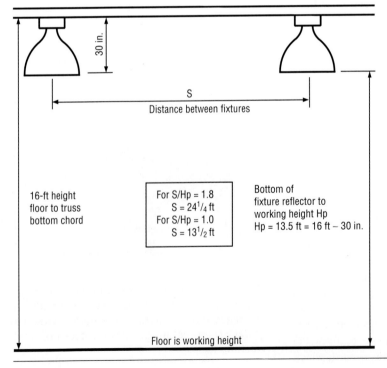

Figure 11.18. HID lamp spacing example.

luminaire manufacturer or lighting supplier can supply the luminaire lighting design parameters for the lamp wattage and reflector design chosen.

LIGHT QUANTITIES AND EFFICIENCY

Lumen (lm) is a measure of the amount of light emitted from a lamp and is used to compare different lamps. A lumen is the amount of light that is radiated in a 1-second period as determined in laboratory testing. Lamp efficiency is determined by dividing the lumen output of the lamp by the electrical energy it consumes in watts (W). Footcandle (fc) is the amount of light striking a working surface where illumination is needed. For light in general, 1 fc = 1 lm/ft^2. For many energy-efficient light sources, such as fluorescent and HID lamps, a ballast energy use must also be included in the efficiency rating. The ballast is used to control the flow of electricity to the gas-filled tube that helps prevent premature burnout.

INSTALLATION CONCERNS

Horse Damage

Light fixtures need to be protected from horse damage and from damaging the horse. This means a high, out-of-reach installation or a fixture protected with a wire cage. A strong glass enclosure is useful for containing a shattered bulb. Likewise, wiring to the light within horse reach (to 12-foot height) needs to be enclosed in conduit to protect from horse damage. (Refer to Chapter 10 for wire protection information.)

Moisture and Dust Protection

Because of the dust and high humidity in horse housing and indoor arenas, install dust- and moisture-resistant fixtures. The common incandescent and fluorescent fixtures used in residential and commercial building applications are not appropriate for the stables, arena, and other high-dust and -moisture areas. In the damp and/or dusty buildings found on horse farms, more rugged dust-proof and moisture-resistant fixtures are needed. A dust- and water-tight fixture for incandescent light is shown in Figure 11.7. It is nonmetallic, has a heat-resistant globe to cover the bulb, and can be rated for up to 150 watt. Because the temperature in these fixtures is higher than in standard fixtures, be sure to use the proper electrical wire that is recommended by the manufacturer. Likewise, fluorescent lights will be enclosed with a nonmetallic dust- and water-resistant gasketed cover as shown in Figure 11.9. A closed fluorescent fixture also assists in cold-temperature operation by increasing the operating temperature of the lamp.

Lamp-Starting Problems

Cold-start or slow-start characteristics plague the most efficient lamp sources, fluorescent and HID, respectively. Selecting the proper lamp and fixtures can easily overcome these deficiencies. All lamps require good electrical connections and properly sized conductors in good condition to further reduce difficulties. Incandescent lamps do not have a warm-up period that HID lamps require.

For cold locations, use cold-start ballast fluorescent lamp fixtures to assure start-up when temperatures dip below 50°F. Special cold-start (electronic) ballasts can light fluorescent lamps down to –20°F. These cost more than the cheap, commonly advertised fluorescent fixtures but eliminate the frustrations of poor lighting. In cold-temperature applications, enclosed fluorescent fixtures increase the lamp operating temperature for higher light output.

HID lamps operate well in the cold (down to –20°F) but under any temperature conditions will take from 3 to 15 minutes to fully light. High-pressure sodium lamps generally start faster than metal halides or mercury vapor. Quick-starting high-pressure sodium lamps cost twice as much as ordinary lamps. HID lamp life is decreased with frequent on-off cycles (less than 3 hour interval). If power to HID lamps is interrupted (even if from a momentary power interruption), the lamp will have to cool for at least a minute before initiating a relight, which again takes several minutes. One practical and recommended solution is to install a separate line of incandescent lights in the HID-lit area so light is immediately available when needed. This allows a quick walk through the area without wasting time and life of the HID lamps.

Lamp Heat

All lamps produce heat, but some produce significant heat that should be included in the building design. Hot-burning lamps create a safety hazard in dusty conditions. HID lights can contribute significant heat to an enclosed environment, which is an advantage during cold weather but a liability during hot weather. A 250-watt unit will produce about 900 Btuh (Btu/hr) and a 400-watt unit produces about 1500 Btuh. For comparison, a 1000-pound horse produces about 1500 Btuh at 70°F, so each 400-watt lamp is functionally equivalent to a horse in heat output. Fluorescent lamps have much cooler bulbs and low infrared light production and therefore do not contribute significant heat to an indoor environment. Incandescent bulbs get hot and should be placed in porcelain sockets when 100 watt or more. Quartz-halogen lamps are very hot in operation and should be kept away from flammable hay, bedding, and dust accumulations.

WIRING LIGHTS

Lighting systems need properly sized conductors and switches that are rated for the application and size of the amperes needed for lamp and ballast loads. Size conductors so that there is no more than a 2% voltage drop between the first and last light fixture. A 5% voltage drop can lead to a 15% lower light output from the lamp. When many HID lights are used to illuminate an indoor riding arena, stagger-start groups of lamps on separate circuits to reduce peak electricity demand rather than starting all the lamps at once. Wire aisle lights separately from groups of stall lights. Outdoor lights should be on their own circuit. Convenience outlets should be on a separate circuit from lights. Use three- and four-way switches for illuminating stairs, entrances, and aisles for "switch-ahead" lighting that allows users to turn off lights after they have reached their destination. (See Chapter 10 for wiring information.)

RELATIVE LIGHTING COSTS

Wiring and lighting in damp and dusty environment require that more rugged construction and noncorrosive materials be used, and these naturally cost more than models made for cleaner residential environments. All luminaires installed in livestock housing, which includes horse housing, are required by the National Electric Code to be moisture tight and constructed of corrosion-resistant materials. Fortunately, lighting technology and manufacture advances typically result in reduced cost, as does bulk purchase.

Operating costs are clearly lower for the more energy efficient lamps. The balance is between energy and purchase installation cost and the cost of

maintaining the system. System maintenance is primarily concerned with lamp and ballast replacement at the high installation height and multiple luminaire locations in riding arena lighting where labor may cost more than materials. Fluorescent and HID luminaires are significantly more expensive than incandescent; however the energy cost savings combined with longer lamp life offset the high initial cost. Where lights are operated for 8 hours per day or longer, a fluorescent and HID luminaire will typically pay for itself in 2 years or less.

Fluorescent and incandescent lamps do not have a higher energy requirement for starting, so that turning them on and off as needed is more desirable than running them for any period of time when not needed. Because of the start-up energy for HID lamps, leaving them on during short periods of unoccupied times saves costs over turning them on and off. Although frequent on–off cycles can reduce lamp life, it is always cheaper to turn lights off when they are not in use. The cost of electricity (even in the cheapest markets) is much more than that of replacing lamps a little sooner.

EXTERIOR LIGHTING

Exterior lighting is to enhance the safety of farm workers, add security against theft or vandalism, and improve the productivity of workers. Use energy-efficient lamps (metal halide or high-pressure sodium) and locate to provide light at building entrances and work areas, such as the manure storage and hay and bedding storage (Table 11.6 provides outdoor lighting recommendations). Low-pressure sodium (LPS) lamps cast such a yellow glow of light that they are not useful in farmstead lighting. For example, under LPS lights the color rendition is so poor that blood and motor oil appear the same. Floodlights (incandescent, quartz-halogen, or HID) on the front, back, and sides of buildings are useful not only for protection but in case of loose animals. These do not have to be lit other than when needed. Outdoor riding arenas may have lights for nighttime riding activities (Fig. 11.19).

Multiple switch control from two or more locations is convenient and recommended. Provide a switch at the residence to allow at least one circuit of the stables' outdoor lights to be lit from the house. Exterior lights should be on a separate circuit(s) from the stable interior lights to keep the failure of one system from interfering with the other.

Table 11.6. Outdoor Lighting Recommendations[a]

Activity	Recommended Illumination (fc)	Typical installation[b] High-Pressure Sodium Lamp 25-feet High
Security lighting	0.2	100 W for 8000 ft^2
General work area	1.0	250 W for 8000 ft^2
Activity area (building entrance, horse loading)	3.0	250 W for 2000 ft^2

[a]Adapted from *Agricultural Wiring Handbook*.

[b]Distance between lamps should not exceed 5 times mounting height. Metal halide may be substituted. Less efficient incandescent lamps of proper wattage may be substituted.

Take care in maintaining good neighborly relations by positioning outdoor lighting and using proper reflectors so light does not glare into nearby homes or at passing vehicles.

One decision with outside lights is whether to run them all night long or until a fixed time, such as midnight, instead of only when needed. For all-night operation, use a photocell to turn the lights on and off. For fixed-time operation, use a photo cell and a time clock to turn the lights on at dusk and off at the specified time. Place a switch in parallel to this arrangement to turn the lights on if needed after the time clock has turned them off.

PHOTOPERIOD CONTROL

It is a relatively common practice in equine industries to birth foals near the standard horse birthday of January 1. Clearly this is out of season for mares that are naturally programmed to foal during the spring season. Mares are long-day breeders. With an 11-month gestation cycle, mare and stallion breeding performance is out of cycle, which is where the out-of-season problem originates. Mares' normal ovarian cycle peaks in May to June.

Provision of 14 to 16 hours of light followed by darkness has been shown to stimulate estrus in the mare. Extending the day length by adding light into the night beyond dusk has been shown to be more effective than preceding the early morning light. In practice, though, addition of lights both before and after the natural day length is used most often. This can be supplied via a timer that automatically turns lights on in the morning and off in the evening. A built-in light detector will turn off the lights if exposed to natural daylight. Start increasing day length 8 to 10 weeks before the desired breeding time frame. For example, start the additional light program on December 1 for a breeding season starting in mid-February. The transition to 14 to 16 hours of daylight can be abrupt on December 1 or incremental by added 30-minute light intervals per week, starting on December 1, until 14 to 16 hours of day length is reached.

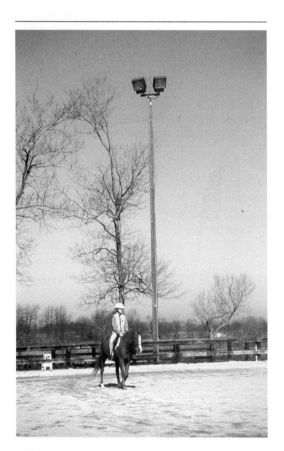

Figure 11.19. Outdoor lighting is desirable in riding areas that get a lot of use.

The minimum amount of light needed to stimulate the estrus cycle is 2 to 10 footcandles (depending on the study). Because about 10 footcandles is recommended for each stall (measured at 2 feet above the floor), this light requirement can be satisfied through stall lights on a timer. Note that this light level is needed at mare eye level, and most studies are recommending the 10-footcandle light level. Day length also influences sperm production in the stallion, with winter production being typically half of the level achieved during the summer breeding season. Off-season breeding of the stallion can be improved by photoperiod control in the same way as the mare estrus cycle. Likewise, mares and stallions confined in a pasture shelter can be similarly lighted.

MEASURING LIGHT

Instruments for measuring light come in a variety of formats that emphasize the wavelengths of light being measured (Fig. 11.20). Various wavelengths of radiation are designated into ranges of interest to a certain application such as visible light, UV light, or infrared.

Most commonly found "light meters" measure visible light, or illuminance, and are known as photometric sensors (approximately 380- to 770-nanometer wavelengths). These meters measure light radiation as perceived by the human eye. Units of measure include footcandle (fc), which is the U.S. system unit of measure, or lux, which is the SI (metric) measure (1 fc = 10.76 lux). Many visible light meters offer display of light readings in both fc and lux. Light intensity meters suitable for use in horse stabling may be found in hardware and agricultural supply catalogs or stores for about $35 for analog and $120 for digital models. More sophisticated sensors provide a choice to display the light intensity on the basis of the light source (e.g., sunlight, incandescent, fluorescent, or HID such as high-pressure sodium and metal halide).

Expose the sensor to the light level of interest. Avoid shading the sensor and keep it level. Tilting the sensor more than 10 degrees beyond horizontal will provide about a 5% error to the measurement of light intercepted by a horizontal surface. It is important to stand away from the sensor because a human body cannot only cast shadow on the sensor but provides a dark surface from which little diffuse light reflects. Place the sensor near the "working surface"

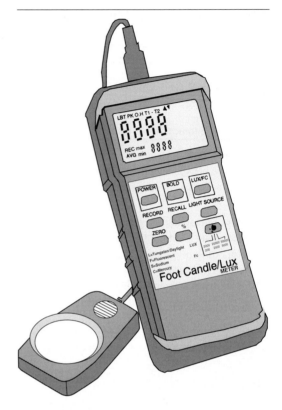

Figure 11.20. Instruments may be used to measure light level at various locations to determine uniformity and overall light level.

to determine light level. The working surface is presumed to be 2 feet off the floor if not otherwise specified as a desktop height, and so forth.

It is important to have a good lighting design to start with. Once installed, it is costly to move fixtures and wiring to improve the lighting system. To evaluate an installed design for potential improvements, take a number of measurements on a grid around the illuminated space. Note what part of the space is the most important to be well lit and have uniform light intensity. Obviously, the light level will be brighter directly underneath and near each luminaire or a natural light source. Take as many measurements as practical with a grid design that captures sites of presumed high light level (right under luminaires) and those that are dimmer (in corners). Improvements can be made with new fixtures, higher or lower wattage bulbs (fixture and wiring circuit needs to safely support higher wattage substitutions), or by changing the type of fixture. For example, more light may be added by conversion from incandescent to fluorescent fixtures while using the same wiring. Natural lighting may be substituted or added to artificial sources.

METHOD TO ESTIMATE PLACEMENT OF LIGHT FIXTURES

Simplified Design Method

A simplified method for estimating the number and placement of light fixtures to provide 10 or 20 footcandles per square foot is given in Table 11.7. Values in the table were developed from lamp manufacturers' data and actual lighting system performance in agricultural settings. (See Additional Resources for detail and original sources of the information.) Incandescent and fluorescent fixtures are used in 8- to 12-foot ceiling height areas, such as tack room, stalls, or stable aisles. HID fixtures are used for higher mounting heights, such as in indoor riding arenas. The spacing between light fixtures is expressed as a ratio of mounting height to spacing distance (s/Hp). This design approach uses a maximum s/Hp ratio of 1.8 to provide relatively uniform light. Ratios less than this will provide more uniform lighting, with ratios of 1.0 providing very good uniformity while minimizing shadows. The spacing criteria needs to be met both between fixtures within each row and between rows of light fixtures if multiple rows of lights are used.

Table 11.7. Indoor Lighting Design Values for Lamp Placement to Provide 10 or 20 Footcandles of Light at a Working Surface[a]

| | | Floor Area per Fixture to Provide | | | |
| | | 10 fc per ft^2 | | 20 fc per ft^2 | |
Lamp Type	Lamp Size (W)	Floor Area Illuminated (ft^2) A_L	Equivalent Diameter of Illuminated Circle (ft) D_L	Floor Area Illuminated (ft^2) A_L	Equivalent Diameter of Illuminated Circle (ft) D_L
Incandescent[b]	100	52	8	26	6
Fluorescent[b] 4 ft long	One 32	87	11	44	7
	Two 32	174	15	87	11
Fluorescent[b] 8 ft long	Four 32	348	21	174	15
HID High-Pressure	150[c]	656	29	328	20
Sodium	250[c]	1128	38	564	27
(reflector + refractor)	400[d]	2050	51	1025	36
HID High-Pressure	150[c]	512	26	356	21
Sodium	250[c]	880	33	440	24
(refractor only)	400[d]	1600	45	800	32
HID Metal Halide	100[c]	250	18	125	13
(reflector + refractor)	250[c]	828	32	414	23
	400[d]	1350	41	675	29
HID Metal Halide	100[c]	201	16	101	11
(refractor only)	250[c]	667	29	333	21
	400[d]	1088	37	544	26

HID, high-intensity discharge; fc, footcandle.
[a]Adapted from *Supplemental Lighting for Improved Milk Production*.
[b]Mounting height = 8 ft above the working surface.
[c]Use with mounting heights of 10–15 ft.
[d]Only use 400 W lamps if mounting height is over 15 ft.

To determine the number of fixtures needed for an area, divide the floor area by the illuminated area shown in Table 11.7. The table also expresses the illuminated area in terms of an equivalent circular diameter of light. Realize that some lamps, fluorescent and HID with rectangular reflectors, provide a more rectangular light pattern on the floor, but for simplicity of the design method a circular pattern is assumed. Check the spacing determined by the above floor area calculation against the equivalent diameter of the light supplied. Some light fixture configurations light only a limited floor area, for example the equivalent of a 10-foot diameter circle, and this distance may control lamp fixture placement. A set of calculations for providing at least 20 footcandles to a riding area surface using two to four rows of HID lights is provided in the following section. When actual manufacturer's data are available on light pattern, then those data should be used. This simplified method is used to screen lighting system designs for potential suitability.

EXAMPLE DESIGN OF INDOOR ARENA LIGHTING PLACEMENT

Set up design conditions:

- An arena of 60 feet by 120 feet has 7200 square feet of riding surface area.
- The sidewall height is 16 feet. Mount light fixtures on truss bottom chord.
- For a riding arena the floor is the important light plane; so if lamps are mounted under the 16-foot-tall truss and the fixture height is about 2 feet, then distance Hp is 14 feet.
- Provide at least 20 footcandles of light; 30 footcandles for bright interior (Table 11.1). Minimize shadows to reduce light and dark patches that may be unsettling to horses.
- Need uniform light with s/Hp of no more than 1.8 with designs to 1.0 desirable to minimize shadows.
- This relatively small 60-foot-wide, but standard, arena size will consider two or three rows of lights parallel to the long sidewall of the building. Four rows of lights are also considered and would need to be evaluated for wider arenas.

Choose various lighting options to evaluate:

- Evaluate all four types of HID fixtures featured in Table 11.7 (high-pressure sodium and metal halide, both with and without reflectors) to see if one offers superior application to the other three.

- Try all three high-pressure sodium wattage fixtures with reflector and refractor; and because of less light output with only a refractor, try only the two larger watt lamps.
- Try only the larger wattage metal halide lamps because the low-wattage lamps illuminate a rather small area for this application.
- Options, calculations, and results are provided in Table 11.8. Each option is assigned a letter-number (A1 through J3) for identification during the example discussion.

Calculate fixture number and spacing needed:

- Determine the total number of fixtures needed. Divide total arena riding area (7200 square feet in this case) by light fixture illumination area (square feet per lamp from Table 11.7) for each lamp type. Fewer fixtures are not necessarily better if light uniformity will not be adequate.
- Calculate the number of fixtures in each row if the arena is provided with two, three, or four rows of lights. Divide total number of lights by the number of rows.
- Determine spacing between rows of lights (D_2 in Table 11.8). Divide the number of rows by the width of arena (60 feet in this case).
- Determine spacing between fixtures in each row (D_1 in Table 11.8). Divide the number of fixtures per row by the row length (120 feet in this case).
- Calculate s/Hp for within-row and between-row spacing of light fixtures. Divide spacing (determined above) by Hp (14 feet in this case).

Check the suitability of spacing for uniform lighting:

- Compare the equivalent diameter (D_L in Table 11.8) of the illuminated area with lamp spacing within and between rows (D_1 and D_2). Spacing greater than equivalent diameter will leave unacceptably large low-light areas on the floor.
- Check if design spacing meets the s/Hp criteria of being no more than 1.8 to provide relatively uniform light.
- To be useful for further consideration, the design has to pass all the spacing checks.

Results and discussion:

- Four lighting design options (A2, D2, F2, H2) provided suitable light uniformity (shown in Table 11.8). These four configurations provided

Table 11.8a. Spreadsheet of Lighting Designs Using High-Pressure Sodium Lamps Evaluated to Provide 20 Footcandles Uniform Illumination to an Example Indoor Riding Arena[a]

	High-Pressure Sodium Fixtures														
	Reflector and Refractor									Refractor Only					
	A1	A2	A3	B1	B2	B3	C1	C2	C3	D1	D2	D3	E1	E2	E3
Lighting Design Options															
Lamp wattage, W		150			250			400			250			400	
Floor area covered, ft² (A_L, Table 11.7)		328			564			1025			440			800	
Number of lamps needed		22			13			7			16			9	
Two rows of lights ($2 \times ...$); fixtures per row	11.0			6.4			3.5			8.2			4.5		
Three rows of lights ($3 \times ...$)		7.3			4.3			2.3			5.5			3.0	
Four rows of lights ($4 \times ...$)			5.5			3.2			1.8			4.1			2.3
Determine Spacing															
Diameter floor area lit feet (D_L, Table 11.7)		20			27			36			24			32	
Distance within row light fixtures apart, feet (D_1)	11	16	22	19	28	38	34	51	68	15	22	29	27	40	53
Distance rows apart, ft (D_2)	30	20	15	30	20	15	30	20	15	30	20	15	30	20	15
s/Hp within row	0.8	1.2	1.6	1.3	2.0	2.7	2.4	3.7	4.9	1.0	1.6	2.1	1.9	2.9	3.8
s/Hp between rows	2.1	1.4	1.1	2.1	1.4	1.1	2.1	1.4	1.1	2.1	1.4	1.1	2.1	1.4	1.1
Spacing Suitability (1 = Yes; 0 = No)															
Meet fixture light spacing within row ($D_1 < D_L$)?	1	1	0	1	0	0	1	0	0	1	1	0	1	0	0
Meet fixture light spacing between rows ($D_2 < D_L$)?	0	1	1	0	1	1	1	1	1	0	1	1	1	1	1
Meet s/Hp uniformity within rows (s/Hp < 1.8)?	1	1	1	1	0	0	0	0	0	1	1	0	0	0	0
Meet s/Hp uniformity between rows (s/Hp < 1.8)?	0	1	1	0	1	1	0	1	1	0	1	1	0	1	1
Design Useful? (needs all "1s" in spacing checks)	0	1	0	0	0	0	0	0	0	0	1	0	0	0	0

[a]Arena 60 ft × 120 ft with 16 ft eave height; floor area 7200 ft².

157

Table 11.8b. Spreadsheet of Lighting Designs Using Metal Halide Lamps Evaluated to Provide 20 Footcandles Uniform Illumination to an Example Indoor Riding Arena[a]

	Metal Halide											
	Reflector and Refractor						Refractor Only					
	F1	F2	F3	G1	G2	G3	H1	H2	H3	J1	J2	J3
Lighting Design Options												
Lamp wattage, W		250			400			250			400	
Floor area covered, ft² (A_L, Table 11.7)		414			675			333			544	
Number of lamps needed		17			11			22			13	
Two rows of lights (2 × ...); fixtures per row	8.7			5.3			10.8			6.6		
Three rows of lights (3 × ...)		5.8			3.6			7.2			4.4	
Four rows of lights (4 × ...)			4.3			2.7			5.4			3.3
Determine Spacing												
Diameter floor area lit, ft (D_L Table 11.7)		23			29			21			26	
Distance within row light fixtures apart, ft (D_1)	14	21	28	23	34	45	11	17	22	18	27	36
Distance rows apart, ft (D_2)	30	20	15	30	20	15	30	20	15	30	20	15
s/Hp within row	1.0	1.5	2.0	1.6	2.4	3.2	0.8	1.2	1.6	1.3	1.9	2.6
s/Hp between rows	2.1	1.4	1.1	2.1	1.4	1.1	2.1	1.4	1.1	2.1	1.4	1.1
Spacing Suitability (1 = Yes; 0 = No)												
Meet fixture light spacing within row ($D_1 < D_L$)?	1	1	0	1	0	0	1	1	0	1	0	0
Meet fixture light spacing between rows ($D_2 < D_L$)?	0	1	1	0	1	1	0	1	1	0	1	1
Meet s/Hp uniformity within rows (s/Hp < 1.8)?	1	1	0	1	0	0	1	1	1	1	0	0
Meet s/Hp uniformity between rows (s/Hp < 1.8)?	0	1	1	0	1	1	0	1	1	0	1	1
Design Useful? (needs all "1s" in spacing checks)	0	1	0	0	0	0	0	0	0	0	0	0

[a]Arena 60 ft × 120 ft with 16 ft eave height, floor area 7200 ft.

illumination and spacing that met the s/Hp uniformity criteria within and between rows of lights and had distance between lamps that was equal to or less than the illuminated diameter of light.

- All suitable designs had three rows of lights with about 5 to 7 fixtures per row with one design using 150-watt and three designs using 250-watt bulbs. The suitable designs represented lamps from the four categories of HID lights evaluated, which indicates that there will be several suitable options for proper illumination of a riding arena environment.
- None of the two-row light designs met the light spacing criteria for uniformity in both within-row and between-row dimensions.
- Illustrations of lamp placement for three designs are shown in Figures 11.21a through 11.21c, with circles representing illuminated area for each lamp. Spaces between circles will have light but with less than the 20-footcandle criteria.
- All four suitable designs effectively covered the arena floor with light. Position lamps to get light into corners of the arena by allowing the circle of

illumination to "touch" the corner. This will overlap some light beyond the walls within the corner of the arena (reflective wall surfaces will help here). This is shown Figures 11.21c and 11.21d.

- Figure 11.21c shows two options for positioning the lamps along the sidewall. The row of lights along the lower sidewall provides 20-footcandle light along the entire sidewall by positioning the lights to overlap the sidewall. The top option has the outer edge of the light circles end at the sidewall, so there will be locations along the wall that receive less than 20-footcandle light in between fixtures. The overlap option on the lower sidewall is preferred because it provides more uniform light at the sidewall where significant riding activity occurs in most riding arenas.
- Other options did not work because of excessive spacing distance between light fixtures. But a couple of these failed options were within 1 foot spacing or close to the 1.8 s/Hp criteria and could be considered further (G1, H3, J2). Design H3 is shown in Figure 11.21d and provides fairly

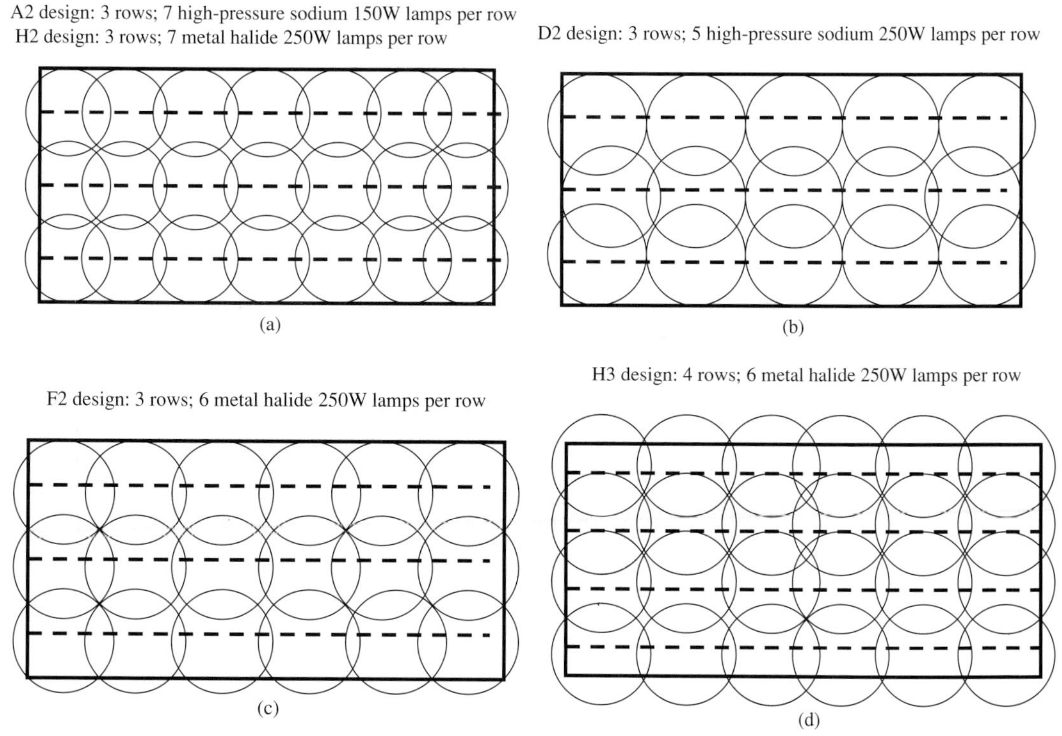

A2 design: 3 rows; 7 high-pressure sodium 150W lamps per row
H2 design: 3 rows; 7 metal halide 250W lamps per row

D2 design: 3 rows; 5 high-pressure sodium 250W lamps per row

F2 design: 3 rows; 6 metal halide 250W lamps per row

H3 design: 4 rows; 6 metal halide 250W lamps per row

(a) (b) (c) (d)

Figure 11.21. Examples of indoor arena lighting spacing of fixtures for uniform illumination to 20 footcandles based on a simplified calculation method.

intensive coverage of the arena with light because there are four rows of fixtures versus three rows in the other designs.

This example showed that more than one lighting design is suitable for illumination of riding arenas. Three rows of fixtures satisfied uniform lighting to 20 footcandles over almost the entire riding surface in this 60-foot-wide arena. Provide light overlap at the edges of the arena surface to get adequate light along the walls where much riding is done. This example considered many more designs than you would logically evaluate without an electronic spreadsheet (which was used in this case) to illustrate how lamp placement can succeed and fail depending on lamp selection and spacing. Professional lighting design with more sophistication than demonstrated by this simplified method is available from lighting manufacturers and consultants. Lighting is important to the successful function of a building and should be given careful attention in the planning stage because it is difficult and costly to correct once installed.

SUMMARY

Good lighting in a stable and indoor riding arena improves comfort and usefulness of the facility. Outdoor lighting improves security and ease of doing nighttime activities. Natural lighting is desirable but is supplemented by electric lighting in most cases. There are many commonly available lighting options to meet the requirements in the various stable areas. A good design usually uses different lamps and fixtures to match the light requirements in different areas. Provide at least one area where good quality and high light level is available for detailed work on a horse. Fixtures need to be rugged and sealed against the high moisture and dust levels found in stabling and arenas compared with the fixtures typical of residential use.

12
Heating

Some stable managers will want to maintain a horse stable as a warm building in the winter. An environment goal may be to just keep the interior above freezing at about 40°F. In northern climates, it is not uncommon to maintain stable temperature at 50°F. Show horses maintained year round with short hair coats and newborn foals will benefit from the warm environment as long as fresh air quality is also maintained in the stable. It is important to resist the temptation to close the stable up tight and use horse body heat alone to heat the stable because this will result in humid, odorous conditions. This chapter describes heating systems that can be used to maintain warm conditions and good air quality in the stable.

Heating involves provision of heat to the building and trying to keep a large portion of the heat not only contained in the building but kept where it provides comfort for the occupants. The three forms of heat transfer are conduction, convection, and radiation. Conduction is heat movement through a solid or from one solid to another; for example, your seat on a cold metal bleacher. Convection heat movement is via moving fluids (gas or liquid); hot air rises to the ceiling of heated buildings, while colder air accumulates near the floor. Radiation is a powerful form of heat transfer between objects that can "see" each other; the closer one is to a woodstove, the more heat is received on the side of your body facing the stove.

COMFORTABLE TEMPERATURES

Horses are tolerant of a wide range of temperature conditions especially down to cold temperatures that humans find uncomfortable (Fig. 12.1). Horses are most comfortable at 55°F compared with the human comfort level at about 70°F. Horses are thermoneutral, or comfortable, in the range of 32 to 85°F. Figure 12.1 shows the wide range of temperatures that horses can tolerate while maintaining a constant body temperature (zone of homeothermy). Horses are tolerant of temperatures

below 0°F if well nourished and acclimated to those conditions (Fig. 12.2).

One solution to keeping both horse and human stable users comfortable is to provide a heated area in the barn where people can warm up or take the horse to work on it. This leaves the stall area well ventilated and at the proper temperature while providing handler comfort in a separate area. Heaters are more often used in separate rooms where people congregate, such as the tack room and lounges. In cold climates, a separate support area with wash, tack, and grooming stations equipped with supplemental heat is a good alternative to keeping the entire stable heated for human comfort.

HEATING SYSTEMS

There are two primary ways to heat a stable interior. One is via space heat so that air within the entire space is heated to the desired temperature. Space heat is provided by a unit heater(s) or central furnace. The second heating system is via radiant energy where occupants of the stable environment are warmed. With radiant use the stable air can be maintained at a lower temperature, yet an individual horse or work area feels warmer. Radiant heat comes in two formats, with one being an overhead, high-temperature unit that provides radiant energy, often to a relatively small area. The second type is in-floor radiant heat that provides heat over its large low-temperature surface area. Both types of radiant heat also provide space heating when used over extended time intervals because air next to the warm or hot surface is heated by conduction and then distributed via convection to warm the room. Each of these heating systems is explained in the following sections and depicted in Figure 12.3. This chapter's discussion focuses on permanently installed heating systems. Portable residential or camping style "space" heaters are not recommended for use in horse stabling because of the fire hazard associated

161

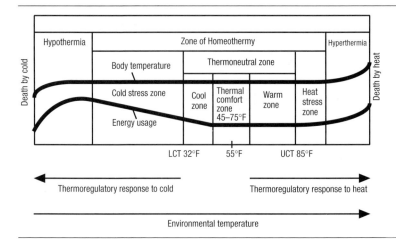

Figure 12.1. Diagram of horse environment temperature ranges relative to thermal comfort and stress. Horses are more tolerant than humans of a wide range and cooler temperatures. LCT, lower critical temperature; UCT, upper critical temperature.

with unattended units and those not designed for use around flammable materials.

Adding heat to the stable environment will entail the addition of more than just the heating unit(s) itself. The heat unit is part of a system that also includes fuel or electricity delivery, controls to detect and maintain the desired temperature, and a way to distribute the heat throughout a space. Heated buildings are insulated to not only reduce heat loss through the walls, but also to keep the interior wall temperature near the interior air temperature (see "Insulation" section of this chapter). Some outside air exchange is necessary in heated stables to remove stale, damp air from the stable and replace it with fresh air.

A stable may employ more than one type of heating system. Space heating via baseboard units may be

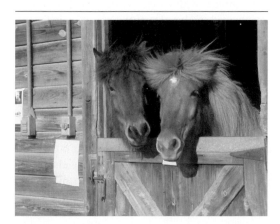

Figure 12.2. Horses adapt to cold conditions and when well nourished will be comfortable at temperatures below 0°F.

used in the tack and feed rooms, while overhead high-temperature radiant heat is used in the wash stall. A centralized boiler can supply hot water to an in-floor radiant heating system of the stable working aisle and to baseboard or overhead unit heaters elsewhere. Zone control is easy with most heating applications, so that heat is supplied only where and when it is needed.

FRESH AIR QUALITY

Heated buildings will usually employ mechanical ventilation to carefully control fresh air exchange. A mechanical ventilation system is composed of a fan(s), planned openings, and controls. Warm stable design typically uses heat and mechanical ventilation during the heating season and uses natural ventilation the rest of the year. Provide one continuously operated fan system for minimum cold-weather ventilation and additional thermostat-controlled fans along with increased inlet opening for mild conditions. (Additional fan and inlet capacity will be needed for hot conditions if the stable is not naturally ventilated during the summer.)

Ventilation will be important during cold weather in warm horse stables to maintain good air quality. Low ventilation rates are used during cold weather to maintain proper air quality and to control moisture buildup. One horse normally respires about 2 gallons of water daily. If this moisture is allowed to accumulate within the stable environment, it increases the risk of condensation and frost formation on building components and provides an overall feeling of dank, odorous conditions. Removal of the moisture will likewise remove odors, ammonia, and pathogens that accumulate in the stable air. One

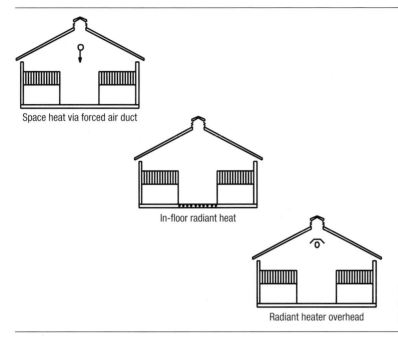

Space heat via forced air duct

In-floor radiant heat

Radiant heater overhead

Figure 12.3. Three heating system applications suitable for stable environment.

of the advantages of heated air in a stable (or tack room, etc.) is that cold outside air is brought into the stable, heated so it will hold more moisture (a natural psychrometric property of air; see Appendix), and then used like a "sponge" to pick up moisture within the heated environment (Fig. 12.4). This warm, moisture-laden air must then be vented from the stable and replaced with fresh, dry air from outside. Realize that ventilation air exchange will be the primary avenue for heat loss from the stable even with the relatively low, controlled ventilation rate recommended for maintaining good air quality within the stable during cold weather. See Chapter 6 for more information on ventilation system designs.

HEAT FOR HUMAN-OCCUPIED AREAS OF STABLE

Discussion in this chapter centers on horse stable applications, but similar heating systems can be used in auxiliary facilities such as a breeding shed or indoor riding arena. Stable office, lounge, arena observation room, and tack room are often built to a more residential construction standard, with heat typically provided via systems borrowed from residential practices (baseboard heat, forced-air system, in-floor radiant, etc.). Remember that even these human-occupied stable spaces will be significantly more dusty and humid than typical homes, and so

equipment corrosion and dust clogging of heater filters will be more challenging. The discussion that follows is for the horse environment built to withstand the rigors of horse activity while providing a high-quality environment for the horse and handler.

SPACE HEAT

The whole stable interior, or portions of it, can be heated to the desired temperature through space

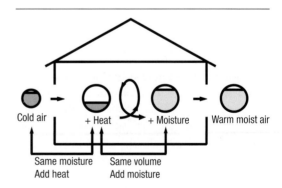

Cold air   + Heat   + Moisture   Warm moist air

Same moisture   Same volume
Add heat   Add moisture

Figure 12.4. Cold outside air with high relative humidity is heated to lower the relative humidity and then used to absorb moisture within the stable. Eventually this warm moisture- and odor-laden air is exhausted with more fresh air brought into the stable.

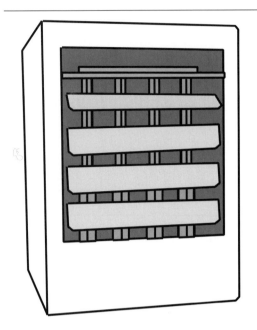

Figure 12.5. Space heat may be provided by an agricultural-quality unit heater that is designed to withstand the higher moisture and dust levels in stables compared with levels found in commercial and residential environments.

heat applications. Individual unit heaters manufactured for agricultural use (Fig. 12.5) are relatively inexpensive and will withstand the humidity, dust, and potentially corrosive nature of horse stable air. (This discussion is *not* about portable space heaters used in homes and offices or in camping environments.) Space heaters will typically be gas-fired for energy cost savings (versus electric). Gas heaters will need fresh air for combustion, which can be provided directly from outdoors, and a vent to the outside for products of combustion. Propane and natural gas combustion products include water vapor, carbon dioxide, and carbon monoxide. The latter compound is deadly but emitted at an extremely low rate with properly maintained heaters that have adequate oxygen supply for complete combustion (another reason for supplying fresh ventilation air). In a well-ventilated space, a space heater does not require a separate vent for combustion products. Provide at least 2½ cubic feet per minute (cfm) of additional ventilation capacity per 1000 British thermal units (Btu) of heater capacity to remove products of combustion. This increases

the recommended cold-weather ventilation rate per horse (25 cfm/horse) by about 10%.

A circulating hot water system may be used for radiators, for perimeter heat pipes in rooms, or to supply overhead unit heaters (it could also supply an in-floor radiant heat system). The boiler or burner may be fueled by gas, oil, wood, or coal. Locate the burner external to the stable to eliminate the need for venting combustion products.

With space heating systems, one of the primary problems is hot air stratified near the ceiling or ridge. Heated air will rise, leaving cooler air near the floor of the stable in the human- and animal-occupied areas unless the heated air is brought back down via ventilation system design or use of ceiling fans. Overhead "ceiling fans" may be used to keep warm air vertically mixed and moving back down to the horse-occupied area. Small circulation fans (8- to 12-inch diameter) may be used to move air horizontally high in the stable to break up stratified air zones. Ceiling or circulation fans should not direct air on the horse during the heating season because the large mass of moving air will provide a convective cooling effect. Some ceiling fan motors can reverse to move air up, thereby bouncing air off the ceiling and back down to the lower stable area without causing high air speeds right below the fan. Ceiling fans can be positioned above the center aisle to minimize moving air over the horse stalls.

Heat Distribution

Without a heat distribution mechanism, the warmest air will remain near the heater discharge area. The unit heaters come with a discharge fan that can throw heated air 10 feet or more, but this is not usually sufficient to thoroughly distribute air within the horse stable. For more even distribution a duct with discharge holes along its length is attached at or near the heater discharge (Fig. 12.6). The duct may be made of flexible plastic, often called a "poly tube" because clear polyethylene is the commonly used material. Alternatively, a solid design using plywood, rigid plastic large-diameter pipe, or sheet metal materials may be used. Either flexible or solid design can work effectively.

The air distribution duct is designed to incorporate several design features. The duct will be long enough to distribute heated air to where it is needed but is usually no longer than 50 to 100 feet to maintain reasonable resistance to air movement. A large heated

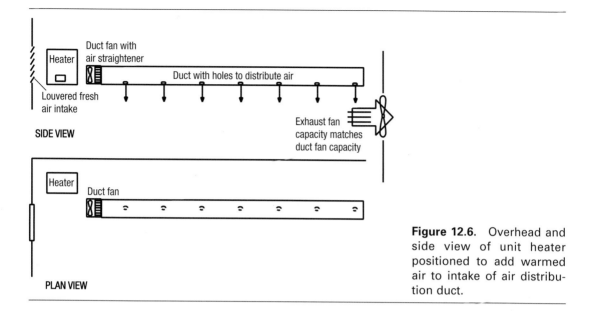

Figure 12.6. Overhead and side view of unit heater positioned to add warmed air to intake of air distribution duct.

space may be divided into zones for heat addition as needed. The maximum air speed in the duct is usually limited to 600 feet per minute (fpm). The cross-sectional area is then determined based on the volume of air that will be distributed: Area (ft^2) = Volume flow rate (ft^3/min) /Air speed (ft/min). Start calculations by providing at least the 25-cfm/horse minimum ventilation through the duct. This fresh air can be heated and delivered throughout the stable as heated fresh air. Additional air capacity may be provided in the duct by adding air already in the stable (recirculated air) or using the duct for both minimum ventilation and higher ventilation levels. Allowing some stable air to be recirculated with the fresh, cold incoming air can temper the duct air temperature to reduce condensation of humid stable air on the cold duct surface. The number and size of the holes are such that the total area of holes is approximately equal to the cross-sectional area of the duct (Fig. 12.7). Table 12.1 lists duct airflow capacity for various duct sizes and options for number and size of discharge holes.

An advantage of the flexible poly tube duct construction is inexpensive initial cost and cheap replacement. However, it is prone to tearing if horses can reach it (less than 12-foot height). A wire is run inside the poly tube for hanging support to keep it in position. The poly tube will deflate between heat additions, unless it is used continuously to recirculate unheated stable air in between

heating cycles. When the poly-tube inflates, it will make a startling noise that ripples along its length as the poly snaps from a loose hanging position into an inflation state as heated air is added. This is a noise that some horses and humans may find unnerving but will likely get used to. Dust and dirt accumulation can be easily seen in the clear poly tube and a decision made to replace it.

Solid ducts for heated air distribution are preferred when heat is added intermittently to the space. Sheet metal and other ducts of light construction will not withstand horse kicking and

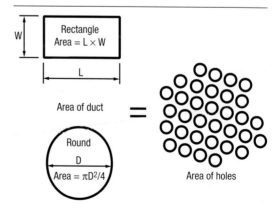

Figure 12.7. Duct cross-sectional area should approximately match the total of all hole areas.

Table 12.1. Duct Sizes and Number of Holes to Provide Selected Ventilation Rate

		Duct Size			Number of Holes of Diameter:					
Ventilation Rate	Duct Area	"Square" Rectangle	Flat Rectangle	Round						
(cfm)	(in.²)	(in.)	(in.)	(in. diam.)	1 in.	1¼ in.	1½ in.	2 in.	2½ in.	3 in.
100	24	4 × 6	3 × 8	6	31	20	14	8	5	
150	36	6 × 6	3 × 12	8		29	20	11	7	5
200	48	7 × 7	3 × 16	8		39	27	15	10	7
250	60	8 × 8	5 × 12	10			34	19	12	8
300	72	8 × 9	6 × 12	10			41	23	15	10
350	84	9 × 10	7 × 12	12				27	17	12
400	96	10 × 10	6 × 16	12				31	20	14
500	120	10 × 12	8 × 16	12					24	17
600	144	12 × 12	8 × 18	14					29	20
700	168	12 × 14	8 × 20	16						24
1000	240	16 × 16	10 × 24	18						34

Note: Duct airspeed approximately 600 fpm.

rubbing abuse. Metal ducts may rust or corrode over time because of the humidity, dust, and physical damage they are exposed to within the stable. Keep less rugged solid duct materials at least 8 feet high to be up out of the horse contact zone. Schedule 40 PVC pipe is a good material for ducts, because it is durable against most horse abuse, is commonly available, and will withstand humidity and dust found in stables. Do not use residential-style fiberglass duct board because it will accumulate dust and absorb moisture. A heated show horse stable is shown in Figure 12.8 that uses a heater (positioned outside the picture in another room of the stable) and PVC pipe to distribute warmed air. Although dust and dirt cannot be seen in a solid duct design, access should be provided for periodic inspection and cleaning of the duct interior.

The position of the holes in the duct can stir debate. Most ducts in horse stables will be positioned high to be up out of the horse contact zone, but fresh and/or heated air is needed in the horse-occupied area. The air discharged from the holes has a high velocity; but with the small air mass involved, the velocity is dissipated within about 5 to 8 feet of the duct. Holes are typically positioned to deliver air straight down, horizontally at the 3- and 9-o'clock position (on a round duct) or at a

slight downward angle at the 4- and 8-o'clock position. Figure 12.9 shows various air distribution duct and hole locations. Consider the primary use of the duct in delivering heated air, fresh cold air, or either of these combined with recirculated stable air. Fortunately, there is no major error in using any of the hole positions, but some guidelines may help in the design. Heated air benefits from being delivered down as low as possible, because hot air has a tendency to rise and will simply accumulate near the ceiling if discharged up high. For this reason, design ducts carrying heated air to discharge air straight down, whether over an aisle or stall area; this small amount of warm air will not cause draftiness as would cold air. For fresh and cold outside air delivery, discharge the air horizontally to mix it with warm air that has accumulated high in the structure. This mixing will not only temper the incoming cold air but also help bring the warmest stratified air back down into the horse-occupied areas.

Example Calculation: Air Distribution Duct

Calculations are presented for delivering air to an area of stable with eight horse stalls. The minimum recommended fresh air ventilation rate of 25 cfm/horse is provided with a second calculation for twice this amount of air exchange. The minimum

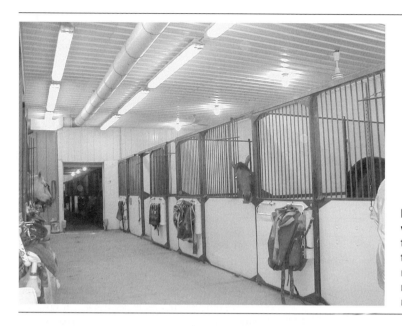

Figure 12.8. Heated stable with overhead rigid duct that delivers warmed air throughout the stable interior. The heater is located nearby in a separate utility room.

fresh air exchange needed is 25 cfm/horse × 8 horses = 200 cfm. Heat may be added to this air and distributed as fresh, heated air. The larger 400-cfm air exchange may be used with a combination of half fresh and half recirculated air during coldest weather and yet can provide all fresh air during warmer conditions. When delivering heated air via the duct, use holes on the bottom of the duct to direct heat down toward the animal-occupied area. If cold fresh air is delivered via the duct, place holes to deliver air horizontally. Table 12.1 is used to select duct size and number and size of holes.

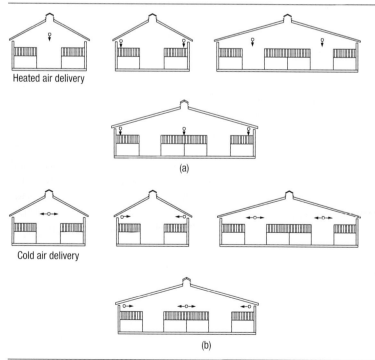

Figure 12.9. Duct location and hole position for heated and fresh air delivery. (a) Heated air delivered downward to get warm air into horse-occupied area. (b) Duct with cold air delivered horizontally to mix with stable air before dropping into horse zone.

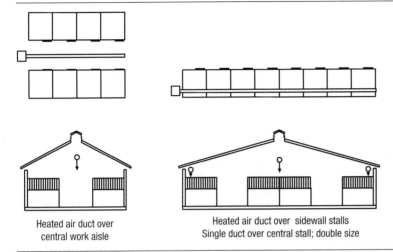

Figure 12.10. Position of heated air ducts for "Air Distribution Duct" example calculations.

Heated air duct over central work aisle

Heated air duct over sidewall stalls
Single duct over central stall; double size

Figure 12.10 shows example duct placement in a stable.

Case 1. Four horses on each side of a central aisle: Duct length will be 48 feet and located overhead the central aisle with holes directing fresh air straight down (heated air) or horizontally alternating on each side of the duct. Using Table 12.1, the distribution duct for 200 cfm can be an 8-inch diameter tube (Schedule 40 PVC will work) and will need fifteen 2-inch diameter holes. Provide sixteen holes 3 feet apart. To provide double the minimum air flow rate to each horse (400 cfm total), use a larger 12-inch diameter PVC tube with either thirty 2-inch diameter holes (spaced evenly every 1½ feet) or twenty larger 2½-inch diameter holes (holes spaced every 2½ feet).

Case 2. Eight horses in one row of stalls: Duct length will be 96 feet and located along the back wall of the line of stalls, with holes positioned to either direct air straight down (heated air) or horizontally on one side of the tube (other side is against sidewall). Provide the minimum cold-weather ventilation rate of 200 cfm with an 8-inch diameter tube with twenty-seven 1½-inch diameter holes or fifteen 2-inch diameter holes. Choose the larger holes and locate sixteen holes 6 feet apart so that each stall has two holes for fresh air delivery. To provide the higher airflow of 400 cfm, a 12-inch diameter tube with twenty 2½-inch holes may be used.

RADIANT HEAT

Radiant heat is used to warm objects that are within sight of the heat source. Radiant heat travels by "line of sight," so that an overhead radiant heater will warm objects directly under it but will not significantly heat the surrounding air (at least when used on a short-term basis). The effect is the same as that of radiant energy from the sun where one feels warm out in direct sunlight, but the radiant heat effect is lost by moving into the shade and out of direct radiant line of sight.

Radiant heat provides energy savings over conventional space heating applications via two physical principles. One is that radiant heat is applied directly to occupants of a space, thereby reducing the overall air temperature that needs to be maintained in the space for the same occupant comfort level. Recall the example of being out in the direct sun versus in the shade. Even though these two places are at the same air temperature, one feels much warmer out in the direct radiant energy. The second energy saving results from the application of radiant heat at the floor and occupied area rather than up high in the building where most stable space heat systems discharge heated air. In-floor radiant heat heats the floor directly. Radiant heaters mounted overhead will heat the floor area that the heater "sees." As air near the heated floor is warmed, it slowly rises. Radiant heaters do not use fans or duct distribution systems and the associated noise and dust movement, but they need to be positioned to radiate heat everywhere that heat is desired.

Overhead High-Temperature Radiant Heaters

Overhead radiant heater applications in horse housing can effectively provide comfort in relatively small but important areas of the stable. They

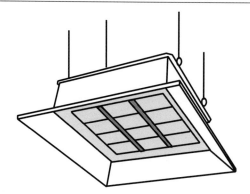

Figure 12.11. Example of overhead high-temperature radiant heater for warming portions of a stable via energy exchange with objects within the heater's "line of sight."

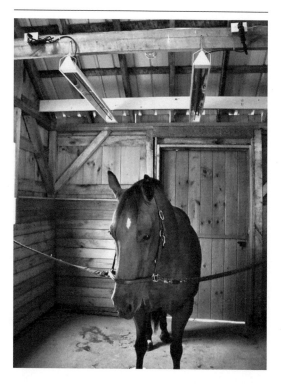

Figure 12.12. Overhead electric radiant heaters used in horse grooming area. Courtesy of Kalglo Electronics.

are powered by electricity or, at less energy cost, natural or propane gas. Radiant heaters have a highly reflective shield around the hot radiant element to direct heat where it is needed and to protect nearby structural elements on the backside of the radiant heater from heat damage or combustion (Fig. 12.11). For additional warmth, a radiant heater is often provided above a wash stall area or over the tacking and grooming area (Fig. 12.12). Radiant heaters work well for warming spectators within indoor arena. They are energy efficient because they directly heat the occupants of the space and are particularly effective for providing warmth immediately. Applications in horse stables typically use overhead radiant heat for the limited time when there is activity at the site. Space heating (forced-air) systems (described in the previous section) are more common when a site needs continuous heat.

Radiant heaters warm any objects they can "see," so that fire safety becomes a concern. Keep flammable materials, such as hay and bedding, far away from high-temperature radiant heat sources. Manufacturer installation instructions provide minimum distances to material of construction (ceiling) above the heater's radiation shield and even greater distance above flammable surfaces where the heat energy is directed. High-temperature radiant heaters can be safely installed well above bedded stalls and flammable indoor arena riding surface materials.

Three Types of High-Temperature Radiant Heaters

Radiant heat equipment suitable for horse housing comes in three designs. The most simple is the individual heat lamp bulb often seen for temporarily providing warmth to a newborn foal. The heat lamp bulb is easily portable but offers a potential fire hazard because it is often hung at a low height. It can be safe if used cautiously when equipped with a metal guard that protects the hot bulb from contacting anything and it is hung such that it cannot reach the ground (and flammable bedding) while plugged in (Fig. 12.13). Hang with a light chain from a hook so the heat lamp is suspended no closer than 3 feet from the stall floor. Mount so that the power cord is at least 1 foot shorter than the floor-to-hook distance, so that if the chain is somehow knocked off the hook, the lamp will unplug before it hits the floor or bedding. Use an "S" hook that is clamped shut for added protection against the lamp being knocked down. Heat lamp fixtures are relatively

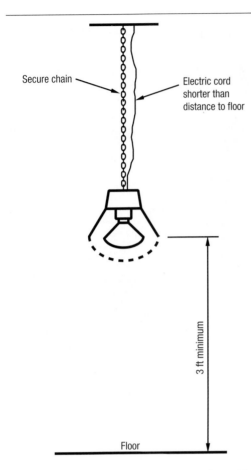

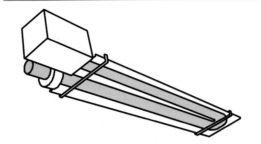

Figure 12.14. Radiant heat may be supplied over a large area by a long radiant tube.

Figure 12.13. To reduce chance of igniting flammable materials, heat lamp bulb should be hung so that it automatically disconnects if knocked off its chain support.

cheap but suffer from being expensive and relatively unsafe to operate, and so they are not used for more general horse stable radiant heat needs.

A second type of radiant heater is an electricity-powered unit that will provide heat to a relatively small area (Figs. 12.11 and 12.12). A wash stall may need more than one unit. Installation is as simple as plugging into a grounded, overload-protected electrical circuit capable of handling the amperage demand of the heater(s). If a person can be in contact with water and the electric power outlet at the same time, a ground fault interruption (GFI) receptacle will be needed. It is recommended to have the heaters on a separate circuit with a switch at the site to be heated. Electric radiant heaters are typically costlier to operate per heat output than gas-powered

units but can be mounted at lower ceiling heights and where venting of combustion products is impractical. Generally, keep electric radiant heaters 3 to 4 feet above room occupants (horse's back), or 8 to 9 feet above the floor. Large gas-fired radiant heaters usually need more clearance. It is important to follow your manufacturer's installation specifications. These values only serve as guidelines for planning purposes.

The third type of overhead radiant heater is a gas-fueled unit. These units range from relatively compact units for heating a small site to long radiant tubes that will effectively warm the entire working aisle of a stable or seating bleachers of an indoor riding arena (Fig. 12.14). The long radiant tube heaters may be seen near the spectator seats in large public horse show venues (Fig. 12.15). Gas-fired units usually cost lower to operate than electrically powered radiant heaters and so are attractive for heating large areas or for long periods of time.

The smaller rectangular gas-fired radiant heaters can be used with unvented combustion products in areas with adequate air exchange. This would be an acceptable application in a stable that follows at least the minimum ventilation guidelines as outlined in Chapter 6. The long-tube radiant heaters are typically 20 to 60 feet long and have an integral air intake and combustion vent. Gas-fired radiant heaters need relatively high mounting heights of at least 12 feet above the floor for high-intensity rectangular units that concentrate heat in a relatively small area. Lower intensity long tubes can be mounted 6 to 14 feet above animal level, with lower capacity units at a lower height.

When a radiant heater is used continuously, it will warm the surfaces that are within its line of sight. A

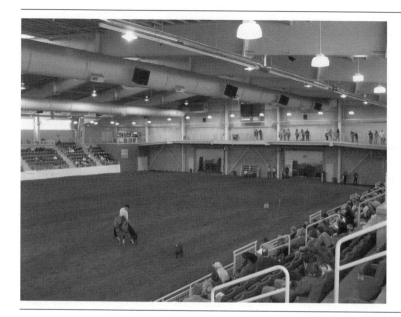

Figure 12.15. Long radiant tubes are positioned (near the overhead lights) to deliver heat to spectator area in addition to space heat supplied by the furnace ducts.

concrete floor is particularly effective in absorbing the radiant heat into its mass and then re-radiating the heat. This provides a warmed surface for heat conduction to those standing on the floor and heat convection to nearby air. Any surface in line of sight of the radiant heater output will behave similarly. Radiant heaters are sized at about 15% less Btu capacity than that for a forced air furnace system with a similar reduction in energy use (this figure is for residential heating; no data for horse facilities were readily available).

Controls

Electric radiant heaters come with controls mounted on the unit and are out of reach in their overhead position in horse stables. For convenience, install a model that has the controls available in a wall-mounted receptacle. A switch on a timer will minimize energy waste because it turns off automatically. Mount the radiant heater switch relatively high to avoid confusion with light switches and to keep it out of reach of children.

Control can be on-off with a simple switch or timer. Electric models offer proportional control with a range of settings from maximum 100% heat to about 20% heat output. Either on-off or proportional control is suitable for intermittent use of a radiant heater, such as in a wash stall or tacking area. A thermostat-controlled radiant heating system is

desirable when the heater will be operated continuously. The thermostat will automatically regulate heater output to achieve the desired set point temperature. Radiant heat set point can be a lower temperature than conventional space heating system set point because the objects within sight of the radiant heater are directly warmed and do not depend solely on surrounding air temperature for warmth. Locate the thermostat so it is out of direct radiation from the radiant heater, or it will record an artificially high reading because of the radiant heat load on the thermostat sensor.

Controls for small rectangular gas-fired units can be via an on-off switch with direct spark ignition or via a thermostat in areas that are to be continuously heated. Long-tube heaters are typically controlled via thermostat, but in locations that are intermittently heated with long-tube heaters (indoor competitive riding arenas used on weekends) a timer or on-off switch can be used. When the high-temperature radiant is the primary source of building heat, then a more efficient design is needed. Because radiant tubes take a few minutes to heat to full capacity, it is most efficient to use them constantly, which assumes full power; so size accordingly. Some long-tube radiant heaters have two-stage operation so that less fuel is used most of the time on the lower power setting, with peak heating demand provided by the larger second heating stage.

IN-FLOOR RADIANT HEATING

Heating the floor in portions of a stable can provide a uniform heat that is considered quite comfortable. It offers advantage in supplying heat low in the structure so that as air is warmed near the floor it rises up and through the structure. This offers advantage in providing heat where it is needed, at human and animal level, rather than being supplied high in the structure as is done with unit heaters and overhead ducts. In-floor heat provides a uniform heat in the area where it is installed without the air movement and associated sounds of unit heater or ducted forced-air heating systems. In-floor heat is considered "radiant heat" because it uses a large heated mass, the floor, in order to store and release the heat (Fig. 12.16)

The warmed floor mass delivers its heat to people and animals standing on it via all three forms of heat transfer. People standing on the warmed floor feel warmth from heat conducted to their feet and also from the radiant heat effect from the surrounding warm floor surface. Additionally, there is convective heat transfer as the warmed air near the floor rises up through the building space. In a cold climate, floor heat will generally not supply enough heat on the coldest days to completely warm an interior, but it will reduce the chill. In the stable's stall area that has many more air changes per hour than human-occupied areas, floor heat will need to be supple-mented with additional types of heat sources in cold climates if the stable temperature is to be maintained well above outside temperatures. An additional advantage is that floor heat will keep floors drier than a similar-sized forced-air heat system.

In-floor radiant heat is used in the human-occupied and working areas of the stable rather than under the horse stalls. A common application is in the work aisle of a central-aisle stable. It can also be used in the wash stall, grooming stations, tack room, feed room, and lounge or office. In-floor heat under a bedded stall loses its primary heating effectiveness because of fresh bedding's insulating value and radiant energy blockage. The warm floor will aid in drying bedding and deposited manure and urine, but at risk of increased ammonia volatilization from the higher floor temperature and potential for dried, crusted manure on the floor. An in-floor heating system has a significant thermal lag time in both accumulating heat for delivery to the heated space and in holding the heat when the system is turned off. It is useful for supplying a continuous amount of heat to an environment.

Hydronic and Electric In-Floor Systems

The two primary types of in-floor heating systems are hydronic and electric. In hydronic systems, heated water is circulated through a manifold of durable plastic tubing embedded in or under the floor.

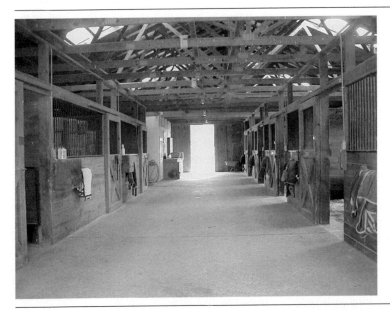

Figure 12.16. In-floor radiant heat may be used in the aisle of the stable to provide warmth for human work activities. Pipes circulating hot water are buried within the concrete floor.

Electric radiant systems have embedded electric cable installed in or below the floor for similar effect.

Electric cable in-floor heating systems, although simpler and usually less expensive in installation than hydronic, suffer from a substantial increase in operating energy cost. Electric systems are typically used on a smaller scale, such as in a single room. Consider electric cable floor heat when the tack room is the only heated space in a smaller stable facility. The most common type of heating cable is covered with polyvinylchloride (PVC), is approved for use embedded in concrete, and delivers from 2 to 7 watts per linear foot. A cable prefabricated in a plastic mesh is available for simplified installation. Cover the cable completely with 1½ to 2 inches of concrete to prevent hot spots.

For the horse stable environment a typical hydronic system circulates 100°F water via pump at velocities of 2 to 3 feet per second (fps) through ¾-inch diameter plastic pipe embedded in the floor. Plastic pipe is flexible, is high-temperature (160°F) rated, and may be made of polyethylene, PVC, or polybutylene. The pipes are laid in a series of loops with one end connected to a supply header and the other end of the loop connected to a return header. The loops may be up to 400 feet long and, when spaced with pipes 1 foot on-center throughout the floor area, will provide approximately 15 Btu/hr per square foot of floor area with 100°F water. For human-occupied areas of the stable facility, the design may be similar to residential criteria with the floor temperature kept at no more than 85°F, which is the average skin temperature for most people.

The floor material for floor heating systems in horse stabling should be a solid construction material that will be durable in an aisle application and suitable in human-use areas and the tack room. Solid or porous (concrete without sand) is recommended in a thickness of 4 inches. (Concrete thickness of at least 5 inches will be needed for strength in an aisle that supports vehicle traffic.)

Hot water for the floor heating system is typically provided by a dedicated hot water heater or boiler in a closed-loop system. The floor heat may be set up in zones. If the system will not be used during the entire cold weather season, an antifreeze treatment is added to the hot water circulation system to lower the freezing point temperature of the installation. Intermittent use is not effective because of the lag time in heating the floor mass for providing radiant heat. The hot water circulation pump may be controlled manually, or for more energy efficiency, via thermostat in the area to be heated. The hot water heat source may be from any type of fuel such as natural gas, propane, wood, or coal. Some boilers can be placed outside to eliminate exhaust vent and fresh air intake construction.

Time and Energy

Understand that the time lag for floor heating is longer than for more conventional heating systems because of the thermal mass of floor that needs to be heated in order to provide detectable warmth. Likewise, when floor heat is turned off, it has a considerable time where it continues to provide heat to the surroundings. Floor heating systems are best used in applications where the heat is needed over long periods rather than an application where heat is needed quickly or for short periods of time. It also works well as a source of minimum heat for an area over long periods of time, so that additional heat (space or radiant) can be added on demand when needed for activities in the area. Floor heating works well in the tack room and human-occupied areas such as an office or a lounge. The aisle of the stable may incorporate floor heating for moderate comfort or designed to provide freeze protection during cold weather.

There is an energy-savings advantage of floor-heated systems over conventional forced-air systems because of radiant heat's ability to put the heat where it is needed at human- and animal-occupied level. Additionally, thermostats may be set 3 to 8°F lower with radiant heat contributing to about a 40% to 60% energy savings than in conventionally heated homes and commercial buildings (data for stables not available). This type of energy savings is likely in the human-occupied areas such as tack room and office. Livestock buildings that use radiant heat (high-temperature overhead units) as the primary heat source realize a 20 to 25% reduction in fuel use versus space heat provided by unit heaters. The larger ventilation rates used in livestock housing and horse stables means that more incoming fresh air needs to be heated as stale air is exhausted, which limits energy savings but assures good air quality in the barn. Radiant heat offers advantage in lower temperature air being exhausted from the building.

Whether insulation is needed under the in-floor heating system will depend on the application design features. Only waterproof insulation, such as rigid polystyrene board, is appropriate. The heating elements should not be laid directly on plastic insulation. No insulation is needed under the heated floor if dry ground can be maintained under the entire structure. This means that groundwater is more than 6 feet below the floor and surface drainage is away from the structure. Perimeter insulation will be needed along the foundation to a depth of 4 feet to reduce heat loss from the heated floor to surrounding ground area. Wet ground is a good conductor of heat whereas dry ground is not. If groundwater is within 6 feet of the floor, install R-10 insulation (2-inch extruded polystyrene) and a vapor retarder below the floor. Foil-faced insulation is not effective under floor as a radiant heat retarder when there is no air space in the assembly. Foil is an effective (but expensive) vapor retarder. Another reason to install insulation under the heated floor is to reduce the volume of material that is heated by the in-floor heating system. Less energy will be needed to maintain heat of a reduced volume and the smaller mass will respond faster to controller changes than a heating system that employs a larger ground mass under the floor. Underfloor insulation will be needed when only a room or two of the stable is heated such as with a heated tack room within unheated stable. Perimeter insulation will be needed to maintain temperature of the heated slab when adjacent to an unheated area.

Proper Design and Installation

A final recommendation is to find a system supplier with experience and/or formal training in radiant design and installation. To generate all the advantages of an in-floor radiant heating system, it must be designed and installed properly. This advice applies for any heating system but is particularly important for in-floor systems because they are less common installations that operate under different principles than traditional forced-air space heating systems.

INSULATION OF WARM STABLES

Insulation is used to reduce heat movement from the warm stable interior to colder outside conditions. Insulation also maintains interior building surfaces near interior temperatures, which will decrease the potential for condensation to form and reduces the radiant heat loss of building occupants to the sur-

rounding cold walls. Although any material has some insulating value, the materials that are commonly referred to as "insulation" have more resistance to heat flow as indicated by their higher R-value. R-value is resistance to heat transfer and has the unit ft^2 °F hr/Btu. Conductivity is the inverse of resistance and indicates how quickly a Btu of heat is conducted through a square foot of material in an hour for each °F temperature difference between the warm and cold side of the material. Heat is transferred from the warm side of a wall (including ceiling or roof assemblies) to the colder side. Three categories of heat transfer are considered: conduction through solids, convection via moving air, and radiation of energy. Most insulation materials are used in wall assemblies to significantly reduce conduction and convection heat transfer. Radiant heat transfer is addressed through the use of shiny foil materials adjacent to an air space in a wall assembly. Table 12.2 lists common building and insulating materials used in horse stable construction.

Materials

Different insulating materials are often used on different parts of the building. A lower R-value insulation is usually used in the walls than in the ceiling. There is greater heat loss through the ceiling (or roof) because of the warmer room air that accumulates there. Provide a minimum insulation in warm stables of R-11 in the walls and R-19 in the roof and the ceiling. Additional insulation often may be easily installed. Perimeter insulation reduces heat loss through the foundation and helps maintain warmer, drier floors. Use 2-inch-thick waterproof closed-pore rigid board insulation a minimum of 2 feet below grade on the exterior of the foundation wall.

Because of the relatively high moisture levels in stables (compared with residential levels), use only insulation materials that do not accumulate moisture. This eliminates the use of loose fill and unprotected fiberglass batts. The insulation property of a loose or batt material is a direct function of the amount of air trapped within the base material. For example, fiberglass batts reduce heat transfer via the air spaces trapped within the fiberglass matrix. The fiberglass itself is a good conductor of heat; the trapped air is a poor conductor. Water is a good conductor of heat compared with air. Fiberglass batts that have been compressed or have a lot of moisture (water) in them no longer have the dry air spaces

Table 12.2 Insulation Values of Common Building Materials and Permeability to Moisture Movement[a]

Description	Conductivity[b] per in. thickness (k) (Btu-in./hr ft²°F)	Conductance[b] for thickness listed (C) (Btu/hr ft²°F)	Resistance[c] per in. thickness (R) (hr ft²°F/Btu-in.)	Resistance[c] for thickness listed (R) (hr ft²°F/Btu)	Permeance[d] (Perm)
Insulation Materials					
Blanket and Batt (fiberglass, mineral wool, glass)	0.29		3.45		30
3–4 in.		0.091		11	
5–6 in.		0.053		19	
6–7 in.		0.045		22	
9–10 in.		0.033		30	
12–13 in.		0.026		38	
Polystyrene					
Extruded					
Cut cell surface	0.25		4.00		0.40–1.60
Smooth skin surface	0.20		5.00		(1 in. thick)
Expanded or molded beads					2.0–5.8
(1 lb/ft³)	0.26		3.85		(1 in. thick)
(1.5 lb/ft³)	0.24		4.17		
(2 lb/ft³)	0.23		4.35		
Polyurethane foam	0.17		5.88		
Polyethylene foam	0.43		2.33		
Building Materials					
Fiberglass Reinforced Panel (FRP)	0.87		1.08–3.26		0.05–0.12
Polyester FRP	0.31–0.48				
Plywood	0.80		1.25		
¼ in. (exterior glue)		3.20		0.31	0.7
³⁄₈ in.		2.13		0.47	
½ in.		1.60		0.62	
⅝ in.		1.29		0.77	
Plywood or wood panel (¾ in.)		1.07		0.93	0.3–4.0
Wood boards					
– Oak			0.8–0.9		
– Softwood			0.9–1.4		

(Continues)

175

Table 12.2 Insulation Values of Common Building Materials and Permeability to Moisture Movement[a] (continued)

Description	Conductivity[b] per in. thickness (k) (Btu-in./hr/ft²/°F)	Conductance[b] for thickness listed (C) (Btu/hr/ft²/°F)	Resistance[c] per in. thickness (R) (hr/ft²/°F/Btu-in.)	Resistance[c] for thickness listed (R) (hr/ft²/°F/Btu)	Permeance[d] (Perm)
Oriented strand board (OSB) (³⁄₈ in.)				0.5	0.75
Hardboard (medium density)	0.73		1.37		11
Particleboard (medium density)	0.94		1.06		
Brick (4 in.)	5.0		0.1–0.4		0.8
Glazed tile masonry (4 in.)					0.10–0.16
Concrete-poured solid (6 in.)		0.75			0.8
Concrete block					
– Lightweight aggregate 2-core (8 in.)		0.46		2.18	2.4
– Cores insulated		0.20		5.03	
Asphalt shingles		2.27		0.44	
Wood shingles		1.06		0.94	
Siding					
Metal					
Hollow backed		1.61	0.0	0.61	0.0
³⁄₈ in. insulated backed		0.55		1.82	
Hardboard (0.4375 in.)	1.49		0.67		
Wood bevel (0.5 × 8 in. lapped)		1.23		0.81	
Wood plywood (³⁄₈ in. lapped)		1.59		0.59	
Gypsum wallboard (½ in.)		2.22		0.45	50
Plastic sheeting (6 mil)				Negligible	0.08
Aluminum foil (1 mil)			0.0		0.0
Tar paper (15 lb)					4.0
House wrap			Negligible		77
Glass	5.00	0.5	0.20		
Double-layer acrylic or polycarbonate extrusion				2.00	
Air	0.16		6.25		

Perimeter Floor (per foot of exterior wall length)

Concrete
- Uninsulated — 0.80 — 1.23
- 2 × 24 in. rigid insulation — 0.45 — 2.22

Air Spaces (¾–4 in.)

Horizontal		0.90
Vertical		1.25
Horizontal with reflective surface		2.20
Vertical with reflective surface		3.40

Surface Coefficients

Inside still air (vertical surface heat flow up)	1.46	0.68
Outside 15 mph wind	6.0	0.17
Outside 7.5 mph wind	4.0	0.25

Doors and Windows

(The following include surface conditions:
Still air inside; 15 mph wind outside)

Door
- Wood solid core 1¾ in. thick — 3.03
- Steel urethane foam core — 2.50

Window
- Single glazed — 1.1 — 0.91
- Double glazed ¼-in. air space — 1.69
- Translucent panel (fiberglass) — 1.2 — 0.83

---

[a]Materials vary widely in heat transfer characteristics and are very dependent upon installation design so use manufacturer data for final design. This table intended for rough estimates only.

[b]Conductance (or conductivity) is the inverse of resistance; a lower value indicates more resistance to heat transfer.

[c]A higher resistance (R) to heat transfer provides more insulation values.

[d]Permeance is a measure of how easily water vapor can move through a material. Lower values are better vapor retarders. Perm is the unit of moisture movement in grains of water per hour per square foot of material with a 1-inch mercury vapor pressure difference.

Source: ASHRAE Handbook of Fundamentals, MWPS handbooks, NRAES Greenhouse Engineering, "Houses That Work" and other builder tables, and manufacturer data.

that provide the insulating properties. To maintain insulation effectiveness, batt and loose fill materials must be protected by a strong vapor retarder (see "Insulation Protection" section).

Suitable waterproof insulation materials include rigid board insulation materials that have closed cell foam (Styrofoam, "blue board"). These materials offer insulation value and are virtually impermeable to water entry, but they are flammable materials. Foil-faced bubblepack insulation is also waterproof but commonly suffers from incorrect applications and deterioration of surface conditions that reduce its heat transfer effectiveness.

Bubblepack insulation with a reflective foil on one or both sides is commonly marketed for agricultural and horse stabling applications (Figs. 12.17 and 12.18). The foil will significantly reduce radiant heat transfer from the shiny metal surface to surrounding objects. Foil installed directly against other materials offers no radiant heat transfer reduction because there is no airspace through which radiant energy exchange occurs; in fact, the foil is an excellent conductor of heat and so offers no help in reducing conductive heat movement. On the interior of a roof, a foil surface will effectively block most radiant heat transfer from the stable interior to the roof or from a hot summer roof into the interior if installed correctly and maintained in a shiny condition. Shiny

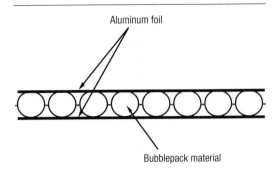

Aluminum foil

Bubblepack material

Figure 12.18. Cross-section of bubblepack insulation with air-filled polyethylene bubbles within a reflective insulation cover.

metal surfaces have a very low (less than 20%) radiant energy emissivity compared with other building surfaces. The radiant energy exchange is purely a surface phenomenon and will apply to any object with a shiny metal surface. The foil must face an airspace in order to provide any radiation heat reduction, and it must remain shiny to maintain its low radiant energy emissivity. Reflective foil facing the interior airspace of the stable will reduce radiant heat transfer as long as dust, dirt, corrosion, and condensation do not foul the surface. Maintaining clean conditions of the foil surface will be difficult in dusty stables, so the effectiveness of bubblepack insulation is reduced to the value supplied by the air trapped in the bubblepack assembly.

Insulation Protection

Vapor retarders (formerly called vapor barriers) must be used with most insulation materials to prevent moisture entry into the insulation. Vapor retarders have a rated permeance to water movement, expressed in perms, with lower values being more resistant to water entry and movement. Perm is an expression of moisture movement in grains of water per hour per square foot of material with a 1-inch mercury vapor pressure difference across the material ($gr/hr\ ft^2\ in.$-Hg). Choose materials with a perm rating less than 1. Polyethylene 6 mil plastic is a common vapor retarder when protected by a stronger material. Use fiberglass or polyester scrim reinforced polyethylene for greater durability when the vapor retarder is not protected by solid building materials. Vapor retarders are installed on the warm side of the wall assembly with attention to sealing all

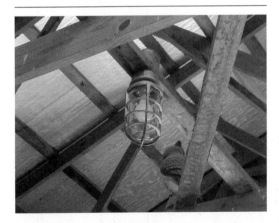

Figure 12.17. Roof insulation is useful even in unheated stables to decrease condensation by maintaining the interior surface temperature near interior air temperature. Insulation with reflective surface is shown, which can provide insulation value if kept shiny and facing an airspace.

gaps around building components and electrical and plumbing components. Rigid board insulation is impermeable to water entry, but gaps between panels need to be taped to reduce moisture migration around each panel. Use vapor retarder on sheet metal ceiling and wall assemblies because joints and fastener holes allow water movement even though the metal sheet itself is impermeable to water movement. Table 12.2 shows vapor retarder materials and permeance of some common building materials.

In areas where horses or riders can come in contact with insulation and/or vapor retarders, protect the insulation assembly with a stronger material such as stall lining boards, plywood, PVC boards, or fiberglass reinforced plastic (FRP) panels. Choose mechanically strong insulation materials (closed-cell boards) where activity may impact sidewalls or roof insulation, such as from balls in indoor polo arenas. Heated rooms in the support area, such as tack rooms and lounges, may be insulated to resi-

dential standards if vapor retarder protection is provided to the insulation materials.

Rodent and bird interest in insulation materials as nesting sites can be considerable. The best protection is an interior liner in addition to the exterior siding and roofing. Be sure to protect the ends of insulation panels and below-grade perimeter insulation. Suitable liner protection materials include FRP or 3/8-inch plywood (below-grade rated for perimeter application). Plywood is not necessarily rat-proof but will discourage most mice. An aluminum foil layer is not sufficient protection against bird and rodent damage.

Condensation

Condensation formation is reduced on insulated building surfaces by keeping the interior surface close to interior temperature. Air next to a cold surface will drop in temperature and lose some of its moisture-holding capacity (warmer air can hold more moisture than cold air; see Appendix). As the air cools, it will

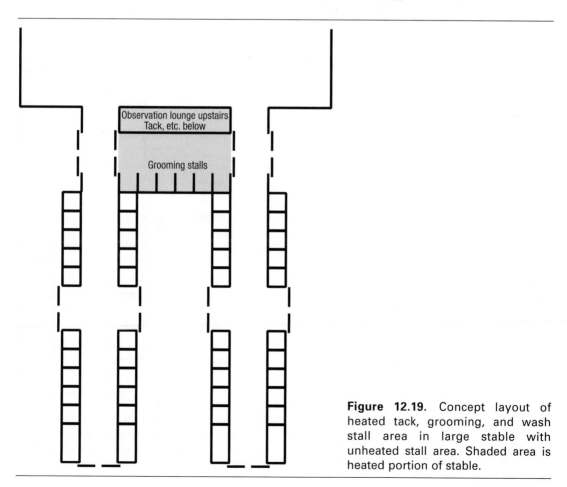

Figure 12.19. Concept layout of heated tack, grooming, and wash stall area in large stable with unheated stall area. Shaded area is heated portion of stable.

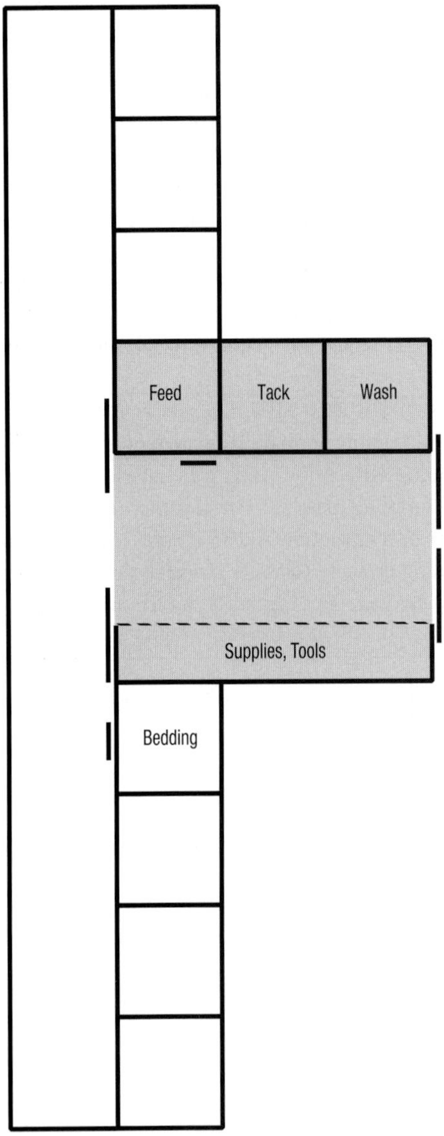

roof and ceiling insulation reduces winter moisture condensation, and the associated dripping water.

Moisture needs to be removed from the stable with winter ventilation; otherwise insulation will absorb condensed water. Moisture-laden insulation solves the dripping problem but results in increased heat transfer because of loss of resistance value of the insulation, degradation of the insulation material, mold formation, and eventually deterioration of the structural components of the building material next to the wet insulation. Do not use insulation materials as a sponge to hide condensation problems that should be alleviated with better ventilation.

SEPARATE HEATED AREA IN STABLE

Mentioned several times in this chapter is the idea of providing a heated working area segregated from the main horse stabling environment. The idea is to

Figure 12.20. Concept layout of separate heated stable work area with stall area unheated in shed-row stable design. Shaded area is heated area.

eventually reach saturation at the dew-point temperature and deposit water on to the cold surface. Frost is formed from condensation on a surface that is below freezing. Condensation prevention also depends on ventilation because fresh air exchange will replace moisture-laden stable air with drier outside air to decrease the potential for interior air to become saturated with water. For unheated stables, even light R-5

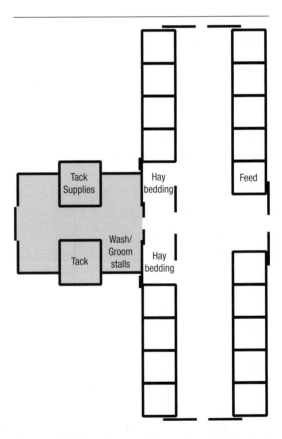

Figure 12.21. Concept layout of unheated stall area with heated grooming, wash, and tack support area in 18-stall stable. Shaded area is heated.

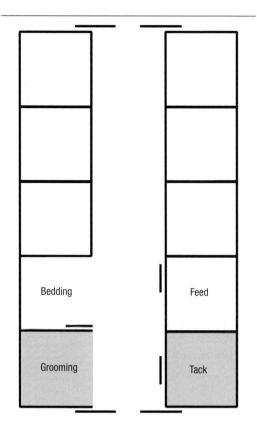

Figure 12.22. Concept layout of small private stable with heated grooming area and tack room with unheated stall area.

accommodate human comfort with a heated working area while providing a comfortable fresh air environment for the stabled horses. This would save fuel by heating less space. The working space will need less ventilation air exchange (and associated heat loss) than the horse stall area. Figures 12.19–12.22 show ideas for large and small stables that incorporate an area that can be heated during cold weather while leaving the stable unheated or heated to a lower temperature. The work area concentrates the functional areas that need heat into one zone of the stable. Keep the tack, grooming, and wash stall sites in the heated portion of the stable. Office and lounge are heated areas but do not need horse access. The heated area is separated from the unheated stable simply by sliding doors to allow easy horse entry and exit. In most cases, feed, tools, equipment, and hay and bedding storage do not need to be in the heated portion of the stable.

CALCULATION OF HEAT NEEDED

A space heating system is sized on the basis of a heat balance on the stable. Calculations of how much supplemental heat will be needed include the heat added to the stable interior from the horse body heat, heat loss via conduction through the building surfaces, and heat loss via air exchange of the ventilation system. As a rough estimate, the recommended supplemental heat for a 40 and 50°F stable environment is shown in Table 12.3. Use these values as a quick estimate, but have someone perform a detailed heat balance to properly size a heating system for a specific stable. A well-insulated stable in a cold climate (R-20 walls and R-33 roof) will need about 5000 Btu/hr per horse to maintain the interior at 40°F when it is –20°F outside or about 6300 Btu/hr per horse to maintain 50°F at the same outside temperature. For a stable kept just above freezing at 40°F, the necessary supplemental heat almost triples for the uninsulated stable (R-5 in roof) compared with a moderately insulated stable (R-14 walls and R-22 roof). Ventilation is maintained during the cold-weather heating season in stables so that some heated air will be exhausted with the stale stable air.

Supplemental Heat Calculation

Size the heating system on the basis of a detailed heat balance of the stable that includes the heat added to the stable interior from the horse body heat; heat loss via conduction through the building walls, ceiling, roof, doors, and windows; and heat loss via air exchange of the ventilation system where warm air is exhausted and replaced by cooler outside fresh air. Part of air exchange heat loss is via infiltration through cracks and holes in the building exterior. The calculations that follow are for space heating system design.

The heat balance format is conceptually described by:

Supplemental Heat Needed =
  conduction heat exchange + ventilation heat exchange + horse body heat

The calculation is set up to automatically describe heat loss as a negative (−) value and heat gain as a positive (+) value. Ignored in this heat balance are solar radiation on the structure, thermal lag time due to heavy masonry construction, and latent heat exchange (moisture evaporation and condensation use and release heat, respectively). Solar gain

Table 12.3. Supplemental Heat per Horse Estimates for Maintaining 40°F or 50°F Interior Stable Temperature with Outdoor Temperature from −20 to 40°F

Interior Temperature (°F)	Outside Temperature (°F)	R Wall R Roof	Uninsulated			Cold-Climate Insulated[a]
			0 5	6 14	14 22	20 33
			Heat Needed (Btu/hr per horse)			
40	−20		15,000	6700	5500	5100
	0		9400	3900	3100	2800
	20		3800	1000	600	500
50	−20		17,800	8200	6800	6300
	0		12,200	5300	4300	4000
	20		6600	2500	1900	1700
	40		1000	400	0	0

Note: Assumptions and design

Center aisle stable design for 8 horses.

Stable size 12 × 12 stalls flanking 12-ft center aisle; 10-foot eave height; 4:12 gable roof slope.

Stable of wood-siding metal-roof frame construction on concrete block foundation.

Window (2 ft × 3 ft) each stall and aisle doors each endwall.

Ventilation rate at minimum 25 cfm/horse; equivalent to 1 ACH for stall volume.

Infiltration ½ ACH.

Insulation values include interior and exterior surface coefficients.

Horse body heat 1800 Btu/hr per horse.

Values rounded to nearest 100 Btuh/horse.

[a]Insulation levels range from uninsulated to fully insulated warm housing for cold climate.

could be added via a sol-air temperature estimate for the stable site. Clearly, solar gain would increase the interior temperature of the stable during daylight hours, but most heating challenge will be at night during the coolest daily temperature. Masonry construction moderates temperature swings inside the building, so the structure mass has a lag time for gain or loss of heat from climate or solar conditions. The calculations with conduction, ventilation, and horse body heat are sufficient to describe conditions within horse stables at a steady-state condition.

In equation form, the heat balance is described by:

$$Q = \Sigma AU(T_o - T_i) + 0.02M(T_o - T_i) - H$$

Definitions of variables:

Q = total heat balance, the amount of supplemental heat added to maintain a selected interior temperature (Btu/hr)

Σ = summation symbol

A = area of each building surface (ft^2)

U = conductivity of each building material (Btu/hr ft^2 °F)

T_i = indoor temperature (°F)

T_o = outdoor temperature (°F)

0.02 = coefficient with standard air conditions for ACH (Btu/ft^3 °F)

M = ventilation rate in (ACH) air changes per hour (ft^3/hr)

H = horse body heat (Btu/hr)

Detail of 0.02 coefficient:

0.02 coefficient
  = specific heat of air 0.24 Btu/lb °F divided by specific volume 13.3 ft^3/lb
  = 0.018 Btu/ft^3 °F

The horse body heat will always be a heat gain to the structure. A 1000-pound horse produces 1800 to 2500 Btu/hr at 70°F. Insulation values are

Table 12.4. Example Heat Balance Calculation of 8-horse Insulated Stable with R-22 Roof and R-14 Walls

Conditions

Temperature inside (T_i)	40.0°F
Temperature outside (T_o)	0.0°F
Number of horses stabled (H#)	8 horses

Ventilation Air Exchange

Infiltration air change rate (ACH_I)	0.5 air changes/hr
Planned ventilation rate (ACH_V)	1.0 air changes/hr

Note: 25 cfm/horse with 1440 ft^3 stall air space = 1.0 stall ACH

Physical Features

Building Dimensions

Length (L)	48 ft
Width (W)	36 ft
Sidewall height (H)	10 ft

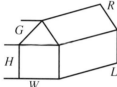

Volume (Vol)	17280 ft^3 = $L \times W \times H$
Eave to gable height (G)	6 ft
½ Roof line (R)	19 ft = sqrt ½ $(W^2 + G^2)$

Window and Door	No.	Height (ft)	Width (ft)	Area per (ft^2)
window (W)	8	2	3	6
door (D)	2	8	11	88

Building Surface Calculations

Window area (A_W)	48 ft^2
Door area (A_D)	176 ft^2
Gross sidewall area	960 ft^2 = 2 $(L \times H)$
Sidewall area (A_{SW})	912 ft^2
(A_{SW} = Gross sidewall area minus window area)	
Gross endwall area	720 ft^2 = 2$(W \times H)$
Endwall area (A_{EW})	544 ft^2
(A_{EW} = Gross endwall area minus door area)	
Gable area (A_G)	216 ft^2 = 2 $(W \times ½ G)$
Roof area (A_R)	1821 ft^2 = 2 $(R \times L)$
Perimeter length (L_P)	168 ft = 2L + 2W

Conductivity Building Materials

Insulation U is inverse of R; $U = 1/R$

Outside surface wind, 15 mph: R_o = 0.17 hr °F ft^2/Btu

Inside surface wind, 0 mph: R_i = 0.68 hr °F ft^2/Btu

R total = R_T

(Continues)

Table 12.4. Example Heat Balance Calculation of 8-horse Insulated Stable with R-22 Roof and R-14 Walls *(Continued)*

Item	Building Material	R	R_o	R_i	R_T	U
		hr °F ft² / Btu				Btu/ hr °F ft²
Roof (U_R)	Metal with R-22 insulation	22.00	0.17	0.68	22.85	0.04
Walls (U_{SW})	½-in. Wood panel with R-14 insulation	14.62	0.17	0.68	15.47	0.06
Window (U_W)	Glass (surface coefficients included)	0.91	Included		0.91	1.10
Door (U_D)	½-in. Wood panel	0.62	0.17	0.68	1.47	0.68
Perimeter (U_P)	Concrete block 3-hole 8-in.	1.11	0.17	0.68	1.96	0.51

Heat Balance Calculations

Temp. diff. (*dT*) $(T_o - T_i) = -40.0°F$

Conductive Heat Exchange Q (Btu/hr) $= AU_T \, dT$
                                       AU value

Roof	80	Btu/hr°F $= A_R \times U_R$
Sides and ends	108	Btu/hr°F $= (A_{SW} + A_{EW} + A_G) \, U_{SW}$
Windows	53	Btu/hr°F $= A_W \times U_W$
Doors	120	Btu/hr°F $= A_D \times U_D$
Perimeter	86	Btu/hr°F $= L_P \times U_P$
Total AU (AU_T)	446	Btu/hr°F $=$ sum (AU)
Total conductive	−17,839	Btu/h $= AU_T \, dT$

Air Exchange Heat Change Q (Btu/hr) $= 0.02 \, M \, dT = 0.02 \times$ Vol $\times$ ACH dT
                              0.02*M* value

Infiltration	173	Btu/hr °F $= 0.02 \times$ Vol $\times$ ACH$_I$
Ventilation	360	Btu/hr °F $= 0.02 \times$ Vol $\times$ ACH$_V$
0.02*M* total (0.02M_T)	533	Btu/hr °F $=$ sum (0.02*M*)
Total Air Exchange	−21,312	Btu/hr $= 0.02 M_T \, dT$

Horse Body Heat Addition

Horse body heat (Btu/hr)   1800–2500 Btu/hr 1000-lb horse at 70°F
Horse heat production (loss) low during cold conditions; use HBH $= 1800$ Btu/hr per horse

Horse heat (HBH$_T$)   14,400 Btu/hr $=$ HBH $\times$ H#

Complete Heat Balance

Complete heat balance $=$ Total conductive $+$ Total air exchange $+$ Total horse heat
$Q_T = AU \, dT + 0.02M \, dT + HBH_T$
$Q_T = -17{,}839 - 21{,}312 + 14{,}400$
Net total heat loss (−) or gain (+) per hour
$Q_T = -24751$ Btu/hr heat loss (−)
Supplemental heat needed at the rate of 3094 Btu/hr per horse

Table 12.4. Example Heat Balance Calculation of 8-horse Insulated Stable with R-22 Roof and R-14 Walls *(Continued)*

Symbol Key				Subscript Key	
	Description	*Unit*		D	door
A	area	ft²		EW	endwall
ACH	air changes per hour	#/hr		G	gable wall
dT	temperature difference	°F		I	infiltration
G	eave to gable height	ft		i	inside
H	height	ft		o	outside
H#	number of horses	#		P	perimeter
HBH	horse body heat production	Btu/hr per horse		R	roof
L	length	ft		SW	sidewall
M	air exchange	ft³/hr		T	total
R	resistance to heat transfer	hr °F ft²/Btu		V	ventilation
Q	heat exchange rate	Btu/hr		W	window
T	temperature	°F			
U	conductivity heat transfer	Btu/hr °F ft²			
V	ventilation	ACH			
Vol	volume	ft³			
W	width	ft			

typically expressed in terms of the resistance to heat transfer R-value, which is the inverse of conductivity ($R = 1/U$).

Table 12.4 shows results of a heat balance on an example stable. A spreadsheet program was used to develop and calculate the heat balance (although it may be done by hand). The program calculates the total supplemental heat or cooling load, total conduction heat loss or gain, total ventilation heat exchange, and total horse body heat contribution on the basis of all the input variables described earlier. The calculation showed that just less than 25,000 Btu/hr of supplemental heat would be needed to keep the stable at 40°F when outside conditions are 0°F. If an in-floor radiant heating system was installed in the 12-foot-wide central aisle, and estimating 15 Btu/hr per square foot of heated floor, then about a third of the heat needed (8600 Btu/hr) would be supplied by the floor.

SUMMARY

Horse stables may be heated for human comfort and to maintain show horses with short hair coat in cold climates. Small portions of the stable benefit from warmth even if the entire stable is not heated. These areas include the tack room to maintain tack condition and an office or lounge where handlers can work or warm themselves. Heat addition requires installation and maintenance of a system of components that provide heat, distribute the heat, and control heat addition. Maintaining good stable air quality, with reasonable moisture levels and low ammonia accumulation, will require that ventilation air exchange be provided. Insulation is used not only to decrease heat loss through building surfaces but also to maintain the interior surface temperature near indoor conditions to reduce condensation.

The two primary heating systems either heat air in the enclosed space or use radiant heat to warm occupants. Targeting the heat application to areas where it is most needed, such as wash stall, tack room, and grooming areas, provides economy in heating system installation and operation while providing the horse housing area with proper conditions. A duct is typically used with space heating to distribute warmed air evenly throughout the stable environment. Radiant heating may be used for spot-heating an area temporarily using overhead high-temperature fixtures or over a long time with large heated mass via in-floor radiant heating. Radiant heat also provides some heating of surrounding airspace but primarily provides comfort by warming objects within its line of sight.

13
Auxiliary Facilities

Auxiliary facilities include those features that are commonly found at horse facilities but are not directly related to the housing and exercise of the horses. They are nonetheless necessary components of for successful horse stabling. Auxiliary facilities covered in this chapter include the feed room, hay and bedding storage, tack room, grooming station, wash stall, tool storage, and veterinarian and farrier work area. A version of each of these facilities is needed in all barns. For example, not all stables will need a wash stall, but there should be some area where a horse can be hosed down, as needed, after exercise or following an injury. Small stables will often have a combination tack and feed room, and others a combination feed and tool storage rather than separate rooms. To avoid repetition, this chapter depends on several other chapters of this book for detailed information. For example, when the recommendation is to provide a concrete floor for the tack room and feed room, the construction of this floor may be found in Chapter 7. The preceding chapters (Chapters 1 through 12) each contain information relevant to design of the auxiliary facilities.

Two common auxiliary facilities, the horse farm office and observation lounge for an indoor riding arena, are not covered here because their design features are more similar to residential construction. Additionally, there is such wide variation in the amenities included in the office and lounge that few common recommendations can be made. Some aspects of their construction that are more unique to their application in horse facilities are scattered throughout other chapters of this book (Chapters 2, 11, 12, and 16). Most relate to the increased moisture and dust levels encountered in horse stabling and riding arenas than in residential construction.

FEED ROOM

Feed room construction in many ways concentrates on exclusion. Exclusion of rodents and loose horses is essential. Features inside the feed room will make it easy to prepare and deliver feed to horses within the stable. In all but the largest stables, horse feed is handled in bags. Large stables employ exterior feed bins.

Exclude Rodents and Horses

Construction for exclusion of rodents requires a concrete floor to eliminate tunneling into the room. Provide tight-fitting interior and exterior doors for rodent exclusion with horse-proof latches for horse exclusion. The nature of horses is to overeat when presented with an abundance of grain feed, leading to major illness and possibly death. Horses cannot regurgitate to relieve the digestive system after an overeating episode. If a swinging door is used, hang it to swing open out of the feed room so a loose horse cannot push it open into the feed room. Sliding doors are more difficult for horses to open wide enough for entry. For human convenience the doors need to have latches that can be opened with one hand.

Size and Location

Typical size for the feed room in many moderate-sized stables is the equivalent of one horse stall (10 feet by 10 feet to 12 feet by 12 feet). The room may be used for short-term storage of hay in addition to feed. A 4-foot-wide door offers room for a wheelbarrow carrying feed buckets to pass comfortably; a 5- to 6-foot door is even better for handling hay bales comfortably or for delivery of a pallet of feed bags. A door in the middle of the feed room wall allows for storage space on both sides of a central working area in the feed room (Fig. 13.1). The room may be heated to maintain feed materials above freezing and for worker comfort with in-floor radiant, overhead radiant, or space heating (see Chapter 12).

Plan the feed storage space on the basis of a known feed routine. As a rough estimate, provide storage for at least 1 and up to 3 pounds of hay

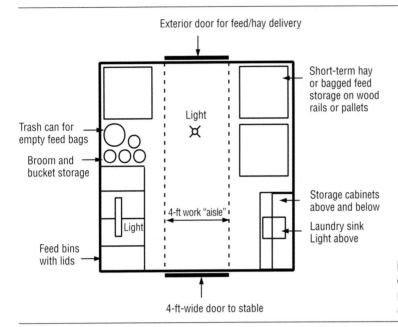

Exterior door for feed/hay delivery

Short-term hay or bagged feed storage on wood rails or pallets

Trash can for empty feed bags

Light

Broom and bucket storage

4-ft work "aisle"

Light

Feed bins with lids

Storage cabinets above and below

Laundry sink Light above

4-ft-wide door to stable

Figure 13.1. Features of centrally located feed room providing a central work aisle.

(includes wastage) and 1 pound of grain per day per 100 pounds of horse weight. Horses consume from 0 to over 2 pounds of grain per 100 pounds of body weight (BW), depending on activity, growth stage, or breeding status. Stocking a 2-month supply of feed in the feed room is reasonable. Most feed grains weigh about 40 pounds per cubic foot. Storage space requirements and density for hay and bedding are given in Table 13.1. As an example of the space needed for feed and hay, consider a 1000-pound horse with 2-month feed supply kept in the feed room and a 6-month hay supply kept nearby with 1 week of hay stored in the feed room. Use 1 pound grain per 100 pounds BW and 2 pounds hay per 100 pounds BW for the estimate. The horse would consume about 10 pounds of grain per day, which requires about ¼ cubic foot of storage or a volume about 7 by 7 by 9 cubic inches per day. A 2-month supply requires 15 cubic feet of space supplied by bags on pallets using a space of 3 feet by 5 feet stacked 1 foot high or feed bin space of 4 feet by 3 feet with a 1¼-foot depth of grain. One week's hay storage in the feed room for this one horse would require almost

Table 13.1. Baled Hay and Straw and Loose Bedding Density for Storage Sizing Estimate

Material	Volume (ft³/ton)	Density (lb/ft³)
Baled		
Alfalfa	200–330	6–10
Non legume	250–330	6–8
Straw	400–500	4–5
Loose		
Wood chips	110	18
Sawdust, fine	110	18
Sawdust, moist	70	28
Wood shavings	200	10

Source: Horse Facilities Handbook.

18 cubic feet of storage using the 8 pounds per cubic foot of grass hay (nonlegume) density estimate from Table 13.1. The horse consumes 20 pounds of hay daily, which occupies about 2½ cubic feet of space 7 days a week. That horse's weekly hay supply may be stored in a 3-foot by 4-foot area at one bale (1½ foot) height. So essentially in this example, one horse's 2-month grain feed storage and 1-week hay storage occupy similar volumes and floor area of feed room space.

For smaller stables a reduced feed room size is reasonable, but allow no less than 4 feet of open workspace "aisle" in the room. This typically means an 8-foot-wide room with a 4-foot depth of feed bin and bag storage and a 4-foot work aisle. Smaller than a 4-foot working width will inhibit moving feed bags and multiple feed buckets.

The feed room is typically centrally located to provide short delivery paths to surrounding stalls. Stall fronts equipped with small doors or holes for depositing feed directly into the feed bucket make for quicker and safer feed delivery for the handler than having to enter each individual stall.

Install a wide door for outside access to the feed room. This allows feed delivery directly into the room without hauling feed bags down the stable aisle to a centrally located feed room. Make the exterior door wide enough to accommodate feed bags delivered in bulk on a pallet.

Feed Storage

Feed bins are common in horse stable feed rooms. Wooden bins, sometimes lined with metal, are constructed with multiple compartments for storage of more than one type of feed or ingredient. A top hinged lid rests back against the wall behind the bin and is shut when not in use. This hinged lid makes it more difficult for a loose horse to get the bin open and comfortably keep a head in the feed bin. Use ¾-inch-thick plywood or 1 by 6 boards in bin construction. A removable liner is useful for periodic cleaning of the bin compartments. Multiple metal trash cans with tight-fitting lids may be used in lieu of a wooden bin with compartments. A hanging scale (10 to 30 pounds) is used to weigh feed materials for more accurate feeding than by volume alone. Leave wall space for hanging clipboards with recordkeeping papers.

Store feed bags on pallets or lumber rails to be off the floor for air circulation. It should be easy to pick up the pallets or lumber to sweep spillage during cleanup. Chapter 7 provides construction recommendations for building a concrete floor that is above groundwater encroachment. Leave space between stacked feed bags and wall for air circulation and cat access to discourage rodents. Cabinets above the stacked feed are useful for storage of various feed additives; use a separate cabinet for cleaning products. Provide a location to hang a broom and cleaning towels. Open feed bags are stored in rodent-proof bins of thick wood or metal (trash) cans. Bins and cans need tight-fitting lids. Rodents chew through soft plastic and thin wood construction.

The feed room is the logical place for storage and provision of feed and water for barn cats and dogs because it is already secured from rodent entry. Of course this means that these animals cannot access their food and water unless allowed into the feed room. To discourage rodents in the stable, remove sources of feed and water. Chapter 3 has a "Rodent Control" sidebar with further information.

Utilities

The feed room will require electric service for light and convenience outlets. A central light fixture will provide overall illumination to the room, but also supply task lighting above the feed bin or mixing area where more detailed work is performed. Hot and cold water supply in the feed room is convenient for cleaning and feed mixing. A laundry-style sink will be big enough to wash feed and water buckets. Provide task lighting above the sink. Provide a frost-proof water supply or heat to the whole room. Enjoy natural light and a view with a window placed above the feed work area, where possible.

HAY AND BEDDING STORAGE

Maintain Quality and Minimize Labor

The two primary objectives of hay and bedding storage are to maintain quality of the delivered material until it is needed and to minimize labor associated with handling the materials. One strong recommendation to reduce fire hazard, with an added benefit of decreasing dust levels in the stable, is to store hay and bedding in a separate building from the horse stable. Chapter 9 contains details of spontaneous hay combustion process and risk. Hay storage above horse stalls in an almost completely isolated loft will offer daily chore advantage while minimizing the dust addition to the horse-occupied area. Hay and bedding need to be protected from rain and snow during storage.

Horse hay comes in baled form, with small rectangular bales being the norm for most stables. Large round bales are used for group-housed, pasture-kept horses. Horses need very high quality hay compared with other livestock that can tolerate more mold and dust. High-quality hay is expensive, and this investment is best protected in a storage structure built to maintain the hay quality until it is fed.

Hay is only harvested during summer months, and long-distance shipment is not usually cost effective. A local supply means that long-term hay storage is needed between when hay is harvested and delivered and when it is fed through the remaining seasons. An alternative is to pay higher prices for hay deliveries throughout the year and forego the cost of long-term storage. Buy only properly cured hay, and monitor new deliveries for bale internal heat increases from postharvest respiration of microbes naturally occurring in the hay. See Chapter 9 for more detail and simple probe (a metal rod) for monitoring hay bale temperature.

Bedding comes in a variety of material-handling formats; for example, bales for straw, bags for wood shavings, and loose for sawdust. Storage criteria for bedding bales and bags will be similar to those for baled hay. Table 13.1 lists the density of common hay and bedding materials for estimating the storage space needed. Storage for loose sawdust will be in a bulk storage with its different handling requirements: delivered by dump truck; removed by hand tools or front-end loader.

It is essential that the storage maintain hay and bedding materials in a dry condition to reduce spoilage from mold formation and subsequent rotting of the material. Sawdust, and other loose bedding, needs to be kept dry or part of its moisture-holding capacity is taken by absorbing rainwater rather than urine in the stall. Maintaining dry conditions means designing and maintaining an airy storage where fresh air can flow through the facility to pick up and remove moisture and heat while the hay is curing.

Minimizing labor for stacking incoming hay and bedding and unloading as needed is the second objective of the storage design. Bulk dumping of loose bedding material clearly saves time compared with stacking hundreds of bales or bags. This savings may be lost, however, if an efficient means of handling the loose material is not used during daily chores.

A tarp may suffice for temporarily keeping rainwater off hay storage, but inexpensive tarps are not waterproof, easily tear providing water leaks, trap moisture and heat within if tightly wrapped over hay stack, and are cumbersome for daily chores.

Stacking Hay

There are plenty of theories about how to stack bales in a storage or mow. Stack for enhanced airflow through and around freshly baled hay to dissipate normal heat and moisture release as the bales "cure." Stack bales with the stems of the cut hay running up and down. This allows natural convection ventilation of warm, moist air up and out of the bale. The greener or moister the hay, the looser it should be packed to allow cooling and curing without danger of mildew formation or combustion. The goal is to allow space for air to flow around the entire stack sides, top, and bottom. In between bales, even a small space can allow moisture and heat to move out and away from each bale. Stack leaving a 1- to 2-inch space between bales on each side even with cured hay. Keep the stack away from solid surfaces such as walls and ceiling to allow airflow around the stack. Realize though that loosely packed bales are more prone to tumbling out of their stacked formation.

Stagger-stack the bales to help stabilize the loose stack configuration, discussed earlier. Stack bales similar to how bricks are laid on a wall. Change the next layer of hay bales to be perpendicular to the layer below. Even within a layer, on occasion change bale direction 90 degrees to tie one row of bales into neighboring rows, similar to timbers perpendicular to a retaining wall that tie the wall into the soil behind it. The practicality of these stagger-stack techniques will depend on how hay is loaded and unloaded from the storage; for example, whether removal is by one horizontal layer of bales at a time or by vertical stacks of bales or some more random method.

Using pallets under the hay stack will allow air circulation and move hay away from any ground moisture. A layer of dry straw under the bottom row is a second option with less risk of providing comfortable housing for rodents within pallet spaces. Pallets may be hard to walk on depending on opening spaces between slats, and they prevent use of mechanized equipment to handle bales.

Account for stacking inefficiencies, particularly for baled hay that is deliberately stacked more loosely than bedding bales, by using no more than an 85% stacking efficiency for estimating space requirements. Bales stacked loosely to allow airflow between bales will take more storage volume than tightly stacked bales. For example, weighing a few hay bales and measuring dimensions results in knowledge that the purchased hay has a density of 8 pounds per cubic foot. A ton (2000 pounds) of this hay would appear to need 250 cubic feet for storage space (2000 pounds per ton divided by 8 pounds per cubic foot). Actually closer to 300 cubic feet will be needed to store this ton of hay (250 ft^3/ton/0.85 = 294 ft^3/ton) when the 85% stacking efficiency is accounted for.

Once moisture and heat are allowed to flow from individual bales, the resulting warm, moist air must be ventilated from the storage structure. Provide full ridge vent for the rising warm and moist air to exit the building. The ridge vent may be a continuous opening protected by an agricultural-grade ridge vent assembly or intermittent openings with larger vent assemblies or cupolas.

Fire Safety

The recommendation to store large qualities of hay in a structure separate from the horse stabling is primarily for fire safety. Once ignited, hay burns at the same rate as gasoline and there is little hope of putting out a hay barn fire. Fire-fighting efforts concentrate on reducing risk to surrounding buildings and eventually suppressing the blaze once the fuel source (hay) burns out. Masonry construction will inhibit fire spread laterally, but their tight construction may inadvertently lead to spontaneous combustion through lack of adequate ventilation. Once the fire event is over, you are left with a masonry building shell but no usable hay or roof. Provide at least 75-foot separation distance between the hay storage and adjacent buildings to reduce spark spread and to allow fire-fighting vehicle access. Good all-weather driveways for heavy trucks are part of good storage design, so access to the storage for the fire equipment should be adequate.

Keep a metal probe in the hay storage for quick evaluation of bale internal temperature. If the probe is handy and hung with directions for use in a visible location, it can be used to check bales during the curing stage and later for those suspected of overheating. Make sure that emergency numbers are posted at the nearest phone. A fire extinguisher seems like a common sense aid; yet once smoke is detected in the storage, the situation needs professional firefighter help. Once flames are seen, a fire extinguisher is of little use. The best defense are the frequent checks (daily) on internal bale temperature during the freshly baled hay curing period so that increasing temperature can be handled before the ignition phase is reached. Having a fire extinguisher handy in a nearby building is more reasonable than expecting someone to enter the smoking hay storage to retrieve one. More about each of the topics discussed in this section is available in Chapter 9.

Long-Term Storage

DIMENSIONS AND STORAGE SPACE

Provide the long-term hay and bedding storage building with a 16- to 20-foot sidewall height and storage bays of 12- to 14-foot width between support posts (Fig. 13.2). Building width typically varies from 24 to 48 feet. Table 13.2 provides storage capacity per foot of building length for a 20-foot sidewall building of various widths. Doors or overhangs that allow semi-truck-trailer and tractor with hay wagon access need to be 14 feet high. The 16- to 20-foot sidewall height recommendation provides room for 4-foot or wider overhang to protect stored hay and still have enough clearance for hay truck delivery. Make a rough estimate of material storage needed with 1 to 3 pounds of hay per day per 100 pounds of horse and 8 to 15 pounds of bedding per occupied stall.

LAYOUT

A hay and baled bedding storage building can be a simple roofed structure with or without solid walls. With no walls, ventilation is assured but at the risk of precipitation contacting the outer layers of stacked hay. A more common version of the open-sided storage is to enclose the endwalls and keep sidewalls open. Figure 13.3 shows three storage layout options including open sidewalls, three-sided with one open sidewall, and fully enclosed. Long eave overhangs are

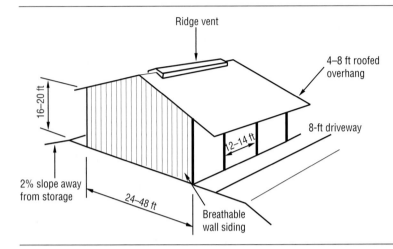

Figure 13.2. Features of long-term hay storage with endwalls of breathable siding and one or two open sidewalls.

recommended particularly along any open sidewall to provide a buffer against rain and snow entry and to discharge rainwater and snowmelt away from the building pad. Long overhangs also provide a sheltered loading area to protect workers and hay being moved to the stable. The roofed structure without sidewalls is sufficient in arid climates and with proper design can work in temperate climates. In a location with abundant blowing snow or rain, this is not a good storage alternative. The perimeter hay bales of the stack will have about 2 inches of weathered, exposed hay that may not be suitable for feeding (horses should not be offered moldy hay). This open design affords plenty of desirable ventilation, access to stored hay and bedding on all sides, and cost-effective construction without the need for sidewall material.

Often the storage has three sides enclosed with large ventilation openings at the eaves of the enclosed long side. A curtain sidewall may be used on the "closed" back wall for easy increases and decreases in ventilation opening. Closed sides constructed of breathable wall (siding boards with narrow air gaps between adjacent boards) offer diffuse ventilation from floor to ceiling along those walls. Breathable wall is the same construction successfully used for over a hundred years on old barn haymows. The open long sidewall is used for loading and unloading the hay and bedding.

One option offering more convenience is to allow access to the storage from both long sidewalls so that hay and bedding can be added from either side as material is removed. In this way, the old, unused hay on the "back" wall is never closed in again by the delivery of a new truckload of material. It can be unloaded from the "backside." This configuration with two sides for delivery and removal of hay and

Table 13.2. Rough Capacity Estimates for a Hay Shed with 20-Foot Sidewall in Tons per Foot Length of Building

Shed Width (ft)	Small Rectangular Bales[a]	Large Rectangular Bales[b]	Large Round Bales[c]
24	1.6	3.0	1.6
30	2.0	3.8	2.0
36	2.4	4.5	2.4
40	2.7	5.0	2.6
48	3.3	6.0	3.2

[a]7 to 9 pounds dry matter per cubic foot; 85% stacking efficiency.
[b]13 to 15 pounds dry matter per cubic foot; 90% stacking efficiency.
[c]9 to 13 pounds dry matter per cubic foot; 60% stacking efficiency.
Source: Horse Facilities Handbook.

Hay Storage Structures Options

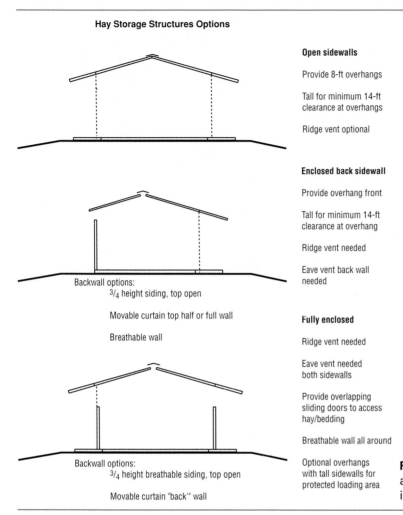

Open sidewalls

Provide 8-ft overhangs

Tall for minimum 14-ft clearance at overhangs

Ridge vent optional

Enclosed back sidewall

Provide overhang front

Tall for minimum 14-ft clearance at overhang

Ridge vent needed

Eave vent back wall needed

Backwall options:
³/₄ height siding, top open

Movable curtain top half or full wall

Breathable wall

Fully enclosed

Ridge vent needed

Eave vent needed both sidewalls

Provide overlapping sliding doors to access hay/bedding

Breathable wall all around

Backwall options:
³/₄ height breathable siding, top open

Movable curtain "back'" wall

Optional overhangs with tall sidewalls for protected loading area

Figure 13.3. Long-term hay and bedding storage building options.

bedding reduces labor by eliminating the need to restack older hay to the front of the storage before the newer hay arrives. The two sides for access can have large overlapping sliding doors in order to access the entire storage while offering rain and snow protection when needed.

Drive-through hay storages offer convenience and risk. A central drive allows the delivery truck to enter the building so hay and bedding can be unloaded to either side. Likewise, the central drive allows a protected location for daily hay and bedding collection for transport to the stable area. Provide a concrete or asphalt floor in the drive area and sweep clean of hay and chaff droppings that can be ignited by hot engine and exhaust parts.

Moving hay and bedding from the long-term storage area to the stable or pasture shelters is best done with some kind of mechanization even if not motorized. Wheelbarrows and other carts that can handle bulky, but not necessarily high-density, loads are useful for smaller farms. Large wheels are easier to move over uneven ground than smaller diameter wheels. All-terrain vehicles and tractors can pull a cart loaded with the daily or weekly hay and bedding supply. In locations of regular rainfall, keep a tarp handy that can be secured over the transported hay and bedding for rain protection if the material is not going to be used right away and risks molding during short-term storage. Provide a covered area where the transport cart can be loaded at the long-term storage and at the stable or pasture shelter to keep the materials and workers out of the rain, snow, or hot sunlight, depending on the climate.

LOCATION

As with all other buildings on the horse farm site, the long-term hay and bedding storage must be placed and/or the site prepared to divert surface water and avoid groundwater. Water is the enemy of proper hay and bedding storage because of the mold growth associated with damp conditions. Make sure the base of the structure, where hay is stacked, is about 12 inches above surrounding grade. The structure will need at least one driveway with access for incoming loads of hay and daily or weekly removal for feed and bedding use. Large tractor-trailers are best handled with a drive-through configuration that eliminates the need for backing. Provide a driveway capable of supporting their weight. Hay storage with ability to load and unload from either side needs a driveway on both sides. Locate the hay storage at least 75 feet away from other buildings. This will minimize fire spread from sparks, allow access by fire trucks, and provide room for hay and bedding delivery trucks.

Short-Term Storage in Stable

Provide short-term storage for up to a week's worth of hay in the stable when a long-term storage is used. Daily movement of hay to the stable is normal for commercial stables with available labor. Weekend movement of hay supply is often a better routine for privately owned stables. Hay is easily stored in an open alcove area off the main work aisle (Fig. 13.4). Locate the storage for convenient delivery of hay coming from the long-term storage and convenient delivery to the stabled horses. Up to 100 square feet of space may be allocated to short-term storage in order to keep a convenient yet modest amount of flammable material in the stable. Short-term bedding storage may be added to the hay area. Locate tools nearby for handling hay and bedding.

In large stables a centralized location is more convenient for daily feeding, with short trips back and forth between the farthest stalls and the hay supply. Short-term storage may be located in the feed room to combine grain and concentrate and forage feeding trips to horse stalls. Whether in the feed room or its own centralized area, provide a wide access door (4 to 6 feet) to the exterior to easily transfer hay from long- to short-term storage. Smaller stables will likely have short-term hay storage near the end of the work aisle for convenience

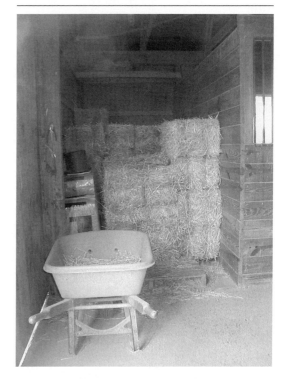

Figure 13.4. Short-term hay storage in the stable with easy access for weekly deliveries from long-term storage and feeding of stabled horses.

in unloading from the long-term storage transport vehicle in an alcove area of 6- to 8-foot width.

Overhead Hay Storage

TRADITION AND DEBATE

The debate of overhead hay storage within horse stables versus separate storage in another building generates strong supporters on each side. Some stable managers indicate that a daily convenience of tossing sections of bales down into the stalls or whole bales into the work aisle can outweigh the dust, mold, and fire hazard of hay storage in the horse stable (Fig. 13.5).

The overhead hay storage tradition comes from barn construction where loose hay was cured in the airy confines of the two-story barn loft with an airy breathable "barn board" construction. With today's big sheathing construction materials, we need to supply more planned ventilation opening to maintain good hay quality with minimal moisture

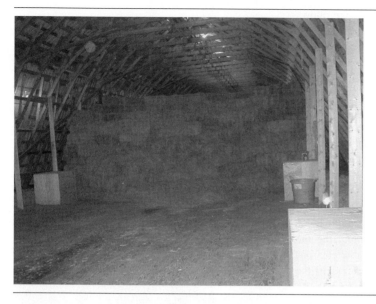

Figure 13.5. Haymow long-term storage that provides air circulation around and over the stacked hay. Plywood boxes cover hay drops to stalls below.

accumulation to discourage mold spore development. Low ventilation increases the risk of spontaneous combustion in the loft area by not removing naturally occurring heat generated from curing hay. The traditional barn loft included a full ceiling over the lower level where livestock, including horses, were housed. One or two large openings in the loft floor allowed forage and bedding material to be dropped down for use in the stabling area. This daily convenience of dropping hay and bedding from storage down to where it is needed remains attractive.

Labor convenience with overhead storage is realized on a daily basis. Build access to the loft via stairs rather than ladder construction to minimize falling injuries. Consider the entire labor for overhead hay storage compared with ground-level separate storage. A considerable amount of labor (or machinery) goes into getting hay and bedding bales overhead, unless topography permits the hay wagon or delivery truck to drive into the loft. So the overall labor savings appear small but can be concentrated into delivery time frames. In locales with considerable snowpack all winter, the convenience of overhead storage is magnified because less effort is needed to shovel snow to get hay out of long-term storage.

DESIGN OPTIONS

Overhead hay storage in horse stables assumes three primary designs. One is a full ceiling with complete separation from the stable environment except for one or more "drop" holes for overhead delivery of

hay bales or sections. Keeping the overhead hay storage isolated from the stable provides for better air quality within the stable. When the overhead hay storage is completely separated from the horse area with a full ceiling, the dust and mold generation can be minimized for the horses except when hay bales are being tossed down on a daily basis and when the loft is loaded with fresh hay. Dust and mold can be somewhat contained in the hayloft, particularly if trap doors to the stall hay feeders are kept closed except when in use.

A full ceiling over the horse stalls compromises natural ventilation of the stalls unless the ceiling is installed to assure good air movement over stall partitions. The goal is to provide adequate space for air circulation and ventilation in the horse stall while keeping the dust, mold, and chaff of hay storage in the hayloft. Provide a stable ceiling, which is the hayloft floor, at least 12 feet high. This allows air circulation within the stable above stall partitions and provides room for fresh air entry and stale air exit at eave vents along both sidewalls. Because stale air can no longer rise up and out of the stable through the ridge openings, larger sidewall openings will be needed to ensure good fresh air exchange. Chimneys may be used to move air from the stable to vent at the ridge (see Chapter 6 for more details).

The second and third overhead storage designs offer partial overhead hay storage with one option for storage over the central work aisle and the other over the stalls. Both will allow dust to rain down on the stabled horses but the over-aisle design allows natural ventilation air movement to horses in their stalls. The over-stall design is highly discouraged because it adds dust and mold from the hay storage to the stable environment and closes in the horse stall for stuffy conditions where there is little opportunity for fresh air movement. Warmed moist air naturally rises from the horse stall where heat and moisture is generated within the stable. An overhead hayloft blocks this natural air movement.

HAY DROP OPENINGS

Horse stable hayloft hay drops should be designed with two goals in mind: minimal dust into the horse zone and safety for loft workers. Minimizing the number of hay drop holes into the stable environment will help achieve both goals. This lessens the area for dusty air exchange and the number of holes in the loft floor a worker can encounter. Permanently open, unprotected loft holes are not acceptable. All loft holes should be protected to make sure that distracted workers cannot step back and fall through a floor hole. Remember that people other than those familiar with the loft organization will be up in the loft. Folks not expected to know or recognize the holes in the floor during busy activity include guest helpers and those invited to help load the loft on delivery day. Tired owners and workers are equally at risk. On gambrel roof barns, the loft openings to the stable can be located near the sidewalls where humans are inhibited from walking because of the low overhead height; yet there is enough height to move hay bales.

Hinged lids on loft openings work well if they are conveniently and consistently closed between hay-feeding events. A pulley system rope attached to an adjacent wall or post allows a quick close-safe hay drop door to be opened for hay delivery and closed automatically. Provide hay drop to two stalls at a time to halve the amount of loft holes needed. One stall gets hay delivery on the right side and the adjacent one on the left side. Figures 13.6 through 13.8 provide an example of how a protected hay drop may be designed in the loft to serve two stalls at a time. The plywood cover over the loft hole serves to keep workers from stepping through and minimizes dust into the horse environment below. Figure 13.9 shows the hay drop from the stall where hay is directed to adjacent stalls. Figure 13.5 shows the mow hay storage and hay drop boxes.

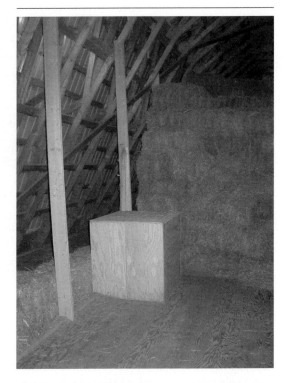

Figure 13.6. Plywood box covers hay drop hole for greater safety than leaving an open hole. Hay can be stacked around and over the box, which is open facing the roof wall.

In some designs the loft ladder access is also the only hay drop hole. This minimizes hay drop holes but offers injury risk with ladder climbing, often while carrying something. Stepping into the unprotected hole while upstairs is additional risk. Provide a 4-foot-tall rail around the loft hole to improve safety. This will not prevent children falling through unless more rails are added.

Overhead hay storage is less risky for stables where the horses are kept outside most of the time. A combined hay storage and stable may be desirable in this case than building two separate structures. Evaluate the cost of construction of both options, because the separate hay storage is a simple and inexpensive building compared with the substantial weight-carrying second story above the stable. The separate hay and bedding storage can serve a dual purpose for machinery storage. Keep machinery and hay storage as distinct as possible to minimize the risk of hot engine and exhaust components igniting the hay litter on the storage floor.

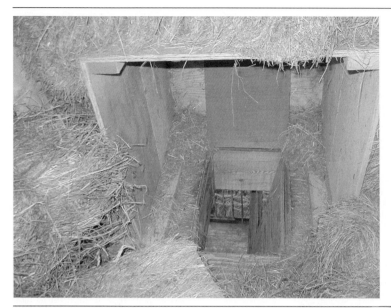

Figure 13.7. Interior of plywood box covering hay drop hole for two stalls below. Hinged lid, toward back of box, can be closed to protect hole further. Hinged baffle is directed to right to send hay delivery to stall on left.

Lighting

Do not use unprotected incandescent or halogen bulbs in the hay storage area. This caution applies to storages whether they are a separate long-term building, a short-term location in the stable, or a loft above the stable. These two types of bulbs have high surface temperatures that can ignite the dust collected on the bulb. Provide lighting in sealed dust and moisture-tight fixtures whether using incandescent, fluorescent, or high-intensity discharge (HID). Appropriate HID lamps include metal halide and high-pressure sodium; low-pressure sodium casts such a yellow light that color rendition is too poor for indoor use. Incandescent and halogen lamps start immediately when switched on. HID lamps take 10 minutes or more to fully light and so are not particularly useful for a storage when there are often short periods of use. Fluorescent will start immediately if supplied with cold-start ballast (electronic) when use is expected in cold weather. The well-sealed incandescent is the

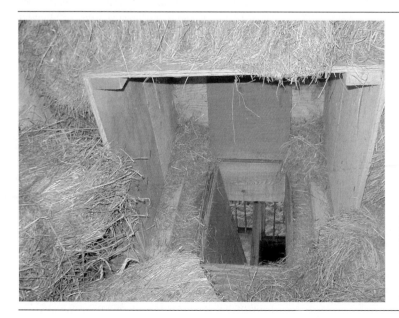

Figure 13.8. Interior of same plywood box shown in Figure 13.7 but with hinged baffle in second position to divert hay delivery to stall on the right.

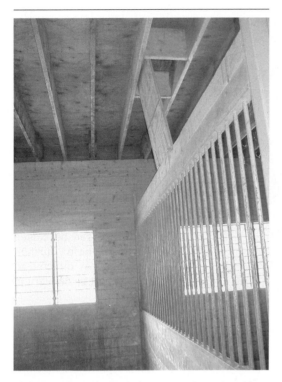

Figure 13.9. View of haymow drop design where baffle board is seen to be hinged from the top of the stall divider.

least costly and most effective light system for long-term and loft storage (see Chapter 11 for pictures of incandescent bulbs in dust- and moisture-tight enclosures). A relatively low light level is needed for simply picking out and loading hay and bedding. Natural daylight can come through open sidewalls, translucent panels along the top of a long sidewall, or movable curtain material for sidewall ventilation. See Chapter 11 for more detail on lighting options.

TACK ROOM

Function

Preservation of tack condition is the primary objective of the tack room environment, while layout focuses on convenient access and organization of the stored tack. For simplicity, tack could be stored in the stable right next to the horses' stall; but although this offers convenient access to the tack, it is not suitable for maintaining tack materials in good condition. Halters and lead ropes are often hung stall-side for quick use.

Leather tack suffers deterioration in quality from overly dry or overly moist conditions. If any room in the stable is going to benefit from being heated in the winter or managed for reduced humidity in the summer, it will be the tack room. Even for small backyard stables, it is recommended that a secured room (or at least a large cabinet or closet) be used for tack storage to preserve the tack from the detrimental effects of a stable's winter humidity, high dust levels, and rodents. The tack and feed room may be combined but with enhanced dust deposition on the tack. The tack room is often located near the grooming stations in the stable layout.

Tack rooms often serve both a storage function and as a social center for the stable. In some ways, the tack room provides an indication of the personality and management style of the facility in being formal or informal, highly organized or relaxed, and so forth. If the room is used as a lounge in addition to tack storage, then indoor climate and room appointments become closer to residential construction. Tack room materials can be more residential than agricultural in construction, but keep in mind that there will be more dust, humidity, and challenge by rodents than in typical residential construction (Fig. 13.10).

Construction and Environment

All tack rooms have common construction features that focus on security against rodents and theft. Provide a rodent-proof floor (typically concrete) and tight construction to eliminate rodent entry (Fig. 13.11). Rodents will nest in piles of blankets or rags. They are attracted to chew on the salty sweat dried into the leather, saddle pads, and blankets. Do not provide pet food and water in the tack room because they attract rodents. The tack room needs a ceiling to seal the room from the stable environment. A lockable door should be installed whether it is consistently locked or not. For storage of highly valuable tack, security increases beyond the lockable door to include barred windows and provision to protect against intruder entry through the ceiling.

Ideal leather tack storage environment is not well documented. Leather conditioning (oiling) can keep leather from drying out, but high humidity should be avoided to minimize mildew and mold formation. Simple guidelines are to keep the room above freezing in the winter, target 35 to 40°F, but ambient temperature will be fine during the summer (in all but the

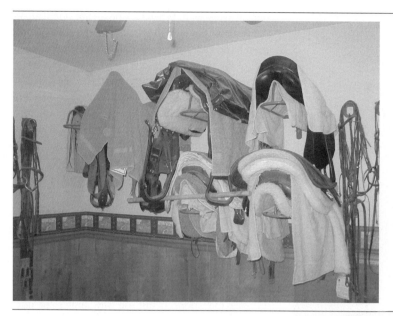

Figure 13.10. Tack is best stored neatly in a room secured against rodent entry and heated in winter to reduce moisture so tack can dry between uses.

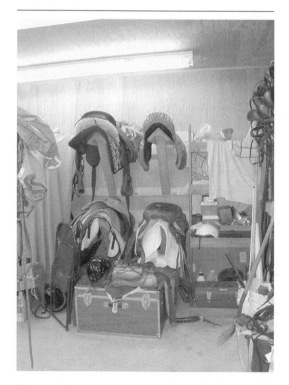

Figure 13.11. Provide a concrete floor in the tack room for easy cleaning and to exclude rodents. Plan room for plenty of shelving and trunks for storing small tack items.

hottest climates). For a heavily used tack room with plenty of wet saddle blankets and sweaty tack to dry, target a consistent 50°F tack room temperature during cold weather with an acceptable range 10°F higher or lower. During cold weather, maintain relative humidity of 30% to 60% in the tack room within the 40 to 60°F temperature range. Supplemental heat added to the tack room allows more moisture to be absorbed by the air to aid drying wet, sweaty tack and saddle blankets. Chapter 12 provides detail on horse stable heater options. Residential humidity and temperature sensors are common and inexpensive, so use one to monitor the tack room environment and ventilate the room to remove moisture or diminish ventilation to increase humidity during cold weather. A residential-style bathroom-sized fan on a switch should be sufficient for the low airflow rate needed to remove tack room moisture.

If a window is installed for natural light, provide insect screening if it will be opened (Fig. 13.12). Fly control is desirable in the tack room because detailed cleaning work is hampered by pests and flies leave behind dirt and specks. Ubiquitous sticky fly paper or other traps may be used.

Utilities

Electric light is needed for the tack room and may be the only available light. Provide at least one overhead centrally-located fluorescent (40 watts) or incandescent fixture (100 watts) per 50 square feet

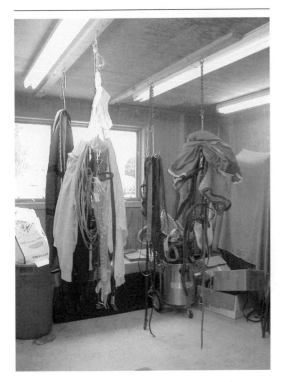

Figure 13.12. Tack room use benefits from plenty of light from both window and overhead electric fixtures. Hangers allow the interior of the room to be used for tack cleaning and storage.

of floor area. Provide higher light level in detailed task area such as near the tack cleaning sink (when provided) on a separate switch. Multiple light fixtures will decrease shadows on the tack that is being cleaned or repaired.

Space electric convenience outlets about every 8 feet around the room, with a minimum of at least one on every wall. When tack boxes are stored along the walls of the tack room, convenience outlets will need to be at a 5-feet height to be above the opened lids of the trunks.

Provide a sink with hot and cold water that is large enough to easily fill small- and medium-sized buckets used for tack cleaning. Do not discard cleaning water on the floor to a drain to decrease the amount of moisture the room's heating and ventilation system must remove. If no sink drain is provided, discard tack wash water in the wash stall or other stable drain system.

Some tack rooms will include laundry washer and dryer for cleaning horse-related items and so will need 110-volt and 220-volt electric service, exhaust vent from dryer, and washer drain. A small refrigerator may be supplied for keeping light snacks and drinks cool. Chapters 10 and 11 provide more detail on the topics of this paragraph.

Space

Tack storage space is highly variable among stables, but some guidelines can help in planning. English and other lighter weight saddles are easy to lift and so can be stored in multiple tiers. Western and other heavier saddles are better stored at hip height to reduce lifting into storage. Saddle brackets attached to a wall provide a clear floor beneath that is easier to clean and/or can be used for additional storage (trunks) than saddle storage on floor racks. See Table 13.3 for guidelines on tack space storage requirements. Tack items accumulate. Make the best estimate you can on how much tack will be stored in the stable and then increase that. The amount of extra tack items beyond those listed in Table 13.3 are substantial, so plan on extra cabinet or hanging

Table 13.3. Typical Tack Dimensions for Estimating Storage Space Requirements within a Tack Room

	Height (in.)	Width (in.)	Front-to-Rear Depth (in.)	Distance Between[a] (in.)
English-type saddle	26–30	22	24	24–28
Western-type saddle	29–36	24–29	26–33	30–36
Bridle	28–40	4	4–6	10
Light harness	70–80	8–10	12	10–12
Tack trunk	24 closed; 48 open	36–48	24–30	

[a]Distance between is centerline to centerline of adjacent saddles or bridles.

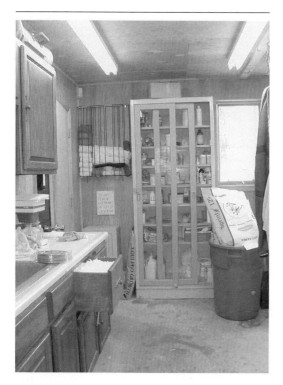

Figure 13.13. The tack room will benefit from a sink with hot and cold water for cleaning and storage cabinets.

24- to 30-inch depth for each boarder. This allows each boarder enough room to position one or two saddles (second saddle rack above lower one) next to two bridle racks with room for a small tack trunk at floor level. Position the tack room door so that there is a clear access aisle into the tack room and so that an interior swinging door does not block tack access. Another option is to store larger tack items such as saddles and bridles and assorted gear in the tack room and provide a cubbyhole in the main aisle for storage of the smaller items, such as riding gloves, crop, and helmet, which are needed just before mounting. The cubbyhole or cabinets can be built into the wall near the grooming area or near entry to the riding arena. In a public stable it is wise to provide space for lockable gear storage.

For the small stable where a separate tack room is not provided, use a tack closet or cabinet to store tack in a dry and secure location that discourages rodent chewing. Seal the closet against rodent entry with close-fitting doors and tight-fitting hardware. But the tack closet will need fresh air movement to dry sweat moisture from the tack. Provide louvered doors screened with $\frac{1}{4}$- or $\frac{1}{2}$-inch hardware cloth stapled to the interior to discourage rodent entry. Even an incandescent bulb kept lit in the closet can provide enough heat to keep the tack warmed in cold winter conditions. (Incandescent bulbs emit most of their incoming electrical energy as longwave heat rather than shortwave light energy.) Install the light low in the closet so heated air rises up over the drying tack and then up and out of the closet. Protect the light bulb from contacting tack items, even those that fall within the cabinet.

Horse blanket storage can take considerable space in tack trunks or other storage locations. They need air circulation for drying when removed from the horse. Particularly wet and muddy blankets need a place to hang and dry. Often a blanket rack is provided on stall fronts or doors. Provide blanket hanging space in a heated room (tack or feed) or large cabinet when rapid drying of damp blankets is needed.

space to accommodate (Fig. 13.13). Use cabinets for storage of accessories such as tack cleaning solutions, sponges, wraps, and small tack items. These cabinets may be provided by residential-style kitchen cabinets.

Provide a well-lit space in the room where a saddle and other tack can be placed on a rack for cleaning with plenty of room for moving around all sides. A portable rack can be used in the middle of the room and then stowed when not in use.

The tack room door needs to be wide enough to easily carry a saddle through and may be a sliding 4-foot-wide door to match other stable doors. Doors less than 3 feet wide are too narrow for comfortably carrying saddles through. Only one door is needed unless the tack room is very large; an outside access door is discouraged to reduce tack theft threat. Doors that easily open and automatically close will discourage fly entry into the tack room.

One quick estimate for boarding stables is to provide about 36 inches of available wall space with a

TOOL AND MACHINERY STORAGE

Horsekeeping involves considerable hand labor. Keep tools convenient to daily cleaning routines, with hanging storage for rakes, brooms, shovels, and forks. This keeps them tidy, in a set location, and up

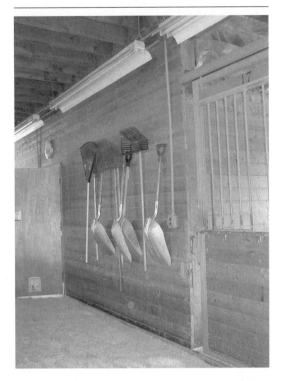

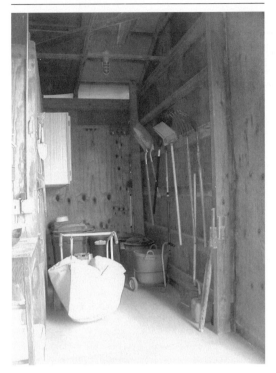

Figure 13.14. Keep hand tools for stall cleaning hanging in a handy location, often in the work aisle of the stable near the centralized work area.

Figure 13.15. Tools and small equipment can be stored in an alcove off the main work aisle to keep the stable's main work aisle uncluttered with items used every day.

out of foot traffic and thus less prone to being knocked over (Fig. 13.14). A storage location near the stable's feed-tack working areas is typical. Tool storage location may be in the work aisle or an alcove storage area. An additional set of tools and a manure collection bucket are often positioned near an indoor riding arena entrance to aid in picking up manure deposited on the arena footing. Some specialized areas may have dedicated tools, such as a cleaning broom kept in the feed room. Also include storage for wheelbarrows, shop vacuums, and similar items. These bigger items are best stored in an alcove, small storage, or inside the feed room if used primarily for feed delivery. A manure-handling wheelbarrow is best stored near the manure-handling tools.

A small alcove of tool and small equipment storage off the main work aisle is useful (Fig. 13.15). An alcove or nook describes an area with no separating doorway between it and the work aisle for unobstructed access. A separating wall with a 4- to 6-foot-wide doorway is an option. Provide a 6- to 8-

foot-wide nook with one wall of hanging tools, room for the wheelbarrow (or similar), and perhaps the all-terrain vehicle. Cabinets and shelves can be hung for storing smaller items. Provide central light fixture with switch at entry to the area. A storage nook may be used for short-term bedding storage and tool storage. Arrange so that manure-handling tools do not contaminate bedding. The disadvantage to this shared arrangement is the conflict in hygiene with hay and manure tools.

Mechanized equipment is often needed for material movement for stall cleaning and feeding activities. Providing covered storage will prolong the useful life for equipment, such as tractors, implements, and all-terrain vehicles, than leaving them exposed to the weather (Fig. 13.16). A simple three-sided shed is sufficient for the larger equipment. A 14-foot clearance will accommodate large-scale horse farm equipment; a 10- to 12-foot clearance will suffice for small farm implements. Provide 12- to 14-feet-wide bays for each tractor or implement needing storage.

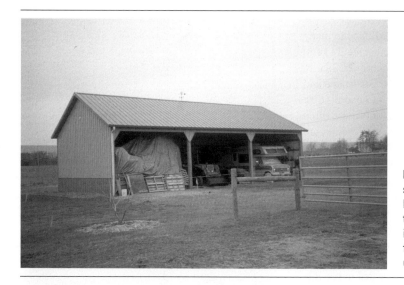

Figure 13.16. A building separate from the horse stable can serve a dual function on a small farm in storing hay and bedding and farm machinery when not in use.

This storage may be added as a large roof extension on an indoor arena construction or as a separate structure.

GROOMING STATION

A grooming station should be provided in busy commercial stables where horses cross-tied in the work aisle inhibit other clients' use of the work aisle. A grooming station is of similar dimension to a 12-foot by 12-foot box stall outfitted with cross-ties for securing the horse. The horse typically faces the open side to the stable aisle. A strong rail can separate adjoining grooming stations. Grooming stations are located near the tack room for convenience because tack is not kept in the grooming station. Flooring may be of any material suitable for horse stalls, with an emphasis on being easily cleanable and durable. Concrete, asphalt, and rubber mats over packed stonedust are common grooming station floor materials. Provide electric convenience outlets on sidewall and posts supporting divider rails between grooming stations. Outlets near the front end of the horse are needed for clippers. When wet floors are anticipated because of light washing or the grooming station doubling as a wash stall, the electric outlets need ground-fault interruption (GFI) for safety against electrical shock. Recommendations for lighting the grooming station may be found in Chapter 11.

Grooming tools and tack will be needed in the grooming station. Shelves for grooming tools and ointments can be provided along a sidewall, preferably recessed or protected by a horse-strong rail. The idea is to provide a reasonably smooth wall surface to prevent horse impact injury or a handler being pinned upon sharp corners. Hangers with multiple hooks hung from the truss or rafters on light chain are a good option to keep lightweight tack (bridle, breast strap, etc.) handy, yet the assembly will give when horse or handler bumps into it. Hanging wire mesh baskets of grooming brushes are a similar option when hung high enough to minimize risk of horse entanglement. When more than one grooming station is provided next to each other, they may be separated by a full floor-to-ceiling wall, partial "kick" wall of about 5-foot height, or single strong rail.

When the tack room and grooming station are close, then a saddle is brought to the horse when needed. Saddles may be brought to the grooming station before they will be put on the horse and need to be set in a convenient location before placement on the horse. Saddles are best kept, even temporarily, on a rack rather than on the floor where they get dirty, bent out of shape, or leather scratched. A wall-mounted saddle rack or portable wheeled model can be located at each grooming station to hold the saddle. A foldaway saddle rack can be stowed between uses. Saddles can be placed on a wood or metal dividing rail between stations when that rail is the equivalent of 4- to 6-inch diameter to support the saddle without it swiveling off. Another option is a 2 by 6 board set flat to use as a temporary narrow shelf for brushes and to hold a saddle until ready for placement on the horse.

WASH STALL

A dedicated horse bathing area is included in many stables where show and competitive horses are kept. A dedicated wash stall is most common, but in smaller stables a simple area may be designated and outfitted with water and drainage to handle horse bathing. Realize that horses being bathed are often animated in response to the water use. Cross-ties are used to keep the horse securely but safely centered in the wash area. Design and maintain the wash stall with limited protrusions that can hurt the horse or a handler who is pushed into the wall. A durable and nonslippery floor is essential for safety. Any electrical outlets in the area need to be GFI (ground fault interrupted) outfitted to reduce the chance of electrical shock.

One wash stall per 20 horses expected to use it is a good starting point for a typical boarding stable. For training facilities with almost daily horse bathing, the number of wash stalls can be doubled. Sometimes, grooming stations and wash stalls are combined for more efficient use of space. In this case, one grooming station and wash stall combination per 8 horses is a good estimate unless current management experience dictates otherwise.

Provide at least one sturdy shelf in the wash stall so that grooming brushes can be easily reached. Additional shelves are desirable for storing wash products and grooming equipment between wash events. Shelving units with sliding, closable doors will minimize clutter and help keep the storage cleaner. Shelves toward the back of the wash stall are out of the way when moving horses in and out. Recessed shelving or a location built into a corner will minimize horse impact (Fig. 13.17). When positioning shelving, consider human and horse safety by visualizing the results of being knocked or squeezed into the shelves by an excited horse.

Water

The water use and discharge from the wash stall will be equivalent to a bathroom shower (see Chapter 10 for estimate). Water disposal must handle substantial hair and manure addition but may still be considered simple "gray water" because it does not contain human waste. The drainage from the wash stall needs a trap so that clogs of hair and manure can be removed before they lodge in piping. Plan on having and removing clogs in the drain; so design accordingly.

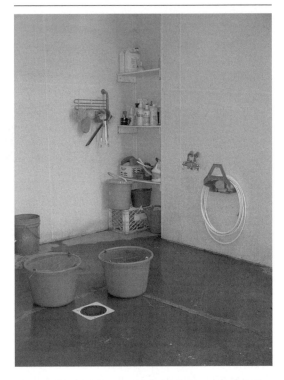

Figure 13.17. Wash stall with recessed shelving in back corner. Wall material is FRP, which is strong and waterproof.

A hose is used to shower the horse with water. Provide a place to stow the hose neatly between horse baths and to get it out of the way for cleanup of the area. For barns maintained below freezing temperatures, provide a convenient way to drain hoses after use. Overhead hose dollies are available that provide similar function to the overhead swinging hoses used in do-it-yourself car washes. Overhead booms have value in getting the hose out from under foot and tangling with the horse. Provide a way to drain the overhead boom in freezing barns.

Both hot and cold water will be needed in the horse wash stall. Freeze-proof fixtures will be necessary in northern climates. Commonly available residential outdoor faucet fixtures may be used when the wash stall is located next to a heated room that can protect this type of plumbing fixture. Within the horse wash stall either recess the faucets to be flush with the wall or shield them with a horse-strong rail if they protrude to protect horses from injury and plumbing from breakage.

Position the water drain along one of the wash stall walls to keep it out from under foot. The assembly consists of a shallow open channel that slopes to a trap drain at one end (or middle) of the channel. Drains along the back wall are most common, but it could be positioned along either side. A drain channel at the front of the wash stall makes sense in a stable that has aisle drainage in this location. Slope the floor with 1% to 2% slope toward the drain (up to ¼ inch per foot). Slope the gutter to the drain at 2% to 4% (up to ½ inch per foot). Provide a strong grate over the drainpipe and a trap area that is easily cleaned each time the wash stall is used. Horses are loath to step on drain grates, so a centrally located drain can be a nuisance and requires more complexity in floor slope than a monoslope floor to one wall.

Cleaning tools will be needed in the wash stall area. Secure a broom and shovel to a wall. Pick up manure as soon as it is deposited to minimize the amount that goes into the drain. Start cleanup by shoveling up as much hair and manure as possible. Sweep excess water and leftover hair and manure toward the drain. The shovel is used to clean accumulated materials from the drain. Provide a nearby disposal basket for the drain contents and collected manure and hair that can be added to the manure stockpile. Another container is convenient for discarded trash such as shampoo bottles and wraps.

Wall Materials

Wall materials will need to have strength against horse impact or kicking and be waterproof. The waterproof material is usually provided to ceiling height because splash from washing can go that high. Horse-strong materials can be to a height of 5 feet as provided in horse stalls (Fig. 13.18). Common wall materials include concrete block (either tile-glazed or painted to decrease water absorption), finished wood (painted or stained to resist water absorption), or fiberglass reinforced plastic (FRP) panels. The FRP panels are thin but strong waterproof panels common in livestock and commercial (car wash) applications for walls exposed to high-pressure washdown (Fig. 13.17). FRP panels are also resistant to mold, mildew, and bacteria growth. The FRP material is available alone or prelaminated to oriented strand board (OSB), plywood, or fluted polyethylene. FRP is also referred to as glass fiber reinforced plastic (GFRP), glass reinforced plastic (GRF), or reinforced plastic (RP). Metal

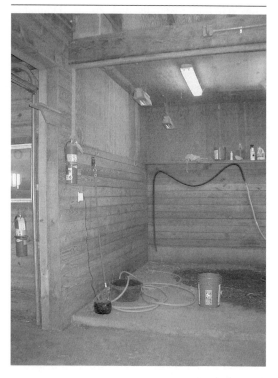

Figure 13.18. Wood kick board liner on lower portion of wall of combination grooming station/wash stall area. Note hanging radiant heaters and sealed fluorescent light fixture.

siding lined wash stalls may resist water but are not resistant to kicking and impact damage.

Heat

Radiant heaters may be positioned over the horse to provide warmth and drying potential. This is a good application of heat for instant warmth for the handler and horse while in the wash stall. If one heater is used, place it directly over and in line with the horse's back. Two heaters may be positioned one to each side of the horse with about a 3-foot distance in between. Manufacturer specifications will advise on radiant heater placement and height to achieve a desired temperature and heat pattern. The heater will have a metal reflective shield above it that directs heat downward and defines the angle of radiant heat that is distributed horizontally. This shield also provides some protection against heat damage of building materials above the heater. The manufacturer will have a recommended distance to mount the heater away from building materials and above flammable materials. Electric radiant heaters are mounted about 3 feet above the horse's back, while gas-fired radiant heaters may need more clearance. Mount heaters so that a rearing horse is not able to accidentally dislodge the heater from it mounting. Heaters should be hung from chain at each end to provide both some flexibility in mounting height and "give" should a horse hit it. Secure the chain at mounting support and at the heater with fully clamped-closed "S" hooks to minimize the risk of the heater falling when struck.

The moisture that evaporates off the horse and wash stall surfaces will need to be ventilated outside, so an exhaust fan or eave-ridge openings in the wash stall area are needed. If supplemental heat is used in the wash stall area, the warmed air is able to hold more moisture. Warmed air provides more evaporation potential than cooler air. If this warmed, moist air is allowed to migrate into cooler parts of the stable, the risk of condensation increases as the air cools and can no longer hold as much moisture. Condensation will form on cold surfaces or may even appear as a fog.

Flooring

The floor of the wash stall is most commonly concrete or asphalt with a nonslip finish. A nonslip surface can be provided with stiff broom brushed concrete finish (that wears smooth over time) or by using larger aggregate gravel in the concrete or asphalt mixture. An alternative is to trowel Carborundum or aluminum oxide chips into the surface at a rate of 1 pound per 4 square feet. Concrete and asphalt are very durable, can be sloped to drain, and provide an easy-to-clean surface. Slope the concrete floor to drain to a wall gutter of the wash stall. Rubber mats with a nonslip finish are also used as wash stall flooring (rubber mats are slippery when wet, so the nonslip finish is essential). A single mat that covers the entire wash stall is preferred to multiple mats (Fig. 13.19). Dirty wash water that gets under multiple mats via joints between mats will need a way to drain, so support multiple mats over a packed gravel or stonedust porous floor. Textured rubber mats can be installed over concrete for cushioning or over worn concrete or asphalt to increase traction. The supporting floor and rubber mat assembly needs to slope toward a drain for disposal of most of the wash water.

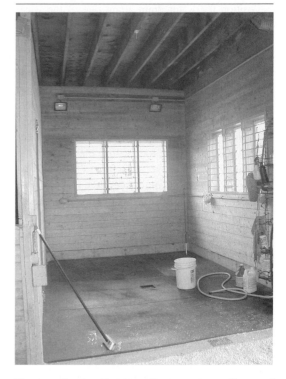

Figure 13.19. Rubber floor mat as floor of wash stall that has stained wood lining, natural light from windows protected by bars, and sealed light fixtures in front (not in view) and rear of wash stall.

VETERINARIAN AND FARRIER WORK AREA

Provide a well-lit and uncluttered area where a veterinarian and farrier can administer treatment and safely work. Ideally this area would be a relatively quiet location, near the parking space (Fig. 13.20) where their supplies and tools are kept, and have easy access to a sink or other hot water source. This area may be part of a work aisle of the stable or a dedicated space in a larger facility. A wash stall can double as the vet or farrier area because it already has a water source and good lighting. Provide cleanup materials such as clean towels, trash bucket, and manure-handling tools. Stocks for horse confinement may be included in this area. A "desktop" is appreciated by the visiting veterinarian for writing notes along with some place to keep supplies off the ground while treating a horse. For example a cart, hay bale, tack trunk, or similar device can be used for keeping suturing supplies handy.

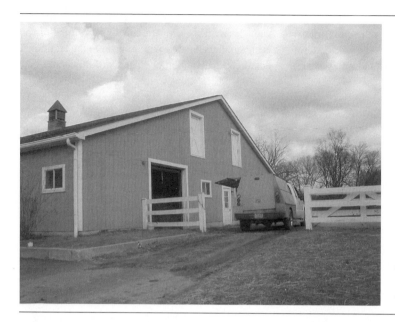

Figure 13.20. Provide a close-by parking area for the farrier and veterinarian near a well-lit work station within the stable.

Provide a light level of 70 to 100 footcandles with incandescent, quartz-halogen, and/or fluorescent light. Reduce glare by mounting lights above eye level and minimize shadows by providing more than one light source for better uniformity. As an example, for a 12-foot by 12-foot area, provide three 40-watt fluorescent fixtures (use cool white bulbs for good color rendition) and at least one duplex convenience outlet on each wall so that power cord lengths can be easily managed. These lights can be on a separate circuit to be lit during the farrier or vet visits (and during grooming station or wash stall use if the location has multiple functions). Position two of the light fixtures above and to each side of the horse position, with the third lamp in front (or rear) of the horse. A location where the horse can be positioned in more than one direction offers advantage in getting light on the subject. Additional, portable task lighting can help when light is needed low or under the horse. Some low light sources can be permanently installed when outfitted with reflectors that reduce glare at human eye level and if sufficiently protected against kicking damage. These low lights would be mounted flush in a wall behind a protective grill. Chapter 11 contains a figure with information on providing good task lighting to a wash stall or vet area.

Veterinarian and farrier evaluations of horse gait for lameness or shoeing decisions will be aided by a flat, hard surface where the horse can trot about 10 strides. An uncluttered stable aisle is often suitable as an indoor site. An outdoor driveway, paddock lane, or parking area may suffice.

CONTAINERS

Consider where to conveniently locate trash and recycling receptacles. Trash containers are likely needed in the feed room (in addition to an empty bag barrel), tack room, wash stall or grooming station, and office. Manure storage buckets for droppings collected outside the usual stall cleaning times should be located in the wash stall to minimize drain clogging and at the indoor arena where picking manure will prolong footing dust-free life. Occasional droppings in the work aisle or grooming station can be swept into nearby stalls or wash stall bucket.

SUMMARY

Several important functions of horse stabling are provided by auxiliary facilities including the feed and tack rooms, grooming and washing stalls, and storages for hay, bedding, tools, and equipment. Tack and feed rooms are constructed to exclude rodents, and it is particularly important that horses are not allowed free access to the feed. Tack is an expensive investment and is best kept in a climate controlled room to inhibit mold and mildew formation or excessive drying of leather. Provide plenty of storage space for tack and accessories, because many items are used for horse care. Hay storage may be in a separate structure or in the more traditional overhead haymow. Modern farms tend to store hay separately to reduce dust and mold in the stable and for fire safety. Wash stalls are a common feature in most commercial facilities and many private barns. This chapter contains information on each auxiliary facility with referral to the additional detail contained in other chapters of this book.

14
Fence Planning

Horse fence can be one of the most attractive features of a horse facility. But not all fences are suitable for horses. Fencing is a major capital investment that should be carefully planned before construction. A fence should keep horses on the property and keep away nuisances such as dogs and unwanted visitors. Fences aid facility management by allowing controlled grazing and segregating groups of horses according to sex, age, value, or use.

Well-constructed and maintained fences enhance the aesthetics and value of a stable facility, which in turn complements marketing efforts (Fig. 14.1). Poorly planned, haphazard, unsafe, or unmaintained fences will detract from a facility's value and reflect poor management. Good fences can be formal or informal in appearance, yet all should be well built and carefully planned. Many experienced horse owners will relay stories about the savings for cheaper, but unsafe, horse fence (barbed wire, for example) eventually being paid for in veterinary bills to treat injured horses.

Often, more than one kind of fence is used at a facility. Different fences might be installed for grazing pastures, exercise paddocks, riding areas, or for securing property lines (Fig. 14.2). Land topography influences the look, effectiveness, and installation of fencing. Consider different horse groups. Stallions, weanlings, mares, mares with foals, and geldings all have different fencing requirements.

Pasture use may range from exercise paddocks (corrals) to grazing or hay production. Paddock layout should allow for ease of management, including movement of horses, removal of manure, and care of the footing surface. Pasture design should allow field equipment, such as mowers, manure spreaders, and baling equipment, to enter and maneuver easily. This will reduce fence damage by machinery and the time needed to work in the field.

This chapter presents information useful in planning fences for horse facilities. The emphasis is on sturdy and safe horse fence.

THE BEST FENCE

Understand the purpose of a fence. The true test of a fence's worth is not when horses are peacefully grazing, but when an excited horse contacts the fence in an attempt to escape or because he never saw it during a playful romp. How will the fence and horse hold up under these conditions? A horse's natural instinct to flee from perceived danger has an effect on fence design (refer to Chapter 1). Like other livestock, horses will bolt suddenly, but because they are larger and faster, they hit the fence with more force. Also, horses fight harder than other livestock to free themselves when trapped in a fence. There are many types of effective horse fencing, but there is no "best" fence. Each fencing type has inherent tradeoffs in its features.

A "perfect" fence should be highly visible to horses. Horses are far-sighted and look to the horizon as they scan their environment for danger. Therefore, even when fencing is relatively close, it needs to be substantial enough to be visible. A fence should be secure enough to contain a horse that runs into it without causing injury or fence damage. A perfect fence should have some "give" to it to minimize injury upon impact. It should be high enough to discourage jumping and solid enough to discourage testing its strength. It should have no openings that could trap a head or hoof. The perfect fence should not have sharp edges or projections that can injure a horse that is leaning, scratching, or falling into it. It should be inexpensive to install, easy to maintain, and last 20 years or more. And finally, it should look appealing.

Unfortunately, no type of fence fits all the criteria for the perfect fence. Often there is a place for more than one type of fence on a horse facility. Stable management objectives and price ultimately determine

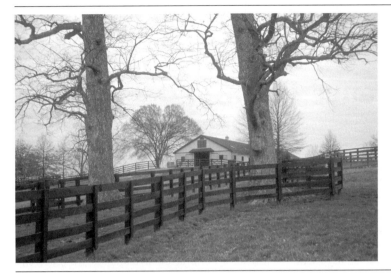

Figure 14.1. Quality horse fence adds value to a property in addition to safely confining the horses. Plenty of options exist for suitable horse fence, including the traditional board fence pictured.

which fencing is chosen. Many new fence materials and hybrids of traditional and new materials are now available. Details of fence materials and construction may be found in Chapter 15.

FEATURES THAT APPLY TO ANY FENCE TYPE

Good Planning Attributes
Planning includes more than selecting a fence type. It is best to develop an overall plan where the aesthetics, chore efficiency, management practices,

safety, and finances are considered. The best planning involves a layout drawn to scale that shows proposed gates, fence lines, where fences cross streams or other obstacles, irregular paths along a stream or obstacle, traffic routes for horses and handlers, routes for supplies and water, vehicle traffic routes, and access for mowing equipment. All these should be in relation to buildings and other farmstead features. Figures 14.3 and 14.4 show attributes of poor and good fence layouts on an example property. Chapter 4 has more detail on integrating the many features of a horse facility into a usable plan.

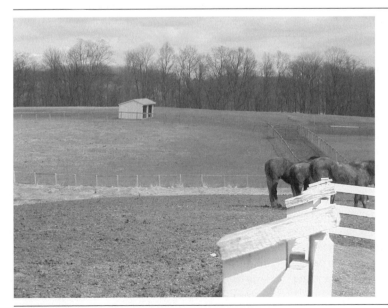

Figure 14.2. Different types of horse fence will likely be used depending on function within the property. Close fence is extra strong and visible in the heavily populated paddock near the stable. Pasture fence in the background will have less intense horse contact. Note useful lanes to get groups of horses to far pastures.

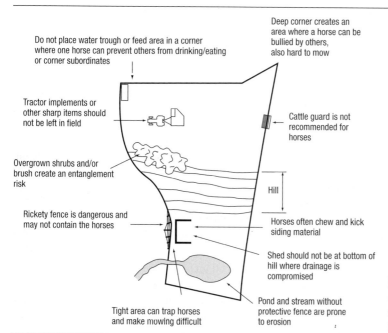

Do not place water trough or feed area in a corner where one horse can prevent others from drinking/eating or corner subordinates

Deep corner creates an area where a horse can be bullied by others, also hard to mow

Tractor implements or other sharp items should not be left in field

Cattle guard is not recommended for horses

Overgrown shrubs and/or brush create an entanglement risk

Hill

Rickety fence is dangerous and may not contain the horses

Horses often chew and kick siding material

Shed should not be at bottom of hill where drainage is compromised

Tight area can trap horses and make mowing difficult

Pond and stream without protective fence are prone to erosion

Figure 14.3. Poor fence layout showing features that can be avoided with better layout and planning.

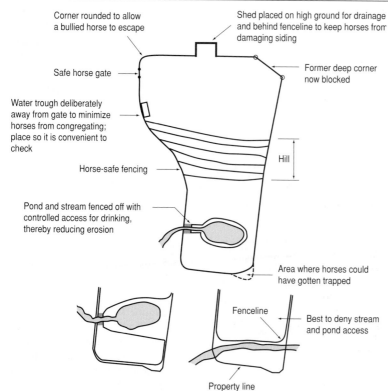

Corner rounded to allow a bullied horse to escape

Shed placed on high ground for drainage and behind fenceline to keep horses from damaging siding

Safe horse gate

Former deep corner now blocked

Water trough deliberately away from gate to minimize horses from congregating; place so it is convenient to check

Horse-safe fencing

Hill

Pond and stream fenced off with controlled access for drinking, thereby reducing erosion

Area where horses could have gotten trapped

Fenceline

Best to deny stream and pond access

Property line

Figure 14.4. Improved fence layout where thoughtful planning has improved function, safety, and drainage, while maintaining water quality.

Select and install fencing that allows easy access to pastures and does not limit performance of stable chores. Gates should be easy to operate with only one hand so the other hand is free. Fencing should also allow easy movement of groups of horses from pasture to housing facilities (Fig. 14.2). All-weather lanes should connect turnout areas to the stable. Lanes can be grassed or graveled depending on the type and amount of traffic that use them. Make sure they are wide enough to allow passage of mowing equipment and vehicles. Vehicles such as cars, light trucks, and tractors can be up to 8 feet wide. Farm equipment needs 12- to 16-feet-wide lanes to comfortably negotiate. Narrower lane widths are acceptable for smaller tractors or mowing equipment. Remember to leave room for snow storage or removal along the sides of lanes and roads.

It is best to eliminate fence corners and dead-end areas when enclosing a pasture for more than one horse. By curving the corners, it is less likely that a dominant horse will trap a subordinate. Round corners are relatively common for board fencing installations and, although more difficult to construct, are highly recommended for wire fences. Chapter 15 contains construction information on rounded corners.

Most wire fencing is installed with the wire under tension as part of the design strength of the fence. This tension may be modest, just enough to keep the wire straight and evenly spaced throughout seasonal temperature changes in wire length, or may be quite substantial, as with high-tensile wire fence. With tensioned fencing, rounded corners may not be as strong or durable as square ones. A slight outward tilt of support posts on curved corners can help resist the inward forces of the tensioned wire. Position the tensioned wire on the outside of the fence post as it travels around the curve, then back to the inside (horse side) on the straight sections. It is possible to build square corners for tension fences and use boards to prevent horses from getting into the corner. This creates areas that limit grazing, requiring regular mowing, but it is cheaper to construct than curved corners.

Good Fence Attributes

Figure 14.5 shows features of a good horse fence made from solid rail material. Horse fences should be 54 to 60 inches above ground level. A good rule for paddocks and pastures is to have the top of the fence at wither height to ensure that horses will not flip over the fence. Larger horses, stallions, or those adept at jumping may require even taller fences. At the bottom, an 8-inch clearance will leave enough room to avoid trapping a hoof yet will discourage a horse from reaching under the fence for grass. A bottom rail with clearance no higher than 12 inches will prevent foals from rolling under the fence. Fence clearance varies with fence types. Higher clearances allow small animals, such as dogs, to enter the pasture. Fences should be built with particular attention to fence post integrity. Several fence material manufacturers

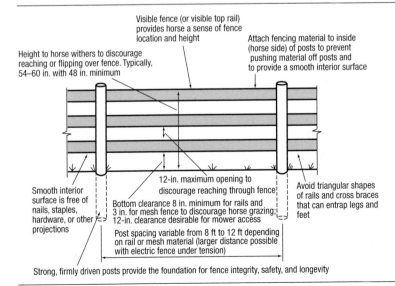

Figure 14.5. Attributes of a good horse fence (nonelectric). No matter what fence rail material is used, horse safety and fence sturdiness are important.

provide good detailed guides to assist in construction and material selection.

Fence openings should be either large enough to offer little chance of foot, leg, and head entrapment or so small that hooves cannot get through. Small, safe openings are less than 3 inches square but can depend on the size of the horse. Tension fences, such as the types that use high-tensile wires, usually have diagonal cross-bracing on corner assemblies. These diagonal wires or wood bracing provide triangular spaces for foot and head entrapment. Good fence design denies horse access to the braced area or at least minimizes hazards if entrapment occurs.

Horses will test fence strength deliberately and casually. Horses often reach through or over fences for attractions on the other side; thus, sturdy fences are essential. Fences that do not allow this behavior are the safest. Keep open space between rails or strands to 12 inches or less. For electric fences, this open distance may be increased to 18 inches because horses avoid touching the fence. With most fence, and particularly with paddock and perimeter fence, a single strand of electric wire can be run 4 to 6 inches above or just inside the top rail to discourage horses who habitually lean, scratch, or reach over fences.

The fence should be smooth on the horse side to prevent injury. Fasten rails and wire mesh to the inside (horse side) of the posts. This also strengthens the fence. If a horse leans on the fence, its weight will not push out the fasteners. Nails and other fasteners should be smooth without jagged parts that can cut the horse or catch a halter.

Visible fences will prevent playful horses from accidentally running into them. A frightened horse may still hit a visible fence while he is blinded with fear. A forgiving fence that contains the horse without injury is better than an unyielding brick wall. Wire fences are the least visible, so boards or strips of material are often added (Fig. 14.6).

FENCE POST SELECTION

The fence post is the foundation of the fence, so its importance cannot be overemphasized. The common element in virtually all successful horse fences is a wooden post. Setting posts represents the hardest work and the most time-consuming part of fence building and is absolutely the most critical to the long-term success of the fence.

Driven posts are more rigid and therefore recommended over handset posts or those set in predrilled holes. Driven posts are pounded into the ground through a combination of weight and impact by specialized equipment. The principle behind driven posts that makes them so secure is that the displaced soil is highly compacted around the post, resisting post movement. Even for do-it-yourself projects, you should contract the job of driving posts. Post

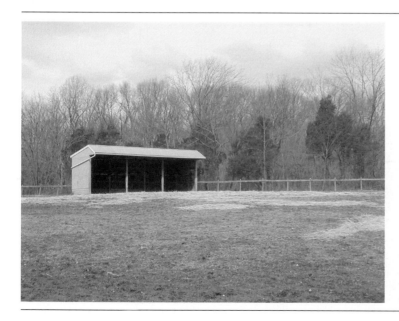

Figure 14.6. Wire mesh horse fence is a safe and sturdy option but benefits from a highly visible top rail of wood or vinyl.

driver equipment may be difficult to rent because of liability concerns. Under some dry, hard, or rocky soil conditions, a small-bore hole will be necessary for driven posts. Chapter 15 has detail of fence post materials, size, and placement.

GATES

Gate Design

Gates should have the same strength, safety, and height as the fence. Gates can be up to 16 feet wide, with a minimum of 12 feet to allow easy passage of vehicles and tractors. Horse and handler gates should be no less than 4 feet wide, with 5 feet preferred. Human-only passages are useful for chore time efficiency.

Fencing Near Gates

Fencing near gates needs to withstand the pressures of horses congregating around the gate, which means it needs to be sturdy, highly visible, and safe from trapping horse feet and heads. Some paddock gates are positioned to swing into the pressure of the horse to prevent horses from pushing the gate open and breaking latches. On the other hand, gates that are capable of swinging both into and out of the enclosure are helpful when moving horses. Additional latches are recommended to secure the gate in an open position, fully swung against the fence and not projecting into the enclosure.

Gate Location

In most horse operation, gates are positioned toward the middle of a fenceline because horses are individually moved in and out of the enclosure. This eliminates trapping horses in a corner near a gate. On operations where groups of horses are herded more often than individually led, gates positioned at corners will assist in driving horses along the fenceline and out of the enclosure. Place pasture gates opposite each other across an alley (Fig. 14.7). Gates that open to create a fenced chute between two pastures will aid horse movement.

Fencing along driveways and roads has to provide room to maneuver vehicles to access gates. Entry driveway surfaces are often 16 feet wide with at least 7 feet on each side for snow removal, snow storage, and clearance for large vehicles. Remember that when driving through a gate while towing equipment, substantial room may be needed to turn between fencelines. A tractor towing a manure spreader or hay wagon will use 16 to 25 feet, respectively, to make a 90-degree turn. The easiest option is to position gates so that machinery can drive straight through the gate. Position gates where good visibility along a road will provide safety for slowly moving horse trailers and farm equipment that are entering and exiting the road. Place gates at least 40 to 60 feet from a road to allow parking off the road while opening the gate.

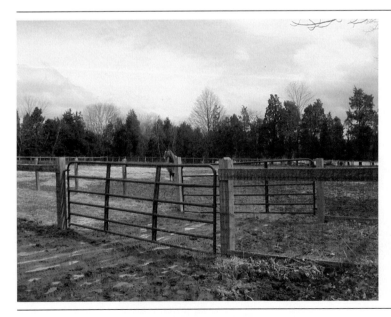

Figure 14.7. Gate top rail should be of same height as horse fence and mounted on sturdier posts than along fenceline. Gates in this double fence are lined up to provide easy equipment access between fields.

SPECIAL FENCE AREAS

Crowded Areas

Strong and safe fencing should be used where many horses congregate or crowd each other, such as near gates, feed and water stations, or shelters. In areas where horses are not often in contact with the fence, such as in very large pastures, a less substantial fence can suffice. Stronger fencing is needed when there are attractions on the other side, such as better grass or equine companions.

Controlled Grazing

Controlled, or rotational, grazing of pasture grasses demands that some areas periodically remain without grazing for regrowth of the grass. If temporary or cross-fencing is used to designate controlled sections, it should be just as safe for the horses as the permanent perimeter fence. Temporary fence does not have to be quite as impenetrable because the perimeter fence will eventually contain a loose horse (Fig. 14.8). A younger or inexperienced horse will need to be introduced to electric fence used in a controlled grazing system.

All-Weather Paddock

A good management tool for horse facilities on limited acreage is to provide at least one all-weather paddock for foul weather turnout. Also known as a rainy-day or sacrifice paddock, this paddock takes the worst wear during unfavorable weather conditions while attempting to preserve the grass of the remaining paddocks. Because turf is easily destroyed during wet conditions, the unfortunate paddock should have an all-weather surface (see "All-Weather Surface" sidebar). It is to be used for those horses that have to be turned out of their stalls despite the weather. This paddock should have safe and sturdy fencing and should be located on well-drained high ground accessible to the stable. Because it will be an ungrassed exercise lot, it is beneficial to locate or screen it away from the more public areas of the stable. Horse contact with the paddock fence is more likely because it is smaller and horses are more likely to be running and playing in it.

Perimeter Fence

Many farms make sure that any loose horse cannot leave the property through the use of perimeter

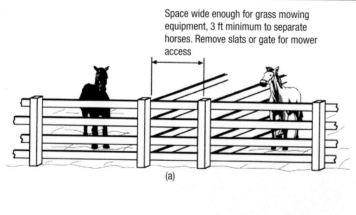

Space wide enough for grass mowing equipment, 3 ft minimum to separate horses. Remove slats or gate for mower access

(a)

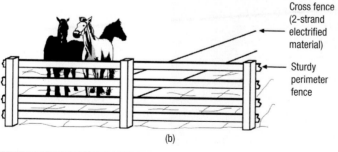

Cross fence (2-strand electrified material)

Sturdy perimeter fence

(b)

Figure 14.8. (a) Double fence to discourage horse activity through and over fence in adjoining paddocks. (b) A simple cross-fence is often suitable for adjacent paddocks used for controlled gazing.

fencing around the entire complex. This fence (and/or gates) fills the gaps at the end of access lanes and often surrounds the public entry side of the facility. Containment of loose horses becomes more important as traffic and neighbors increase around the horse facility. Sometimes the perimeter fence functions to keep human and canine intruders away from the horses. Perimeter fence does not have to be of the same construction as paddock or pasture fence because it should have limited contact with unsupervised horses, but it should be visible and strong.

Double Fence

An alternate fencing scheme favored by some farms is to double fence so that each paddock has its own fence with an alley between (Fig. 14.9). Gates can be positioned across from each other in each of the double fencelines to allow a direct transfer of horses between paddocks when both gates are opened across the alley between (Fig. 14.7). Double fencing is almost always used with stallions and particularly valuable stock. Other applications include boarding or training facilities where horses are worked and stabled individually so they are not allowed to socialize. Social and antisocial activity over the fence may be virtually eliminated with double fencing. A combination double fence and perimeter fence may be used where human contact with

horses is discouraged, such as along public roads and residential boundary lines. The first fence keeps the horse in, and the second fence keeps unwanted visitors away from direct horse contact.

Terrain

Some sections of the site may be too steep or rocky for pasture use, or the soil may be unsuitable for adequate grass growth. Soils that do not drain readily will cause wet areas that become eyesores. It is suggested to fence horses out of unsuitable sites, including swampy areas and streams. Contact the U.S. Natural Resources Conservation Service or your local Cooperative Extension office for soil information on your acreage and recommendations for types of pasture vegetation to use on the site. *Pasture and Hay for Horses* provides good information and recommendations (see Additional Resources).

Fence for Stream Bank Preservation

As population density in rural areas grow, more attention is paid to environmental impact. Good land stewardship is essential to the health of the environment and positive public perceptions of agricultural endeavors. Pollutants such as animal waste and sediment from small streams find their way into larger waterways and bodies of water. Stream banks within pastured areas are very susceptible to erosion if not properly protected. Pastured animals that

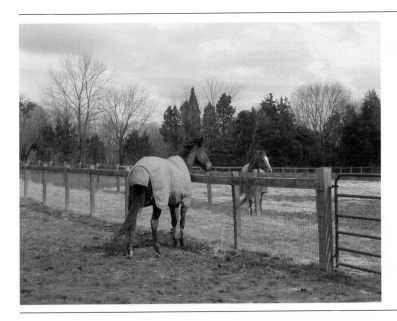

Figure 14.9. Example of double fence with room for grass maintenance in lane between.

travel along the bank kill the vegetation that is desperately needed for soil support. If left unsupported, the bank itself will begin to crumble and flood damage (erosion) will be intensified. The small silt particles in the soil, which make up a large percentage of stream pollutants, can be carried by the stream for miles.

It is recommended that stream banks be fenced off at least 15 feet from the stream on each side to allow a protective vegetative strip to grow. The fence prevents animals from trampling the banks, thereby reducing bank erosion and sedimentation downstream. This vegetated strip acts to stabilize the stream bank while filtering water runoff and trapping sediment, pesticides, and excess nutrients. Animal access for drinking and crossing can be provided through stream crossings or access sites. Planned crossings provide suitable access to the water while minimizing the risk of injury to the horse (Fig. 14.10). To minimize erosion, a gentle ramp is cut into the stream bank at a specific slope (maximum 4:1 to 6:1, depending on footing). The ramp floor is made with a 6- to 12-inch layer of packed rock or crushed stones and may be terraced with railroad ties to help contain the footing. The walls of the ramp that parallel the stream must also have a gentle slope (less than 2:1) to slow the speed of water runoff and prevent footing from being washed away. The length of the ramp depends on the height of the stream bank in relation to the streambed. The greater the difference, the longer the ramp will need to be.

Each stream crossing is different and should be engineered for that particular crossing. Individual design incorporates many important factors that will aid in the longevity and functionality of the crossing. Financial assistance for design and construction may be available through foundations dedicated to protection of watershed quality. Stream bank crossings may require a general permit. The local conservation district can be contacted for information about obtaining this permit. (See phone book's blue government pages under "State Government.")

Trees

Trees should be fenced off. Horses usually strip off tree bark left within their reach, and dead branches pose a safety hazard. Some trees are poisonous to horses, while dead limbs can impale them.

Buildings

It is best to fence horses away from contact with buildings. Horses kicking, chewing, and scratching on exterior siding will damage the building materials. For metal-sided buildings there is risk of the horse being cut on exposed metal edges or from kicking through. Regardless of this, metal siding is easily dented by even casual horse contact. Providing a fence rail around pasture shelters located in the middle of a field is recommended (Fig. 14.11), but remember to provide access for mowing and/or weed-trimming equipment. Locating the shelter within the fenceline is another good option (Fig. 14.12). A human-sized fence gap will allow entry to check shelter conditions without need for a gate. Chapter 15 presents sizing for human fence gap construction options.

COMMON FENCING QUESTIONS

How Much Area Needs to Be Enclosed?

Horses may be kept inside most of the time and only turned out for exercise a few hours daily. In some cases, horses are turned out individually rather than

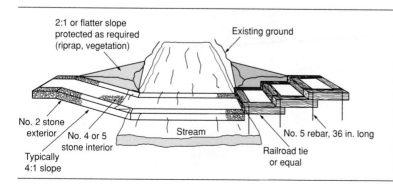

2:1 or flatter slope protected as required (riprap, vegetation)

Existing ground

No. 2 stone exterior

No. 4 or 5 stone interior

Typically 4:1 slope

Stream

No. 5 rebar, 36 in. long

Railroad tie or equal

Figure 14.10. Examples of stream bank crossings that protect stream from erosion and provide safe passage for horses. Each crossing needs to be evaluated on the basis of specific site characteristics.

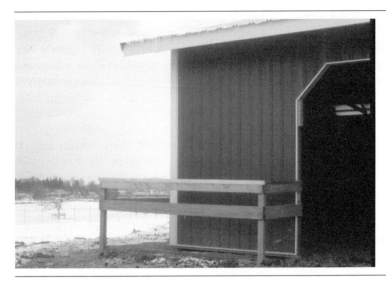

Figure 14.11. Fence horses away from contact with building exterior unless it is designed for horse contact. Metal-sided buildings need to have horses fenced away from the sheet metal that is easily dented by horse activity ·and will not withstand kicking abuse.

in groups. This means more, and perhaps smaller paddocks, are required, which increases the amount of fencing. An all-weather paddock may serve to exercise several horses, in succession, each day. Moving horses between turnout and stable should be convenient.

Rectangular areas are more relaxing for a group of horses. Square pastures take less fencing. For example, 800 feet of fencing is needed for a 200-foot square area, versus 1000 feet of fencing needed for a 400-foot by 100-foot enclosure of the same area. Straight fences on level ground are faster to build and easier to maintain than fencing covering rough terrain.

Plan an average of 2 to 5 acres per horse for grazing without supplemental feed. This prescription works well during the grass-growing season of the northeastern United States. Most horses are provided supplemental feed and do not depend entirely on pasture grazing, so acreage per horse becomes less relevant. Acreage needed then depends on the size of turnout paddocks for exercise, and space for riding areas and stables.

In overstocked and overgrazed pastures, topsoil erodes as the vegetation is trampled away. Additionally, horse manure is easily transported into nearby areas via water runoff. It is important to

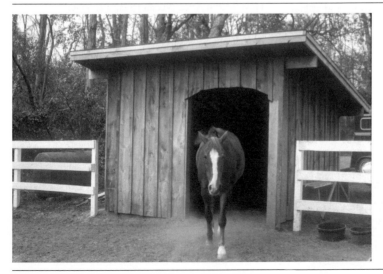

Figure 14.12. Install pasture shelters flush with the fence-line for simple protection of the shelter's exterior building components. A small human-sized gap between fence and shelter wall allows easy access for checking conditions within the shelter.

contain this runoff so that it does not cause pollution. If topography permits, vegetated areas around the perimeter of ungrassed paddocks may be enough to filter and absorb runoff. Substantial grading of the site will be needed to divert, and possibly store, runoff from large, ungrassed lots. Daily manure removal from the paddocks for storage elsewhere will reduce the concentration of potential pollutants in the runoff.

Why Is the Horse Outside the Fence?

Horses are herd animals, usually desiring other equine companions. They can test fence strength in an attempt to join neighbors, especially when a horse is kept alone. Other social pressures and overstocking instill a similar desire to get to the other side of the fence. If the grass really is greener on the other side, expect horse attempts to get to it. Strong, solid-looking fences usually provide adequate protection. Make sure the horse cannot climb the fence, and social and antisocial activity over the fence will not lead to injuries. Preventing this activity is recommended, but realize that most fence will suffer damage from even innocent horse pastimes such as scratching, chewing, pawing, and playing. Loose wires or boards make it easier for a horse to escape. Maintenance should be factored into the total cost of a fence installation. When electric fencing is chosen, make sure that horses are safely contained during times when the current is off.

How Much Is Reasonable to Spend on Fencing?

Attractive fences tend to be more expensive. In general, safer fencing is also higher in cost. Some types of fence have a higher initial cost but significantly less maintenance cost and a long life. Some savings are gained by placing the aesthetically pleasing fencing along the public side of the property, while less attractive, yet equally functional, fencing can be used in more remote locations.

Save costs by installing fence yourself, buying fence materials in large lot sizes or shopping for reasonably priced and locally available materials. Availability and prices for materials vary widely. Keep in mind that some types of fencing are difficult to install properly without specialized equipment, such as wire stretchers and post drivers. Books and fence material manufacturers' literature are available to explain details of construction.

New fencing materials are appearing on the market every year. Price and warranty can vary among manufacturers and installers. Shop around to learn the benefits and drawbacks of different fences. Ask for references from both fence dealers and installers to determine whom to contact for future fence problems. Visit farms with different types of fencing, and talk with the manager about impressions and concerns. A well-designed and carefully selected fence will increase the amount of time you spend with your horse compared with time spent mending the horse and fence.

FENCE LAYOUT EXAMPLE

Start fence layout planning with a scaled drawing of the farm and its current features. Include overall distances and special features that need to be fenced around. An affinity diagram allows a perspective on what features need to be near other features at the facility (Fig. 14.13). This part of the planning process is not concerned with exactly where fences and gates will be, but it emphasizes general areas of use on the site. In the figure, note that turnout paddocks are conveniently located near the stable, while larger pastures may be farther away. Include a service area that contains manure storage and other

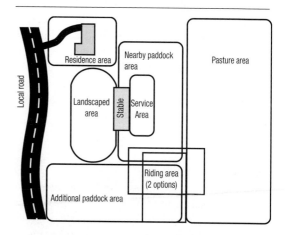

Figure 14.13. An affinity diagram is used to plan location of features that need to be near each other for efficient stable function. Plan for nearby turnout paddocks that have multiple sessions of exercising horses. Pastures or paddocks with horses turned out all day, or longer, can be farther away from the stable.

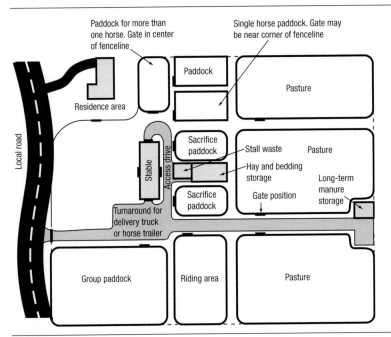

Single horse paddock. Gate may be near corner of fenceline

Paddock for more than one horse. Gate in center of fenceline

Paddock

Pasture

Residence area

Local road

Sacrifice paddock

Stable

Access drive

Stall waste

Pasture

Hay and bedding storage

Long-term manure storage

Sacrifice paddock

Gate position

Turnaround for delivery truck or horse trailer

Group paddock

Riding area

Pasture

Figure 14.14. A public stable fence layout may include an option for perimeter fence and plenty of space for visitor's vehicle access. Because the horse population may change frequently, fencing should keep horses that are unfamiliar with each other in separate paddocks and double fencing should be used where horses will be kept in adjacent paddocks. Typically, a residence is separated from the commercial facility for enhanced privacy.

features that are not generally considered attractive. Locate the service area away from public view, if possible, and close to the stable for chore efficiency. Chapter 4 has more detailed information on using affinity diagram.

Private and public stables have different fence layout objectives, particularly in relation to vehicle traffic flow and access to the residence. Figures 14.14 and 14.15 take the features from Figure 14.13 and provide a layout appropriate for public and private stable sites, respectively. Both figures show fenceline positions and gate locations for convenient access to the stable.

All-Weather Surface

Grassed paddocks will not survive under all-weather conditions. Horse weight on sharp hooves tears even the best sod under soggy ground conditions. Sandy soil and high-traffic areas are impossible to keep in grass. Some paddocks will likely need to be sacrificed to all-weather use; hence the term "sacrifice paddock" or more appropriately "all-weather paddock." Mud used to prevail in these unfortunate grounds but an all-weather surface is a better

alternative for horse well-being and owner satisfaction. The paddock is designed to remain dry and mud-free under all-weather conditions.

An all-weather paddock provides a well-draining surface material over a base that can shed water. Not all paddock locations can serve this purpose. Choose paddocks on higher ground; buildings and riding arenas will likely be located on the best drainage locations. Where possible, locate all-weather paddocks away from public view because they will not be pleasantly grassed. They resemble an outdoor riding arena surface when well managed and so are not as unsightly as a muddy paddock.

Most topsoil and all sod is removed from all-weather paddocks to allow delivered stonedust, coarse sand, or fine gravel to be supplied as the surface. Slope or crown the base to shed water and divert any incoming water from the all-weather paddock(s) area. Provision of a geotextile layer between the delivered material and original base material is useful to keep the layers separate. Do not expect significant water to drain through the geotextile (because it clogs), and so slope base surface to drain accordingly. Apply a 2- to 4-inch layer of delivered material

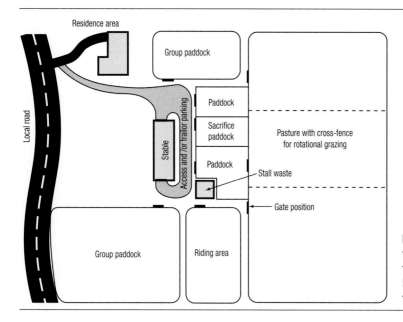

Figure 14.15. A private facility will often have less fluctuation in population of horses so that horses can be turned out together.

as the paddock surface. *Pick up manure droppings to prolong the useful surface life without manure mud and decomposed manure dust. A grid or paver assembly may be added to help hold the surface material in place in especially high-traffic areas, such as near the gate. See "Pavers for Mud Control" sidebar in Chapter 4 for more information.*

The all-weather paddock is valuable for allowing horse exercise at liberty during all weather conditions because it will not be muddy-slick or frozen into potholes of nonnegotiable mud formations. If daily turnout of horses is needed under intensive conditions, then all-weather paddocks are needed. For some farm management situations, the all-weather surface may only be needed near areas where many horses congregate, along horse or light vehicle travel lanes, where managers need to walk, or in enclosures that provide access to multiple pastures from a common shed or feeding location. Locate gate and feeding area on high ground relative to the rest of the all-weather paddock.

SUMMARY

The most time-intensive part of fence building takes place before any ground is broken. Thoughtful fence planning and layout will help make daily chores and routines more efficient. The best fence differs from facility to facility and even within a horse property; different fence types are used to meet the objectives of the enclosure. Good fence design emphasizes a proper foundation, or post integrity. By taking the time to understand a facility's fencing needs and expectations, you can provide a safe, functional fence that will provide years of service and enhance the property's value.

15
Fence Materials

CHOOSING A FENCE TYPE

Fences may be categorized by type or style of construction, such as board, mesh, and strand. These categories are helpful when considering fence function and how it looks. Traditionally, fences have been discussed in terms of materials. Common fences often incorporate one or more materials such as wood, steel, "plastic," and rubber or nylon. In addition, electricity, although not a material, is a component of several successful fence types. Many modern and safe horse fences are hybrids of traditional and new technology materials.

Horses are capable of destruction of virtually any type of fence. Destruction may be casual with normal horse behavior such as leaning over the top, reaching through for grass, trying to jump the fence, rubbing an itch, kicking at a horse in an adjacent paddock, pawing in frustration near a gate, or running into the fence during play or in fear. Horses are large, strong animals and not many fencing materials are truly strong enough to contain all this activity. Conversely, almost any fence is capable of injuring the horse when he leans, reaches, kicks, paws, rubs, or runs into the fence. Good fence design and construction tries to minimize the amount of damage to horse and fence during normally expected activity. Horse injuries from fences seem to occur when new individuals are introduced into the paddock population. Reestablishment of social order creates enough chaos that chasing and chased horses end up tangled in fencing.

An early decision in selection of fence type will be whether electric shock or substantial fence construction will be the primary fence design feature for enclosing the horse. In the past, substantial fences were the norm; now trends are shifting to electric shock as a primary or an added feature of horse fencing. The incorporation of electric shock as an integral design feature is to teach the horse to "respect" the fence, which essentially means to not contact the fence in any fashion, thus eliminating the long list of normal behaviors that destroy fencing. Even some of the most substantial fences incorporate one or two electrified lines to keep horses at a distance from the fence.

OVERVIEW OF FENCE OPTIONS

Wood board, or estate, fence is the classic beauty of horse fencing, while post and rail is a more rustic alternative. Other fence types incorporate wood as posts and visibility boards at the top. Wood fence is the first choice for many horse facilities owing to its safety and aesthetics. With new preservative treatments, wood fences can last longer with less care than they used to. A drawback of wood is that it can splinter and injure a horse. Properly installed, however, a wood fence generally poses little threat to the horse that it confines. Be aware that the horse may pose a threat to the fence if he is a confirmed wood chewer. Most horses chew on wood and can substantially damage wood fences. Horses are especially fond of soft wood such as spruce, fir, and pine and tend to chew less on hard wood such as oak. Wood chewers can be deterred with an electric wire strand or lumber protected by metal (without sharp edges) or plastic guards on the edges.

Metal horse fencing options include wire mesh, wire strands, steel pipe, and cable. Electric fencing also falls into this broad category. Although not an option with all metal type fences, keeping the fence "hot" (electrified) often discourages contact and decreases the incidence of injuries of wire strand fences. Metal fences, such as horse mesh, comprise some of the safest horse fences, and other types, such as barbed wire, are among the most dangerous. Barbed wire should not be used with horses because of the severe injury caused by horse entanglement. A frightened or fleeing horse may not be deterred by wire strand fence. Strand fences generally lack visibility, and most horses will fight if entangled. Some newer wire-based fence designs provide enhanced visibility through the combination of wire and other more visible synthetic materials. The common, woven wire stock fences, with 4-inch or greater squares, should not be used for horses in small paddocks because of the danger of entrapped legs and the associated lacerations.

Synthetic fence products are increasing in number and quality as new applications and materials are identified. Synthetic fences come in many formats including those made of rigid material that simulates the look of traditional wood board fence or of woven fabric-like materials that incorporate electric wires. Some synthetic fence designs offer a secure and safe fence that is attractive to look at, often with reduced cost, compared with more traditional horse fencing materials. Proponents point to enhanced visibility compared with metal fencing and maintenance-free materials compared with wood. Vinyl and other "poly" fencing products had initial problems with designs that allowed the normal temperature expansion and contraction of materials to pop rails out of the posts. Early rigid poly fence rails shattered into sharp pieces when broken. For rigid vinyl fence material, some discoloration and brittleness occurred with exposure to sunlight; squeaks during breezy conditions spooked unaccustomed horses. Look for ultraviolet (UV)-stabilized synthetic products for longer material life. These are points that should be discussed with synthetic horse fence manufacturers. Design, manufacturing, and material improvements have overcome many of the problems discussed earlier.

Comparing Fences

Shop around to learn the benefits and drawbacks of the fences you may be interested in installing. Arrange to visit farms with different types of fencing and talk with the manager about their impressions, concerns, and advice. A well-designed and carefully selected fence will increase the amount of time you spend with your horse, not doctoring the horse and the fence. Prices and warrantees vary between fence material manufactures and installers. Be sure that you know whom to contact in case you should have a problem with the fence in the future. Ask for references from both the fence dealer and installer if you are not installing the fence yourself.

The most time-intensive part of fence building takes place before any ground is broken. By taking the time to understand your fencing needs and expectations, you increase the chances of having a safe, functional fence that will provide years of service. Chapter 14 covers aspects of fence layout in relation to facility management and safety. Sizing and placement of gates are covered more thoroughly in that chapter.

BOARD-STYLE FENCE

Wood Board

Board fences grace some of the most attractive horse farms in the country. They are highly visible and relatively safe. Many variations on this fence exist depending on board thickness, board number and spacing, type of posts, species of wood, and color. Figure 15.1 shows attributes and overall dimensions of safe and sturdy board-style horse fence. They can be painted white or black or left to naturally weather. Painting or staining every few years maintains the condition of board fences; otherwise a properly installed board fence is fairly maintenance free. Board fence is an expensive fence to build and one of the most time consuming to install properly. It is also one of the safest fences. Black creosote is cheaper than white paint, and a black fence under repair usually looks better than a white fence of similar condition.

Fence strength depends on the wood species and lumber dimensions and how the assembly is fastened together. For example, hardwoods are stronger, for the same size, than softwoods. Fence posts can be square, round, or partial round in cross section (see the "posts" selection of this chapter). Board thickness is usually 1-inch rough-cut for hardwoods such as oak or 2-inch nominal for pressure-treated softwoods. Weathered oak boards are very hard and when broken tend to splinter into long jagged pieces. Pine boards break more cleanly and are therefore preferred for fencing young stock. Protect softwoods with an electrified wire strand or edge protection because horses easily chew through softwood boards, which compromises fence strength, is unsightly, and costly for frequent board replacement. Board width of 6 inches is common and looks most balanced. Board spacing based on increments of this width is the most pleasing to the eye: space boards 6, 9, or 12 inches apart (Fig. 15.2). Usually, all rails are the same distance apart. One attractive variation positions the top two rails closer together. Do not use diamond or cross-patterned rails because these provide narrow angles to catch feet and heads.

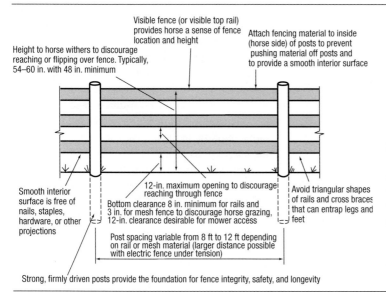

Visible fence (or visible top rail) provides horse a sense of fence location and height

Attach fencing material to inside (horse side) of posts to prevent pushing material off posts and to provide a smooth interior surface

Height to horse withers to discourage reaching or flipping over fence. Typically, 54–60 in. with 48 in. minimum

Smooth interior surface is free of nails, staples, hardware, or other projections

12-in. maximum opening to discourage reaching through fence

Bottom clearance 8 in. minimum for rails and 3 in. for mesh fence to discourage horse grazing, 12-in. clearance desirable for mower access

Avoid triangular shapes of rails and cross braces that can entrap legs and feet

Post spacing variable from 8 ft to 12 ft depending on rail or mesh material (larger distance possible with electric fence under tension)

Strong, firmly driven posts provide the foundation for fence integrity, safety, and longevity

Figure 15.1. A safe, sturdy horse fence has attributes described here. Electrified fence construction is more variable with larger open spaces between wire strands or flexible synthetic material strands and much longer distances possible with strands under high tension.

Posts are set such that fence panels are about 8 feet long. Boards are positioned on the inside (horse side) of the fence post. This discourages horses from scratching on posts, which loosens them. Rails nailed on the inside mean that horse pressure on the fence works with fastener strength rather than pushing them out. Nails that protrude are a safety hazard of board fence design. A face board on top of the nailed ends provides increased strength and safety by prohibiting board ends from becoming loose projections. Board length is usually 16 feet so that they span two fence panels. Post spacing of a couple of inches less than 8 feet allows for board ends to be trimmed for a finished look. Boards are staggered so that alternate boards end at each post.

A three-board, 9-inch spaced board fence is adequate for mares and geldings. The smaller size of foals and ponies demands a fourth, lower board and

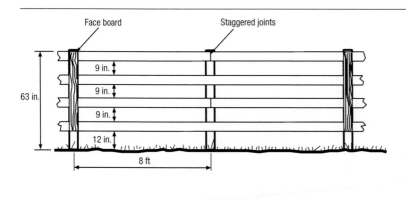

Face board

Staggered joints

9 in.

9 in.

9 in.

12 in.

63 in.

8 ft

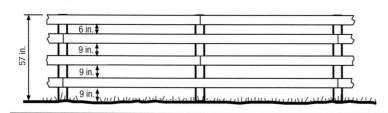

6 in.

9 in.

9 in.

9 in.

57 in.

Figure 15.2. Wood board fence dimensions. Board width of 6 inches appears balanced with spacing between boards of 6, 9, or 12 inches. Board length of 16 feet allows post spacing up to 8 feet apart.

6-inch spacing. Fence height should be no less than 4 feet for placid animals. Stallions require at least a 5 feet high, five-board fence. Some horsemen feel that board fencing is not as suitable as horse mesh wire fencing for breeding stock, including broodmares, who can become aggressive or protective at times. Mares kicking or otherwise defending territory across board fence can become entrapped or injured.

Rigid Polymer Board

High-grade polyvinylchloride (PVC) has a long life span, with companies offering 15- to 25-year warranties. Many designs resemble whitewashed plank fence and are manufactured specifically for horse use (Fig. 15.3). It has virtually no maintenance because it does not require periodic painting, staining, or tightening. Horses will not chew on it; decay and insects will not destroy it. PVC fence semirigid material is very strong, yet it will absorb some of the impact of a horse hitting it. If it does break, horse fence grade PVC does not splinter. PVC and other polymer fence materials, such as high-density polyethylene (HDPE), needs to be treated with UV light inhibitors to resist discoloration and brittleness, either during or after molding into fence post and board stock. For all these features, PVC has the most expensive purchase price of all fences. However, when construction, material, and maintenance costs are considered over a 5- to 20-year period, the PVC fence becomes cost competitive because of its minimal maintenance.

Although the material itself is strong, the PVC fence post and rail assembly does not withstand normal horse activity, and so it needs to be protected with an electrified line(s) to discourage horse contact. Generally, PVC fence should be used for decorative purpose and is not recommended for enclosing horses or livestock unless electrified.

The PVC fence is built in 8-foot sections. The boards (1½ inch by 5½ inch or 1½ inch by 6 inch) and posts (5 inch by 5 inch) are usually hollow-core PVC with dimensions similar to wooden boards. Posts are often set into concrete, which increases installation time and cost. The PVC material expands and contracts, and hence changes length, with temperature fluctuation; therefore this must be taken into consideration during assembly. Boards are set in sleeves with a gap between them, rather than being nailed onto the post. This loose assembly is what allows horses to dismantle the fence. Variations in PVC fence stock exist, so that rails can be round rather than board shaped or in colors other than white.

Post and Rail

Wood post and rail fences have a rustic attractiveness that is highly visible (Fig. 15.4). They are sturdy and yet will yield a bit on impact. They are relatively

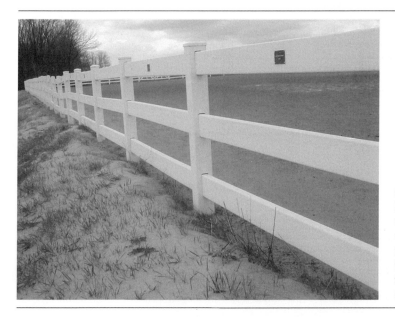

Figure 15.3. PVC rigid board fence is manufactured with the appearance of white board fence. PVC offers a low-maintenance fence but needs an electrified strand to withstand horse use.

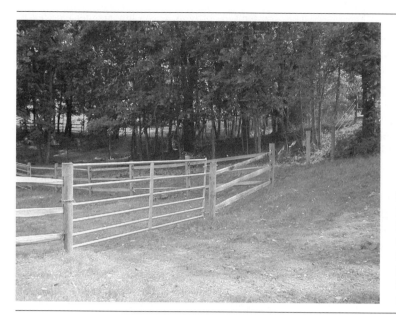

Figure 15.4. Wooden split rail fence offers a safe, visible fence that is particularly attractive in rustic or rough topography. It benefits from an electrified strand to keep horses from working the rails loose.

easy to install, have low maintenance, and are fairly expensive. With their more rustic appearance, they provide a nicely finished fence even on rough topography where the straight-line construction of a board fence may accentuate the ups and downs of the uneven terrain. Their construction eliminates the hazard of protruding nails in wood board fence.

Like board fences, they need at least three rails to contain horses (Fig. 15.5). For foals, the bottom rail should be no higher than 12 inches off the ground. Fence height should be at least 4 feet, and up to 5 feet, for jumpers and stallions. Fence panels are typically 8 to 10 feet long. Pressure-treated lumber and cedar may be used.

Much of post and rail fence safety and strength depends on proper installation. The posts have to provide firm, undisturbed support over the lifetime of the fence; otherwise rails will work loose as the post changes position. Soils that experience frost heaving or settlement will not be suitable for this type of fencing. Rails are placed into the appropriate holes in the post, and then the posts are tamped firmly into place. Rather than using nails to fasten the fence together, post and rail fence depends on juxtaposed pressure of two rails in one hole. The rails need to be installed tight enough so that the ends will not come out upon horse impact or contact. Loose rails present a hazard similar to a spear.

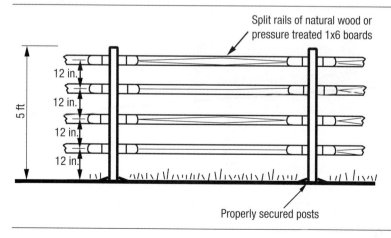

Split rails of natural wood or pressure treated 1x6 boards

5 ft

12 in.
12 in.
12 in.
12 in.

Properly secured posts

Figure 15.5. Split rail or slip rail fence with four rails at 12-inch open spacing satisfies horse fence height (48 inches) and rail spacing requirement.

Slip Rail

Wood slip rail fences are a hybrid of board and post and rail. Posts have holes that accept boards instead of rails. This provides a fence that is more forgiving on impact than board but does not have the spear-like quality of the rails. Slip rail fencing is constructed in the same manner as a post and rail fence. Boards are placed between the posts and held in by juxtaposed pressure. No nails are needed to secure the boards. A properly installed slip rail fence is very attractive and may be painted, creosoted, or left natural. One safety feature is that the fence can be taken apart to rescue a cast horse. But this same feature allows the horse to more easily work the boards out. Wooden shims can secure the assembly with increased friction against movement. Sometimes nails are used to secure the slip rails if they loosen over time. To minimize injury risk, they may be nailed from the outside (non-horse side) of the fence assembly. Screws are a more secure alternative.

MESH FENCE

Wire Mesh

Wire mesh fencing designed for horse use, with a top board for visibility, is considered to be among the safest horse fencing (Fig. 15.6). Wire mesh fence construction falls into the substantial fence category because it does not depend on electricity to contain the horse. It can range from intermediate in cost to one of the more expensive depending mainly on the type of wire. It is a low-maintenance fence, with care limited to wood treatments, and is relatively easy to install with the proper equipment. Opinions vary as to its attractiveness; the well-built varieties have an understated beauty. It is excellent for keeping most interlopers, such as other animals and humans, away from the horses. On a breeding farm, wire horse mesh fence offers protection for foals who cannot roll under the fence and risk injury when trapped between the ground and lowest board.

Horse-variety wire mesh is manufactured in diamond or rectangular design pattern (Fig. 15.7). The diamond, or triangular, mesh is nearly impossible for a horse to get a hoof through. A 2-inch by 4-inch triangular mesh is commonly available. The horizontal wire is typically of heavier gauge (10-gauge) than the vertical wire (14- or 12½-gauge). Wires that wrap around the wire intersections are preferred to welded wire intersections, which come undone. At least one manufacturer offers an interwoven wire where mesh junctions are part of the continuous weave. A straight rectangular mesh ("turkey wire") with upright openings 2 inches wide and 4 inches high is not quite as safe because these openings are big enough for a pony- or foal-sized striking hoof to pass through. The wires then form a trap around the ankle when the horse tries to escape. Another rectangular mesh for horse applications starts with lower openings that are narrow in width but increase in size with the fence height. This prevents hooves from getting through the bottom of the fence but

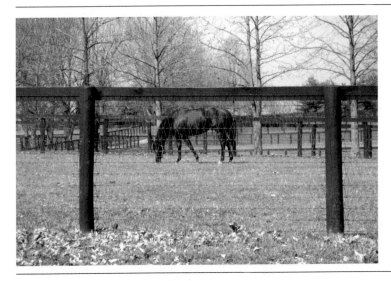

Figure 15.6. Wire mesh fence designed for horses with a top board for visibility is considered one of the safest designs because horses cannot reach head, feet, or legs through.

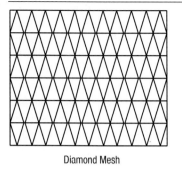

Diamond Mesh

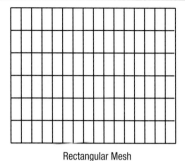

Rectangular Mesh

Figure 15.7. Two examples of wire mesh fence pattern suitable for horse fence, because each prevents horse hooves from going through the approximately 2-inch by 4-inch mesh openings.

provides a more open appearance toward the top of the fence. Mesh fence will not cut a horse, which falls against it. It is sturdy and yet has some give, and it is virtually breach-proof if installed correctly. Some horses have caught shoes and halter buckles in the mesh of even the safest wire mesh fences.

The better wire mesh fence installations include a top board to increase fence visibility and to keep the top, unsupported wire portion from sagging because of the pressure of horses leaning over it (Fig. 15.8). This board is positioned overlapping the top 1 to 3 inches of the mesh to provide a fence height of 54 to 60 inches, including the top board. Mesh material height is typically 50 or 58 inches, but 42-, 60-, and 72-inch mesh heights are available. In some cases, the top board can be economically replaced with an

electric wire strand or polybraided wire rope positioned 4 inches above the mesh to discourage fence leaning. The top board provides important visibility and presents little danger to the horses compared with a wire strand on top. Visibility boards are similar to those used on board fences and would be 1-inch by 6-inch rough-cut or 2-inch by 6-inch nominal boards; these demand a nominal 8-foot post spacing for board attachment. An option is use of plastic rail or wide polybraided ribbon. These products, installed with tension springs, would offer visibility but not protection from horses leaning over the fence (unless electrified).

Correct installation calls for the wire mesh to be strung tightly between posts. This requires a fence stretcher. Mesh is then stapled securely onto square

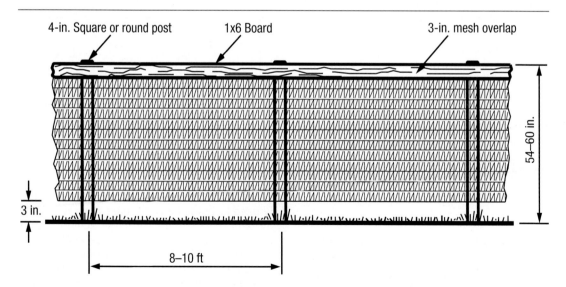

4-in. Square or round post   1x6 Board   3-in. mesh overlap

54–60 in.

3 in.

8–10 ft

Figure 15.8. Because wire fences of all types can be nearly invisible from a distance, a top board is added to increase fence visibility for the horse and to discourage reaching over the top.

or round posts spaced 8 to 10 feet apart. The mesh wire is not attached to the top visibility rail. Wire is installed on the same side as the horses to present a smooth surface that prevents hooves and heads from becoming trapped between wood and wire. The wire requires very little maintenance and rarely sags once stretched onto the posts. Wire mesh fence goes up faster than board fence. Check with your fence dealer or installer for the proper clearance under the mesh. Many mesh fences are installed flush with the ground or with about 3 inches of clearance underneath to discourage grazing under the fence. Grazing pressure damages the appearance with distorted metal mesh pushed out at the bottom. This low height will inhibit grass mowing activity.

Many mesh fence materials sold as general farm fencing suffer from material weakness and improperly sized mesh openings for safe horse use. The larger mesh size (4 inches by 4 inches or greater) increases the risk of a horse leg becoming entangled. Wire fence for general farm use must be heavier than 12-gauge wire to be strong enough for horse use. (Remember that the lower the gauge number, the heavier the wire.)

Plastic Mesh

Plastic mesh fencing combines the safety of a wire mesh fence and the visibility of colored plastic or vinyl. Unlike the metal, however, the plastic will not have sharp, protruding edges should a section of the fence be damaged or broken. The material used to make the fence comes in a variety of widths and can have added benefits such as providing a windbreak or shade. Installation of plastic mesh fencing follows the same guidelines as wire mesh. Make sure that mesh spaces in the fencing are of appropriate size for the horse it will be containing. As in metal mesh fencing, larger openings increase the probability of a horse becoming entangled in the fence. A top board to prevent horses from leaning on the fence and damaging it is also recommended. A variety of colors are available.

Chain Link Mesh

Chain link fence is common in residential and commercial applications but not so in agricultural settings. It is relatively expensive and does not maintain its original attractiveness if abused by horse contact. Unless well supported, edges tend to sag and sway. Unprotected chain link edges have looped metal pro-

jections that can catch halters and cut horses. It could be a suitable fence for suburban or urban horse facilities where one objective is to discourage humans and their pets from interacting with the horses. Features that discourage human entry, such as being difficult to climb over or through, can be found in more conventional horse fence, such as wire mesh. Chain link can be easily built to heights beyond those normally encountered with farm fences. It is fairly visible and sturdy while yielding on horse impact.

Adjacent stallion runs have been fenced with 7-foot high chain link. For any horse application, all piping supports should be at least 3 inches in diameter. The top and bottom of the fence should be finished: the top with pipe and the bottom with a pressure-treated 2-inch × 10-inch board positioned with its bottom edge 2 inches below the wire and attached to the inside (horse side) of the fence (Fig. 15.9). Keep the bottom board fence edge at least 8 inches above ground. One common problem with chain link is from pawing horses loosening and pulling shoes when caught in the edge loops. The low board prevents this and also discourages grazing horses from pushing under the fence. Another option is to bury the lower edge a few inches into the ground to cover the bottom edge loops. The lower fence portions will

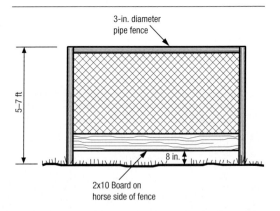

Figure 15.9. Chain-link fence is not commonly used as horse fence because it is rather easily bent out of shape by horse activity, but it does provide opportunity for extratall fence. Protect horse against injury from metal loops at edges of the chain-link material with a top pipe and bottom board. Bottom board also prevents bending of bottom mesh from pawing or horse reaching under fence.

suffer bending and dents from horse hoof activity, but even small intruders will be excluded.

STRAND FENCE

Conventional Smooth Wire

Five to seven strands of smooth wire on wooden posts make the least expensive fence. Once posts are set, the fence installs quickly. Wire fence is potentially the most dangerous horse fence; but with top rails for visibility and electrified wire(s) to discourage contact, it can be cautiously used for quiet horses. It is often used for cross-fences that divide a large enclosure for rotational grazing or for very large pastures where horses are infrequently in contact with the fence. However, horses should not be pastured in adjacent pastures with this type of fence. Social or antisocial behavior over or through the wires can result in serious injury.

The wires of a strand fence must be stretched tight (using a stretcher) during installation, and maintenance mainly involves keeping things tight with spring-loaded tension units. Maintenance involves patrolling the fenceline for downed branches and trees resting on the wire fence. High vegetation will inhibit electric fence function. Individual strands may need to be tightened periodically as the wire stretches with age or warm temperature. Loose wire is a hazard for horse entanglement, as is a horse reaching through the fence.

Wooden fence posts are recommended for smooth wire fencing. These can be set up to 15 feet apart, but wood visibility boards will be long and difficult to attach (Fig. 15.10). Alternatives are to use white plastic pipe or a ⅜-inch plastic wire cover on the top strand for visibility. Polybraided rope or tape (see later section of this chapter) may be used as the top rail along with additional strands for their increased visibility and ability to carry electricity. Steel and fiberglass posts make connection of visibility boards difficult, and these posts can impale a horse attempting to jump the fence. Fences with only two electrified strands on fiberglass or steel posts have been successfully used as cross-fences, which may be portable, in rotational grazing applications. Always use a plastic cap or sleeve on metal "T" posts to reduce the danger of horses impaling themselves on this type of fence post. Horses may entangle themselves and be cut in a smooth wire cross-fence.

High-Tensile Wire

High-tensile wire fence uses wire of 11 to 14 gauge with a tensile strength of up to 200,000 pounds per square inch (psi). (In comparison, conventional galvanized, type I fencing wire has about a 55,000-psi tensile strength.) The fence can withstand livestock contact and low-temperature contraction without losing its elasticity. The high elastic limit reduces common stretch or sag associated with conventional smooth wire. Wire tension is set at 200 to 250 pounds at installation and is maintained by permanent in-line stretchers or tension springs. Electric versions are possible and highly recommended.

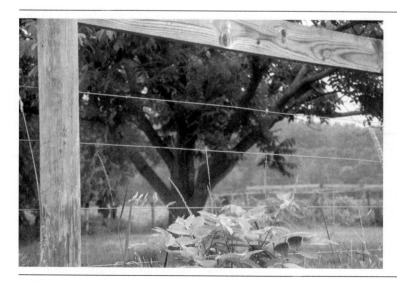

Figure 15.10. Wire strand fences suffer from poor visibility to the horse, so adding a top board or a thicker and bright material will improve safety. A top board offers the advantage of discouraging reach over the fence but limits the post spacing distance.

Horses must respect this type of fence. Wire fences can be very dangerous if horses are to be pastured on both sides of it simultaneously. The stretched wire will act as a paring knife and cause serious cuts for horses reaching or kicking through it.

Wires are held in tension along sturdy posts spaced up to 60 feet apart (Fig. 15.11). End posts must be well braced (Fig. 15.12). Battens or light posts can be used in between posts to maintain wire spacing. High-tensile wire fence is most suitable to flat or gently rolling terrain to take advantage of the long, straight-line distances between support posts. It is no more difficult to build than other fences. Each wire is tightened with a ratchet in-line stretcher. Once end posts are solidly set and braced, the wire installation proceeds rapidly. Features, limitations, and cost are similar to a conventional smooth wire fence. *High-Tensile Wire Fencing* (see Additional Resources) provides more detail for this type of fence installation.

Electric Wire

Smooth wire, of conventional or high-tensile variety, is connected to an electrical charger to provide a reminder to horses to stay away from the fence. The electric shock provides a degree of respect that a plain, smooth wire fence cannot always provide. A single electrified strand is often used with more

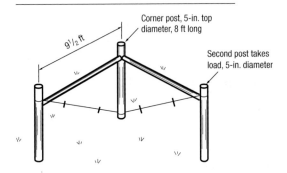

Figure 15.12. Corner bracing of wire strand or mesh fencing distributes the fence's tension load through the three-post assembly.

substantial horse fences to discourage horses from contacting the fence. Simple wire two-strand electric fence can serve as a cross-fence for rotational pasture management; this is not a suitable horse fence as the primary perimeter fence. The electrified strands, one at least 42 inches and the other 18 to 22 inches off the ground, can be positioned on posts set 20 feet apart. It is good practice, and the law in most states, to identify electric fence with signs placed about 200 feet apart. Electric wires and insulators should be installed on gates so that the charge goes off when the gate is opened.

Electric fences, like all wire fences, suffer from lack of visibility and the potential for severe cuts to horses entangled in it. Electric fences can be successfully constructed from more visible products such as multiple strands of wire incorporated into a woven plastic tape, rope, or ribbon (Fig. 15.13; see "Polybraid and Polytape" section). These materials offer advantage in being forgiving of horse impact and will not cut the horse. Another option to enhance visibility of wire fencing is to attach strips of colorful plastic or cloth to the wire to create contrasts and movement for increased visibility. However, this may short out the fence and decrease attractiveness.

Maintenance of electric fence requires removal of heavy vegetative growth at the fenceline. Vegetation can conduct electricity and act as a "ground" for the current, which will short the electricity in the fence. Check fence voltages at different points along the fenceline using a meter to check for voltage leaks due to grounding and weed growth. Inspect fenceline after heavy wind and rainstorms to clear away fallen trees and debris that can inhibit fence function.

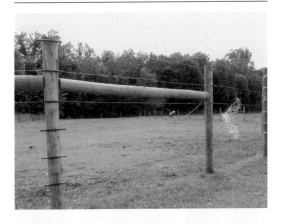

Figure 15.11. High-tensile wire fence offers the advantage of wider post spacing than conventional wire fence, shown here. Without electrification, several wire strands will be needed to contain horses, such as the six-strand fence shown here.

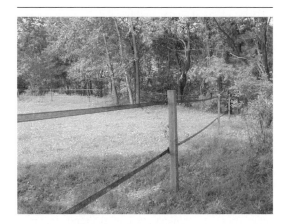

Figure 15.13. An electrified polytape fence may have as few as two strands in applications where horses will have limited time and access for fence contact, such as shown here in a large pasture in rural setting.

Electric Charger and Grounding Systems

Many types of plug-in or battery-powered electric chargers (fencers) are offered, for example low impedance, high voltage, and short-impulse models, which are considered to be the most appropriate. Shock duration is about $\frac{1}{400}$ of a second with 45 to 65 shocks per minute and about 1000 to 3500 volts per shock. Solar-powered chargers require adequate time to charge the battery before the first use. Many problems associated with solar charger longevity are due to a failure to allow the battery to come to full charge prior to its first use. Heavy-duty batteries designed to withstand a deep discharge before recharging are recommended for use. Some models are capable of electrifying up to 50 miles of wire, while others may only have enough power to electrify up to 2 miles.

Older "weed-burner" chargers, which claim to burn weeds growing over the wire, are not recommended with horses. They put out a higher charge at intervals that can burn or electrocute horses and could start brush fires. The new low-impedance chargers claim to not set grass fires even though wires may touch vegetation. In some states weed-burner fencers are illegal. Do not electrify barbed wire because children and animals can become entangled and be repeatedly shocked.

Electrical grounding is very important with modern chargers. This is because conductive bodies (horse, human, plant, etc.) will act as receivers for the electrons and will complete the circuit (shock) if the fence is not properly grounded. Over 95% of all problems with electrified fencing can be ascribed to poor grounding. Do not use an existing household grounding rod. Place the grounding rods for the fence at least 50 feet away from water lines and other grounding systems. This will prevent signal interference in electrical, phone, and digital lines in the house.

For grounding each charger, select an area that tends to stay moist or wet, and place four driven copper ground rods 6 foot long at least 6 feet apart or three rods 8 foot long at least 10 feet apart (Fig. 15.14). Rods should be installed in a square or triangular pattern or in a straight line perpendicular to the fence. Another grounding option is to provide a minimum of 20 to 50 feet of buried pipe or an existing steel culvert. Use additional grounding for each 3000 feet of fence in areas where soils tend to stay moist.

Dry, rocky, and sandy soils or soils that commonly have freezing conditions reduce the efficiency of chargers because dry ground does not effectively conduct electricity to complete the circuit. In these types of climates, running nonelectrified stands back to the charger helps to increase its effectiveness by creating a better "ground." By making one strand of fence electrified (positively charged) and another grounded (negatively charged), anything that connects the two oppositely charged strands completes the circuit and will receive a shock. For long stretches of fencing, more grounding rods may be required using this method.

Grounding can be checked by carefully placing your hand on the top of the grounding rod and

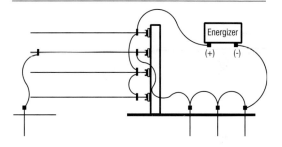

Figure 15.14. Example of wiring necessary for grounding system of electric fence charger. Adapted from Electrobraid product literature.

slowly touching a patch of grass. If you can lay your hand completely on the grass without receiving a shock or feeling a tingling sensation, the fence is effectively grounded. It is best to cover the tops of the grounding rods and mark their location to help prevent injury and equipment damage, as well as preventing breaking or disconnecting the rods and wires.

Poly-Bonded Wire

Poly-bonded wire is a hybrid fencing material consisting of a thin (about ⅜-inch) vinyl coating (PVC) surrounding a 12½- gauge wire (Fig. 15.15). The wire is best kept under tension similar to conventional wire fence. It is recommended that the vinyl be bonded to the wire because vinyl has a larger amount of expansion and contraction during temperature changes than does the wire. If the vinyl is not bonded to the wire, and merely coats the wire, it expands beyond the wire causing bubbles in the coating during hot weather, then shrinks, exposing the wire during cold weather. Unbonded fencing allows water to penetrate between the coating and the wire that, over time, erodes the wire.

Poly-bonded wire fence can carry an electric charge but will not shock animals because the metal is embedded in the nonconducting vinyl coating. Some manufacturers offer a coating with strips of conducting carbon material so it can act as a traditional electric fence. Another option on a multiple-strand fence is to alternate electrified wire for shock with bonded wire for visibility. Strips of plastic coat

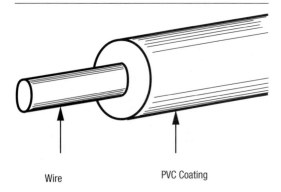

Wire   PVC Coating

Figure 15.15. A bonded PVC jacket surrounding a wire for increased visibility with ease of installation of wire strand.

may be added to an existing fence wire. Poly-bonded wire fence combines the improved visibility of PVC with the strength and ease of installment of wire strand. It comes in different colors, mainly white, brown, and black.

Polybraided Rope and Tape

Polybraided wire fence is more visible than wire strand and can be electrified. Braided fence material may look like ⅜-inch diameter rope or a flat ribbon fabric ½ to 2 inches in width (Fig. 15.16). The fence material is braided polyester, polyethylene, or similar flexible fabric-like material with metal (copper, stainless steel, etc.) strands incorporated into the weave. This allows electrification, while preventing crimping and breakage of the wires. The braided material is forgiving to a horse that runs into it and will not break. The flexible fabric material creates a slippery surface that will allow a hoof or head, which may have gotten through the fence, to be removed easily without cutting the skin. Select UV-resistant materials. Currently, the polybraided fence materials have a 10- to 15-year life expectancy, with some companies offering a 25-year warranty. Manufacturers offer detailed information about installation of these types of fences.

The success of various designs, which vary in strand spacing and post distance, is still being determined with this newer fence material. Generally, in most situations other than cross-fencing in rotational grazing systems, three electrified strands are recommended to keep horses from going over the top, through, or underneath the electrified fence installation. Some installations of ribbon strands have suffered from wind whipping of the material resulting in faster wear in fence material and hardware. An open weave tape design allows some air passage to reduce wind effects. Fence post spacing can be 50 to

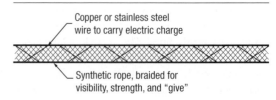

Copper or stainless steel wire to carry electric charge

Synthetic rope, braided for visibility, strength, and "give"

Figure 15.16. Metal wires are braided into a synthetic rope for increased visibility of stand while providing electric shock capabilities.

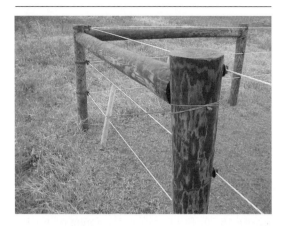

Figure 15.17. Polybraided wire and polytapes provide a visible, safe horse fence at lower cost than more traditional board and mesh fence installations. Photo courtesy of Jennifer Zajaczkowski and R&R Fencing.

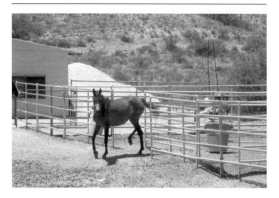

Figure 15.18. Metal pipe and cable fences are sturdy and affordable alternatives to wood board fence in areas of limited lumber supply.

100 feet, with the shorter distances recommended for ice holding capacity in regions with freezing rain. The fence has provided good safety and visibility for horse use (Fig. 15.17).

PIPE AND CABLE FENCES

Steel pipe fence tends to be used in areas where wood is less available or is quickly damaged by insects. Pipe fence is extremely sturdy and visible but usually has a high labor cost to construct because welding may be required. At least one manufacturer offers a design where the rails slide through holes in the post for easier assembly. Pipe fence requires little maintenance if properly treated during installation. It is successfully used for paddocks, round pens, and riding arenas with height and rail spacing similar to board fence construction (Fig. 15.18).

Cable fence makes a good, sturdy horse fence with more give to it than pipe fence. Steel posts use welded rings to position ½- or ¾-inch diameter cables, and wooden posts have drilled holes. Post spacing is up to 20 feet with good corner posts. Cable tension is maintained by high-tensile wire-type tensioners. Cable fencing has been associated with abrasion and puncture injury. A pipe top rail above three to four strands of cable is an option. Another combination pipe and cable fence places two strands of cable equally spaced between a top and middle pipe rail with two addi-

tional cables spaced in between the middle rail and the ground.

FLEXIBLE RAIL FENCES

Flexible Vinyl

A flexible synthetic rail replaces wood boards for the look of "board" fence with the flexibility of high-tensile strand fence (Fig. 15.19). This hybrid fence combines high-tensile wire strands, which provide support and form the edges of the fence rails with a flexible covering of PVC. This is a very strong fence that absorbs impact and rebounds when horses hit it.

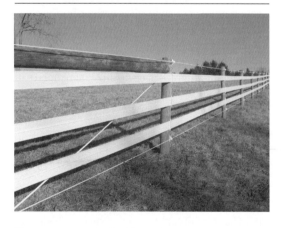

Figure 15.19. A flexible vinyl rail installation that mimics the appearance of board fencing is proving to be a safe and low-maintenance alternative with some installation savings with wider post spacing.

The flexible rail fence is considered a very safe and sturdy horse fence even without being electrified. It overcomes one of wire fencing's major drawbacks in that it is highly visible. It also maintains PVC fence's low-maintenance features. Cost for materials and installation is more than for an equivalent high-tensile wire fence yet significantly less than for rigid PVC board fence. The "rails" come in varying widths, with 4 to 5 inches being typical. There are options for "lighter" 1- to 2-inch-wide rails.

Flexible PVC fence is assembled similarly to high-tensile wire fence. Tensioners are used to keep the rail assembly tight (also see "High-Tensile Wire Fence" section). The number of wires in each PVC strip (usually 2 or 3), strip width, and color options vary by manufacturer. The material can be attached to wooden or synthetic (PVC or recycled plastic) fence posts. The corner and end posts must be sturdy to maintain the approximately 250 pounds of tension in the wires.

Rubber or Nylon

Reprocessed tires and conveyer belts form the raw material for rolls of nylon and rubber fence "rails." It is one of the less expensive fencing options but is being replaced by interest in the flexible plastic rail installations (discussed earlier). Nylon and rubber fences can be used for paddock and riding arenas. They are visible and sturdy, and yet they yield upon horse impact, thus making them safer fences. They can sag under pressure. Digestive impaction problems can result if curious horses chew strands off the fence. Modern materials and careful installation have eliminated frayed threads, hazardous loose strands, and problems with material deterioration. But, when enclosing young horses or confirmed chewers, rubber or nylon is probably not the best choice because horses may still try to eat the material.

The rubber fence construction follows a conventional four- or five-rail wooden format with 4-inch top round poles spaced 8 to 10 feet apart (Fig. 15.20). The $3/8$- to $5/8$-inch-thick and $2^1/2$- to $3^1/2$-inch-wide rubber or nylon material is attached with nails or staples. The strips of rubber or nylon are stretched tightly between posts, so corner and end posts need bracing. The minimal maintenance amounts to periodic tightening of any sagging rails. If the manufacturer has not sealed the material to prevent frayed ends, use a propane torch to shrivel the nylon along the edges.

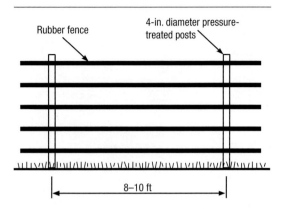

Figure 15.20. Rubber or nylon fence materials provide a visible fence offering decreased injury upon impact or entanglement than with board or strand fence. Similar features of flexible vinyl rail have displaced some rubber fence use.

FENCES TO AVOID

Selection of fencing needs to take management style into account. Some fences are more suitable for one facility than another. However, some fences are not suitable for any horse under any management style.

Barbed Wire

Barbed wire was designed to keep placid cattle within bounds on large tracts of land. The majority of horses never learn to stay away from barbed wire despite severe cuts from fence encounters. Veterinary bills will negate savings in initial fence cost. Barbed-wire fencing is definitely not recommended for use with horses.

Stone Walls

Despite their elegant and traditional look, stone walls are unforgiving of any horse who tries to go through or over them. The cost of constructing new walls is prohibitive, especially to a height suitable to contain a horse.

Snake Rail

Zigzag wooden enclosures may be picturesque, but they are easily pushed over because of their loose construction, or jumped over because of their low height. Pointed projecting rail ends and multiple corners are hazards, especially to horses cornered by pasture-mates.

GATES

Gates can be bought or built in as many styles as fence but do not have to be the same style as the fence. Gates need to be the same height as fence material to discourage horses from reaching over or jumping the gate. Chapter 14 has information on gate location and width.

The most common and recommended gate materials are wood and metal tubes. Easy-to-assemble kits for wooden gates are available with all the hardware, including fasteners, braces, hinges, and latches. The kits can be bought from farm, lumber, or hardware stores. Horse-safe tubular pipe steel gates (often 1⅜-inch outer diameter pipes) have smooth corners and securely welded cross-pipes to minimize sharp-edged places for cuts and snags (Fig. 15.4). Metal horse gates with a thick wire mesh on the bottom is even safer because horses cannot paw through it. By contrast, channel steel or aluminum stock livestock gates are not recommended for horse use because of their less sturdy construction and numerous sharp edges. Horses often paw at the gate in anticipation of being brought inside the stable or prior to feeding.

Avoid gates with diagonal cross-bracing. Although this strengthens the gate, the narrow angles can trap legs, feet, and possibly heads. Cable-supported gates offer a similar hazard to horses congregating around the gate. If gate supports are needed, a wooden block (short post) can be placed under the free-hanging end of the gate to help support its weight and extend hardware life. The use of a cattle guard (rails set over a ditch) instead of a gate is not recommended because horses do not consistently respect them. Horses have been known to jump them or try to walk over them, which results in tangled and broken legs.

Gates are hung to swing freely and not sag over time. The post holding the swinging gate maintains this free-swinging action, necessitating a deeply set post with a larger diameter than that of fenceline posts. Gate hardware must withstand the challenges of leaning horses and years of use. A person should be able to unlock, swing open, shut, and lock a properly designed gate with only one hand so that the other hand is free to lead a horse or carry a bucket, for example.

POSTS

Posts are the foundation of every fence. Setting posts is the most time consuming part of fence construc-
tion, but improper installation will shorten fence life and compromise fence safety. Driven posts are highly recommended because they are more secure than hand-set posts or those placed in a pre-drilled hole.

Wooden Posts

Wood is recommended for most horse fence posts. The best buy is a pressure-treated post from a reputable dealer. The preservative must be properly applied to be fully effective. Initially, treated posts are more expensive than untreated ones, but they last four times as long as untreated ones. Depending on soil conditions and preservative treatment quality, a pressure-treated post can last 10 to 25 years.

Suitable wooden fence posts are similar for board, mesh, and flexible rail fences. High-tensile wire and other strand-type fences require similar posts, but distances between posts are often much longer than for board or mesh fence. Post distance on high-tensile wire fence depends on wind influences and topography. Round wood posts are stronger and accept more uniform pressure treatment than square posts of similar dimension. Attachment of wooden rail boards to round wood posts is improved when one face of the post is flat (Fig. 15.21).

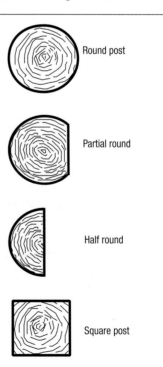

Round post

Partial round

Half round

Square post

Figure 15.21. Wooden post cross sections of use in horse fence construction.

Setting Wooden Posts

A properly installed post can support fencing for 20 years or more; a sagging post means stretched wire, torqued-off boards, and taking out the fence sections on either side of the bad post to reset it. Soil packed tightly around the post keeps both water and air away, so the post bottom resists rotting. Driven posts initially have about five times the holding strength of hand-set posts. Posts may be driven without a pilot hole for more strength. The ability to do this depends on the type of soil, soil moisture content, presence of rock, the amount of soil compaction, and the amount of force delivered by the post driver. By pounding the posts in with a driver, the soil directly under and around the post is tightly compacted, which prevents rot and adds to post stability (Fig. 15.22). When pilot holes are drilled, they need to be the same diameter as the post or up to an inch smaller. If the pilot hole is larger than the post, the soil will not be tight enough to support it and prevent rot.

How deep to set the post for structural stability varies considerably with soil conditions. Soil characteristics play a major role in determining the longevity and maintenance requirements of a fence. Some soils remain wet and can quickly rot untreated wooden posts. Posts in sandy or chronically wet soil will need to be set deeper and perhaps supported by a collar of concrete casing. Other soils tend to heave with frost and can loosen posts that are not

driven deep enough. Fences under tension, such as wire strand or mesh materials, will require deeply set posts to offer long-term resistance against tension. A typical line post depth is 36 inches. Corner and gateposts are required to handle greater loads and are about 25% larger in diameter and are set deeper, often to 48 inches.

Wood Preservatives

The post is the foundation of every fence. Wooden posts are the most common and are also among the safest for horses. However, if not properly protected, wood has a lot of natural enemies (insects, molds, fungi, microbes) that will shorten its useful life span. Even if naturally rot resistant species, such as Osage orange, western red cedar, western juniper heartwood, or black locust heartwood are chosen, sealers and preservatives can add years to the useful life of the wood.

Wood sealers and preservatives can be topical (paints and formulated water-repellent agents like sealers, stains, etc.); however, topical remedies only treat the surface of the wood and may offer only a few years of protection. Topical protection will offer no benefit if the wood cracks or pits after the application. The first coat of paint on a fence lasts about three years with the second coat lasting five to seven years, depending on weather conditions. The most important part of the wood to protect is the open end-grain.

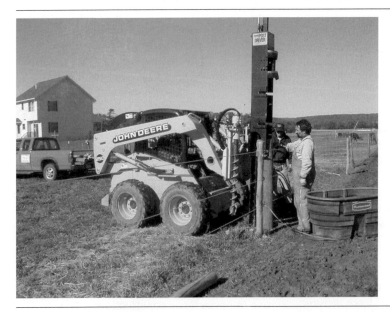

Figure 15.22. Driven posts offer stability from compacted soil around the post as it is driven into the ground. Photo courtesy of Jennifer Zajaczkowski.

Other preservative options include copper cromated copper arsenate (CCA), pentachloropheno (penta), copper naphthenate (CU-Nap), and creosote. Posts treated with CCA are readily available almost everywhere. These are the greenish pressure-treated posts. CCA offers a broad range of protection and should penetrate the entire post. Penta is another preservative commonly found in pressure-treated wood. Unlike CCA, penta is an oil-based preservative. In general, oil-based preservatives offer better protection for wood than their water-based counterparts, but this fact is highly dependent on penetration and retention rates. This penetration, unlike topical applications, protects the wood if the post should crack or develop surface checks and is chemically fixed to the wood to prevent leaching. When selecting pressure-treated posts, choose posts with the highest retention value. The retention value is the amount of preservative retained (in pounds) per cubic foot of wood. The higher the number, the more preservative is present in the wood. CCA-treated posts may not be a good selection for chewers and cribbers, because ingestion can be harmful. One alternative for cribbers and chewers is CU-Nap. Posts pressure-treated with CU-Nap have limited availability in most areas. CU-Nap can be purchased as a topical treatment for residential decks and applied to fence posts. Unlike CCA and penta, CU-Nap has not demonstrated a health risk if ingested, but the treatment's longevity is unknown. It has been claimed that protection lasts 10 to 20 years; however, this is highly variable and correlated to retention.

Creosote offers the best protection from both pests and weather effects. Creosote is an oil-based treatment that uses diesel fuel as a solvent carrier. Creosote needs time to cure and during the curing process the solvent carrier volatilizes, sometimes carrying the creosote with it. When this happens, it is called "bleeding." The fumes from the solvent volatilizing can pose a health risk. This is one of the reasons creosote can only be applied by licensed handlers. However, creosote also has an offensive odor that seems to discourage horses from chewing and cribbing on it. Once the creosote has cured, it poses no health risk to those around it and the preservative is mechanically fixed to the wood and will not leach out.

A classic method of protecting the grain on the top of the posts is to cover it with a "sacrificial" piece of wood. Attaching a "cap" of board material can shield the grain and help prevent water damage on the top of the fence post.

Metal and Synthetic Posts

Exceptions to wood posts are allowed for horse-safe steel posts typically used on chain link fences, pipe posts for welded fences, and rigid PVC fence post. Hollow posts require top caps to cover the ragged top edge or should be designed such that the top fence rail covers the top of the post. Recycled plastic, 4-inch-diameter solid posts are suitable for horse fence but require a small-bore pilot hole before driving. Metal and fiberglass T posts are slightly cheaper but pose a serious risk of impalement and are not recommended. They are also not strong enough to withstand horse impact without bending. With a plastic safety cap installed on the top, T posts may be cautiously used in very large pastures where horse contact is rare. One electrified fence option uses T posts covered entirely with a plastic sleeve for protection and support of electric wires (Fig. 15.23).

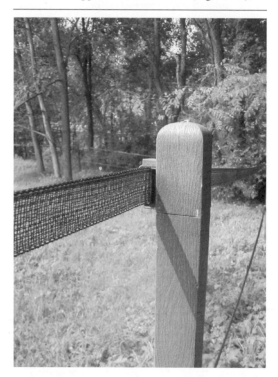

Figure 15.23. A more suitable option than unprotected metal T posts is one with a full plastic sleeve for protection against horse injury and ability to easily connect electrified strand materials.

Hand-Set Posts

For placing one or two posts, hiring a post driver may not be feasible; so knowing how to hand dig and set a post is useful. The hand-set posthole should be at least twice but not more than three times the diameter of the post. If the hole is too narrow, there is limited room to tamp effectively, and too wide means there is too much tamped soil to provide the most secure post. Figure 15.24 shows the steps for a hand-dug post placement.

Once the placements of the posts are established, dig a hole. An absolute minimum depth of 2½ feet is needed to set a line post securely, and 3 feet is preferable. Posts supporting more weight or tension, such as a corner or gate, will need to be deeper at about 4 feet. In particularly wet, heavy soil, a chemical treatment of the wood, such as creosote, will retard rot. In wet soil, fill the bottom 6 inches of the 3-foot posthole with sand and/or gravel to promote drainage and keep water away from the base of the post.

The post is lined up on two different planes before tamping begins. The post must be vertical and on a line with the other posts. Once the drain material, if any, has been placed and the post is properly positioned, the tamping routine begins. Because the objective is to have this post stand up and stay up for up many years, about 25% more dirt should be tamped into the hole than was removed. Extra dirt will be required.

The most important part of setting posts is tightening the soil in the ground around the post. A tamping tool, or "digging iron," of heavy metal or wood is used to impact the fill dirt. Dump loose dirt into the bottom 6 inches of the hole around the base of the correctly positioned post and tamp it down until the dirt is so solidly compacted that it cannot settle later. The tamped area will be much more solidly compacted than the surrounding soil. Push in another 6 inches of loose dirt and repeat. The noise the tamping rod makes when contacting completely tamped dirt approaches the sound of a steel rod pounding concrete. Do not fill in the entire hole and then tamp from the top because the appropriate force will not carry down through the full 3 feet of dirt. With improper tamping, water will cause the earth around the post to loosen and crack and the post will loosen and sag.

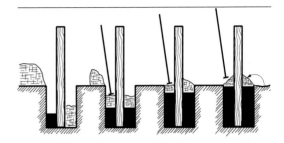

Figure 15.24. Process for installing hand-dug fence post.

SPECIAL FENCE APPLICATIONS

Fenceline rounded corner

Figures 15.25a through 15.25f show the dimensions for positioning posts on 8-foot interval, such as used with board-style fence construction, to make a sharp fenceline corner into a rounded corner.

Human-Only Passages

Figure 15.26 shows two designs for easy human-only passage without the use of a gate for quick entry and exit from fenced areas. A simple gap in the fence can also work but is typically of narrower dimension (12 to 14 inches clearance) than the designs shown.

SUMMARY

Fence materials function together into a type of fence that safely contains the horse. Initial fence material selection will begin with choosing between electrified and substantial fencing options that contain the horse via shock and physical strength, respectively. Many successful horse fences incorporate both physical strength and electric shock. Mesh fence materials are considered very safe horse fencing when horse-type mesh is used that has openings that cannot allow a hoof to pass through. Mesh fence prevents a horse from reaching through the fence, which is behavior that injures both horse and structural integrity of the fence. A top board for visibility and to discourage horses from reaching over completes the mesh fence's safety design. The classic horse fence that most people envision has wooden rails of rough-cut hardwood, dimension lumber, split rail, or slip rail design. These remain attractive and safe horse fences but suffer from relatively high installation and maintenance cost. Many of these rigid

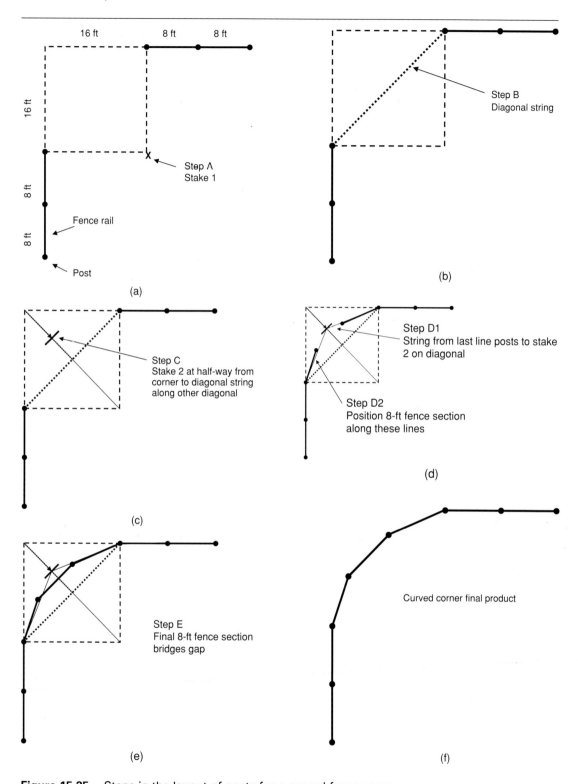

Figure 15.25. Steps in the layout of posts for a curved fence corner.

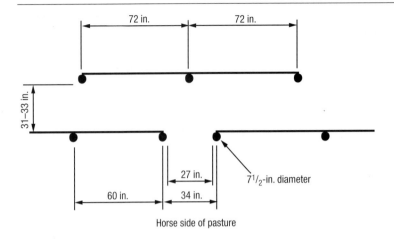

Horse side of pasture

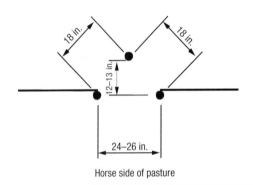

Horse side of pasture

Figure 15.26. Dimension for human-only passages for easy entry and exit of fenced areas.

board fences have an electrified wire to keep horses away. Synthetic material manufacturers have tried to duplicate the look of classic wooden horse fence with maintenance-free materials. Applications using flexible vinyl rails similar in size to lumber offer an attractive, lower –maintenance, and safe alternative to wooden board fence. An evolution in rigid PVC fence material composition and installation design has overcome some initial longevity and safety problems, although this fence design is not considered horse-proof and needs protection via electrical shock. Great improvements have been made in strand fence design for horses. Previous applications of multistrand high-tensile or conventional smooth wire suffered from poor visibility, leading to horses running into the fencing and subsequent lacerations from entanglement. Manufactured strands of braided rope and webbing incorporate electrified wire to discourage horse contact with the fence. The increased material greatly improves visibility and virtually eliminates lacerations from wire entanglement. Finally, underlying every great fence is the post. Proper selection and installation of posts will have the most impact on long-term success of the fence.

16

Indoor Riding Arena Design
and Construction

Indoor arenas are a welcome addition to most riding stable complexes (Fig. 16.1). They extend riding season into cold inclement weather months and ensure that even rainy days do not spoil riding opportunities. In fact, a bright and airy indoor arena is one of the goals as few people enjoy riding around within a dark, dank interior. Despite the fun and usefulness of indoor arenas, they are an expensive investment and are another item to add to the facility maintenance list. Their construction is often a once-in-a-lifetime undertaking for their owners; consequently it makes good sense to follow sound rules of site preparation and construction. Initial short cuts most often play out as long-term problems with continual maintenance cost and headache.

SITING THE INDOOR ARENA

Site the arena reasonably near the stable. Direct connection is not necessary and is a disadvantage for fire suppression and natural ventilation purposes. Yet, easy access from the barn is desirable, especially for inclement weather. Convenient location may be compromised in relation to challenging site topography. Obviously, when less site grading is needed, then arena site preparation will be less expensive. Topography will affect drainage, building location, access routes, and exposure to wind and sun.

Excess water is the enemy of a good arena site. Surface water needs to be diverted away from the indoor arena site and direct roof rainwater away using gutters and downspouts. Do not build in a "hole," which includes low or flood-prone areas. The arena site will have its topsoil removed so that subsoil is graded and firmly compacted. Initial grading and site work for drainage serves as the foundation of the surface upon which your horse will work (see "Site Preparation" and "Surface Construction"

sections of this chapter and "Features of Outdoor Arena Construction" in Chapter 18).

ARENA CONSTRUCTION

Indoor Arena-Stable Configuration

The recommended arena-stable configuration is provision of separate buildings, as shown in Figure 16.2. The next acceptable alternative is to have a breezeway or work area connection between stable and indoor arena (Figs. 16.3 and 16.4). Designs where the arena and stable are more fully integrated into one shared air space tend to compromise air quality in both environments, provide risk for fire loss of both buildings, and, in some configurations, offer unreasonable conflict between riding activity and horse stable function. Figures 16.5 through 16.7 provide more information about the challenges of some arena-stable configuration along with construction alternatives to improve the design.

The recommended configuration is provision of separate buildings for indoor riding arena and horse stabling.

Indoor Arena Framing and Siding

An indoor riding arena is actually a relatively simple structure. It is a shelter over a riding surface. Its immense size in height, length, and width is what contributes to structural material cost. Selecting common framework sizes that are easily transported to the site and that can be handled by typical construction equipment can minimize cost. Clear-span structures are used where either trusses or rigid frame support a gable roof (typical) structure (Figs. 16.8 and 16.9) without interior posts. Steel, wood, or combinations of the two are used. Hoop

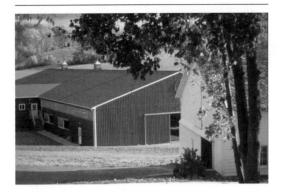

Figure 16.1. Indoor riding arenas need careful construction and site preparation but offer great convenience in extending riding times into darkness and through inclement weather.

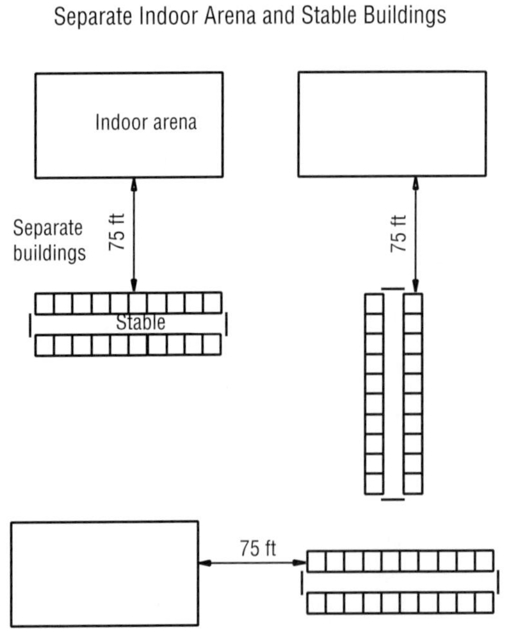

Separate Indoor Arena and Stable Buildings

Figure 16.2. An arena separated from the stable is recommended for improved indoor environment within both. A minimum 75-foot separation distance between buildings is recommended for vehicle and equipment access and for fire safety. This distance provides fire-fighting equipment access and reduces spark spread. (Not to scale.)

Breezeway Attached Arena and Stable

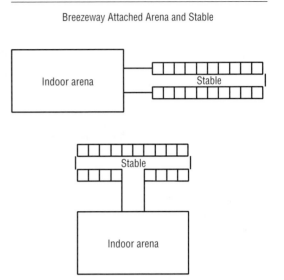

Figure 16.3. Consider a breezeway connection between stable and indoor arena to separate the two environments while providing weather-protected access. Arena endwall connection option is preferred to sidewall connection for improved ventilation of both buildings. (Not to scale.)

structures also provide clear-span interiors using pipe frame construction with a durable material cover (Fig. 16.10). Exterior visual appeal of such a large building should be considered in the overall site plan as the indoor arena will have a commanding impact on farmstead aesthetics.

Interior material selection will affect the look and feel of the riding environment. All-metal building interiors often have a cold and industrial feel to them compared with the more natural atmosphere of a wooden structure. Wood framing is maintenance free in terms of surface care; staining of wood siding may be desirable. Of course, many combinations are possible. For example, a clear-span structure can be made of heavy wood arches with a metal roof, and similarly a wooden truss structure can be clad with metal siding and roof. Sheet metal surfaces that will potentially be in contact with horses need to be lined with wood to minimize dents to the metal and injury to the horse (see "Rider Guard" section). Provide opportunity for natural light entry. Light colors of walls, roofline, and footing surface material will brighten the interior (see "Light" section).

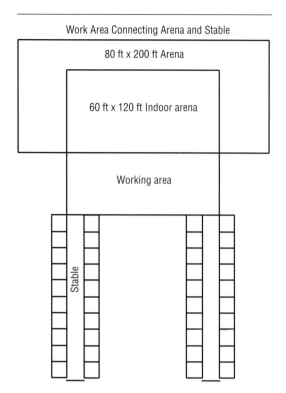

Figure 16.4. The indoor arena may be conveniently linked to the stabling with a working area that includes tack room, grooming stations, observation lounge, and wash stalls. This arrangement groups spaces that may be heated during cold weather, while the arena and stalls have more fresh air exchange and remain near outside temperatures. (Not to scale.)

Size and Structural Support

Arena size is primarily determined by two features: intended use and cost. Often the riding or driving discipline of intended users will indicate which basic features are most important. Table 18.1 provides guidance for competitive arena size. Indoor arena size is often smaller to limit construction cost unless the arena is designed for competitive use. Two typical indoor arena sizes have evolved: the 60 foot wide × 120 foot long and the 80 foot wide × 200 foot long. Indoor arena clear-span structures 100 to 200 feet wide are necessary for group riding or driving horses and competitive events. Length is more variable among arenas and less expensive to add than a comparable arena width. Lengths less than 120 feet inhibit obtaining any speed on horseback before a corner has to be negotiated.

Most private and smaller commercial indoor arenas are of wood truss construction. The standard 60-foot × 120-foot indoor arena with a 16-foot sidewall height is a product of standard construction practices. It is not so because a 60-foot × 120-foot arena is the perfect riding size but because it is a cost-effective riding size. Sixty-foot trusses are commonly manufactured and relatively easy to truck to site, and contractors can handle their erection with common building techniques. Stretch to an 80-foot-wide truss and trucking costs increase (wide and long load restrictions often apply) and special skills are demanded of the construction crew in handling and placing these longer trusses. Stretch to a 100-foot truss, and the work really begins. But this larger size may be exactly what you need based on anticipated arenas activities.

Metal or wooden rigid frame construction allows for wider arenas than truss construction at 100 feet and greater. The open interior roof structure is visually appealing in its uncluttered design and bird

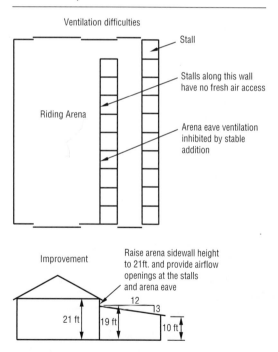

Figure 16.5. An arena directly attached to the stable along a long sidewall compromise ventilation and air quality within both buildings and is not recommended. An improvement allows room for eave ventilation along the common wall of arena and stable. (Not to scale.)

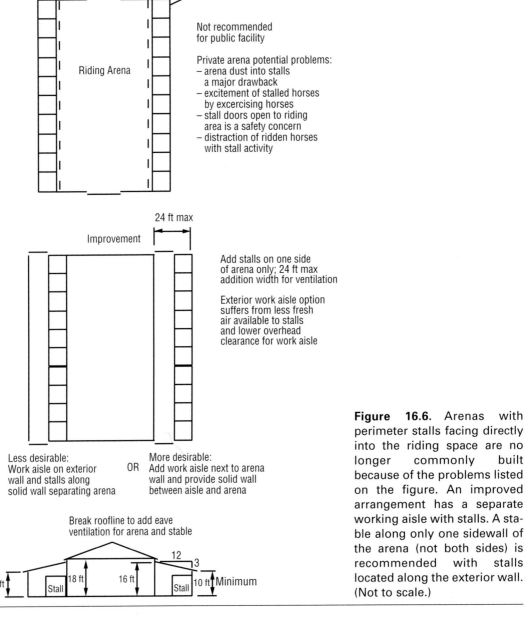

Figure 16.6. Arenas with perimeter stalls facing directly into the riding space are no longer commonly built because of the problems listed on the figure. An improved arrangement has a separate working aisle with stalls. A stable along only one sidewall of the arena (not both sides) is recommended with stalls located along the exterior wall. (Not to scale.)

roosting is less of a problem than with wooden trusses. (Bird netting material on underside of truss construction discourages bird activity inside building.) Transportation to site is simplified by frame pieces being delivered rather than a truss that spans the entire width. Generally, smaller arenas (60 to 80 feet wide) are more commonly and economically built of trusses, while larger arenas (over 100 feet wide) benefit from the economy of rigid frame construction. Locally available materials, building manufacturers, and construction companies will have a great impact on midsize arena economics.

Arenas less than 80 feet wide are more commonly and economically built of trusses, while arenas over 100 feet wide typically benefit from the economy of rigid frame construction.

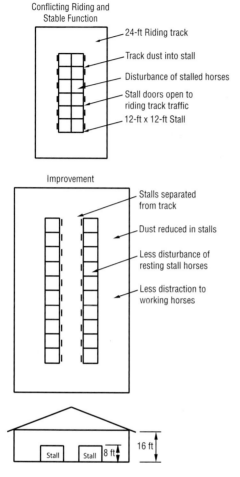

Figure 16.7. On center-aisle stable design where horses will be exercised around the perimeter track (in addition to "hot walking"), improve riding and working conditions with a central aisle to separate these functions.

Arena visual appeal is often dictated by roof line shape and trim details. Most private arenas use gable roof shape for simplicity of construction. Large arenas benefit from more complex roof shape or other features, such as cupolas, clearstory, or attached spectator lounges, to add some architectural appeal.

Height

The minimum recommended sidewall height in a riding arena is 16 to 18 feet. The trend in construction is toward the 18-foot height. This provides a good, airy riding environment where jumping and

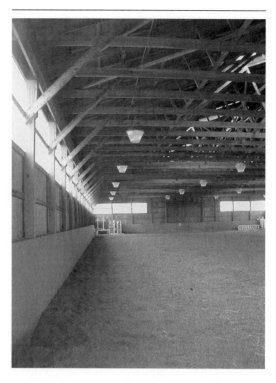

Figure 16.8. Trusses are used for clear-span construction in small- to medium-sized indoor arenas.

rigorous activity can be enjoyed. Generally a 24-foot pole, set 5 feet deep, can be used for an 18-foot sidewall that is not significantly more expensive than the poles used for a 16-foot arena height. Glu-lam techniques (wood layers are laminated together with glue for a strong composite wood construction member) allow for poles with pressure-treated lumber on the bottom portion and less expensive untreated lumber above ground level. Higher arena height (20 feet and more) is desirable for large and wide public arenas. Minimum head clearance for horse and rider is 14 feet, with 12 feet minimum at doorways.

Final arena height is the distance from the top of the surface footing material to the lowest object that could be hit (or reached) by a horse or rider, such as the truss bottom chord, suspended light fixtures, or an automatic watering system sprinkler. Remember to account for objects that hang below truss height when planning on final arena headroom clearance. Light fixtures hanging on the lower chord of a truss hang about 6 inches and 30 inches below the truss

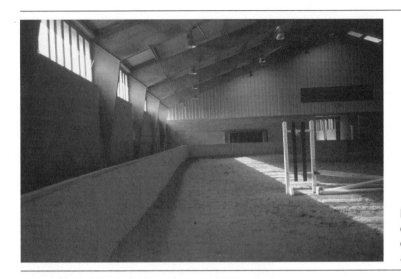

Figure 16.9. Rigid-frame clear-span construction is common in larger indoor arenas.

for fluorescent and high-intensity discharge (HID) lamps, respectively (see Chapter 11 for more detail).

Final arena height is the distance from the top of the surface footing material to the lowest object that could be hit (or reached) by a horse or rider.

Doors

Arenas need a direct access to the outdoors that is usually provided by endwall doors of considerable size. Often another large door provides direct or breezeway access to the stable.

These doors need to be high enough to allow safe horse and rider access. Doors should be 12 to 14 feet tall and wide enough for surface maintenance equipment such as a pickup or tractor and harrow. Door width of 16 feet is recommended. Trucks delivering footing material will need access for initial installation and during footing replenishment or replacement every 5 years or so. Horse and rider doors of 12 feet × 12 feet and 14 feet tall by 16 feet wide equipment doors are typical on private riding arenas. Doors may be single or double and open by swinging or sliding. Overhead doors may also be used. For sliding doors, provide a track at

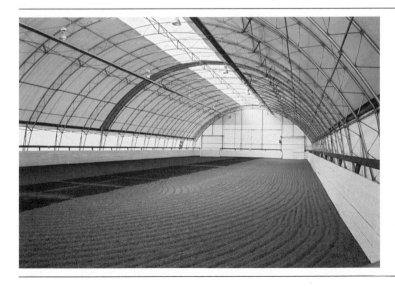

Figure 16.10. Hoop structures covered with a flexible material offer clear-span construction. Courtesy of Coverall Building Systems.

top and bottom guides to keep the door square and solid from the influences of wind, snow accumulation, and footing material that may work its way into the door frame. Once big doors are opened, gates should be available to maintain the arena guide rail fencing. Provide separate doors for human-only access so that a large door does not have to be wrestled open for pedestrian entry. For fire safety, and by code in some locations, a door will be needed about every 200 feet within a large structure and is a good idea for convenience or as an emergency exit for other reasons.

Extra Space

The area occupied by the building itself, or footprint, is supplemented by the space needed to access the arena with maintenance equipment, such as a tractor and harrow for footing maintenance. All-weather access lanes are a must for commercial facilities where vehicle access of boarders, visitors, and competitors is necessary. Indoor arenas benefit from enough space around the exterior perimeter to provide convenient access by vehicles, maintenance, snow removal (Fig. 16.11), water drainage, and perhaps landscaping. Fence pastured horses from contacting the arena siding to lessen dirt, chewing, and kicking damage.

Plan space for short- and long-term storage of training aids used in the arena, such as jumps or barrels and maintenance equipment. Dedicate a small sectioned-off area for short-term storage of training aids that is out of the way. Barrels, jumps, and equipment stored in a jumble in an unprotected arena corner pose a safety hazard for the hapless rider thrown and landing on them. See sections in this chapter on common arena design features.

INDOOR ENVIRONMENT

Indoor riding arenas can be as simple as a roof over a riding ring. This provides sun and rain protection in warm climates. In northern climates, more protection is sought from winter wind and cold, and so sidewalls are required. The goal of an indoor arena is to provide a better environment than that available outdoors, because of excessive cold, wind, heat or precipitation. This requires attention to arena environment conditions. The bigger the difference between desired indoor conditions and outdoor weather, the more complex the environmental control will become. In most cases, the interior environment is usually kept to within a few degrees of outdoor temperatures so simple natural ventilation is adequate. Consider site layout in relation to prevailing seasonal winds (Fig. 16.12). Some arenas are heated or evaporatively cooled at additional expense. Ventilation is needed in all weather conditions to remove excess moisture during cold weather and excess heat during hot weather. Of particular importance is maintaining fresh air and dry conditions during cold weather when indoor arenas

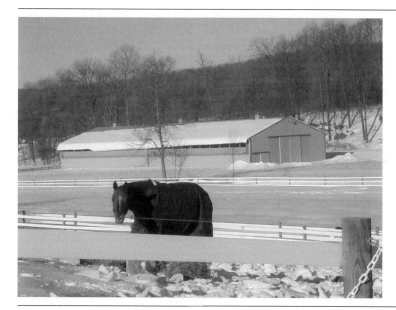

Figure 16.11. Provide enough room around the indoor arena exterior for maintenance equipment traffic, snow storage, drainage, and perhaps landscaping.

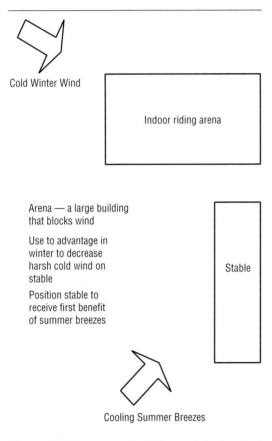

Cold Winter Wind

Indoor riding arena

Arena — a large building
that blocks wind

Use to advantage in
winter to decrease
harsh cold wind on
stable

Position stable to
receive first benefit
of summer breezes

Stable

Cooling Summer Breezes

Figure 16.12. Large buildings disturb wind airflow patterns for 5 to 10 times their height downwind. For a typical indoor arena with 18-foot sidewall and 3 in 12 or 4 in 12 roof slope, its total height is about 35 feet. This will disrupt airflow 175 to 350 feet downwind.

are more heavily used than during mild weather. More detail of ventilation principles and methods of air movement is provided in Chapter 6.

The goal of an indoor arena is to provide a better environment than what is available outdoors. This requires attention to arena environment conditions.

Cold Weather Ventilation

Ventilation is needed during cold weather to maintain good air quality in the arena and to remove excess moisture. Moisture comes from horse and human respiration, sweat, and evaporation from the riding surface. Arena moisture levels are an order of

magnitude greater than in most commercial, industrial, or residential environments.

Indoor arena environments have been found to be more humid than outdoor conditions during cold weather. Evaporation of water from arena footing material is thought to be the primary cause. Water is commonly applied to the footing material for dust suppression and replenished frequently because of evaporative loss from the footing material. Arenas attached directly to the horse stable environment can be even more humid than unattached arenas because of the migration of moisture from the stable to the arena. If the temperature in the arena is lower than in the stable, which is usually the case, considerable condensation can form in the arena as moist, warm stable air drops in temperature upon entering the arena (and hence, as it cools, cannot hold as much moisture anymore; see Appendix). Arenas attached to heated or underventilated stables are not recommended. Use an open breezeway to dissipate moisture if connection of stable and arena is deemed necessary.

Indoor arena environments are more humid than outdoor conditions during cold weather, which will make them feel damp without adequate ventilation.

Air exchange needs to be provided or condensation and damp, clammy conditions within the arena will decrease riding enjoyment. Natural ventilation, where wind (primarily) causes air to enter and exit the arena, is most often suitable. Mechanical ventilation using a fan and inlet system can be used for more control of air exchange rate, which is particularly useful during cold weather in a heated arena. Openings are needed in the arena structure for proper air movement for both mechanical and natural ventilation systems (see Chapter 6 for more detail about ventilation system design features).

OPENINGS FOR NATURAL VENTILATION AIR EXCHANGE

Effective natural ventilation of an indoor riding arena requires two sets of permanent openings: one high at the ridge and the other low at the eaves. These openings will provide the ventilation needed during cold winter months when excess moisture and stale air removal is the objective. These "fixed" and permanently open vents provide some modest air exchange at all times. Positioning these openings along the eave soffit and ridge eliminates drafts on arena users than having large openings at rider level. During warmer weather when more openings are needed to reduce heat buildup in the arena, large adjustable doors, wall panels, and/or sidewall curtains are opened to supplement the fixed-size cold weather inlets.

OPENING SIZE

Sizing of the fixed ridge and eave openings is for winter air quality and moisture removal. These openings are kept open year round and provide the minimum ventilation of the arena. Ventilation openings will be similar to those recommended in Chapter 6 for horse stable air quality. On arenas up to 80 feet wide, provide permanent openings no less than 2 inches wide along the entire eave on both sides of the arena. The absolute minimum ridge opening is 4 inches along the entire length. Preferred and recommended are 4-inch openings at each eave and 8-inch openings at the ridge. Proportionally wider openings are needed on arenas wider than 80 feet. Typically, the ridge opening is equivalent to the sum of all eave openings for this minimum opening size that is used during cold weather. This amount of opening, or more, will provide modest air exchange for moisture removal. Horse exercise increases respiratory and sweat moisture that is added to the arena air. Heavy equestrian activity during winter in indoor arenas, such as frequent group riding lessons, competitions, or polo, will add enough moisture to increase normal winter ventilation openings to 6 inches at each eave and 12 inches at the ridge (larger openings for arenas wider than 80 feet).

Provide permanent ventilation openings 4 inches wide along the entire eave on both sides of the arena with an equivalent ridge opening of 8 inches along the entire length.

EFFECTIVE OPENING SIZE

These opening recommendations are the "effective" opening area. Often, a wire mesh or 1-inch by 2-inch hardware cloth is used to cover eave openings to discourage bird entry, but an unprotected soffit is simpler and provides unobstructive airflow (Fig. 16.13). Obstructions to airflow through the

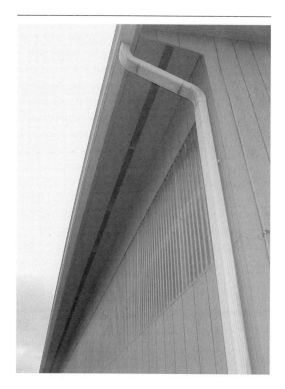

Figure 16.13. Provide eave openings along entire arena sidewall length. Protect opening from bird entry with nothing more restrictive to airflow than 1-inch square hardware wire mesh.

eave, such as when using wire mesh, should be accounted for by increasing the opening area by 10% to 20%; increasing the open area by twice this amount will account for dust accumulation. Chapter 6 contains a summary of soffit covering effectiveness related to the recommendations that follow. Do not use residential-type window screening or metal soffit vents to cover the ventilation opening as they do *not* provide adequate opening. Soffit vents designed for residential attic ventilation are unfortunately seen on many metal-sided horse stables and arenas, but they do not allow adequate air exchange. The small, pinhole-sized openings do not provide an adequate "effective" open area and they will quickly clog with dust, thus allowing no airflow. If soffit mesh is used, it may be placed in a vertical position to discourage bird nesting, which can be a problem on horizontal soffit screening. Likewise, the ridge opening may be screened with hardware cloth (or equivalent) to discourage bird entry.

OPENING LOCATION

The permanent ventilation openings are best provided on a continuous basis along the entire building length. This way, fresh air can enter and exit with equal opportunity throughout the building, which will decrease the chances of stale air zones. An alternative is to provide the same total opening area with evenly distributed intermittent openings. Ridge opening can be provided with a simple continuous opening, continuous ridge vent assemblies, cupolas, or intermittent ridge openings. For example, rather than providing 4-inch continuous ridge opening along the entire 120-foot length of an arena (4 inches wide times 120 feet long = 5760 square inches or 40 square feet of ridge opening), ten 6-inch-wide by 8-foot-long chimneys or ridge vent assemblies can be substituted to provide the same ridge opening area. Equally distribute the intermittent chimneys or vents along the ridge.

Choose commercial ridge vent assemblies designed for agricultural applications that provide an unobstructed airflow path as air moves through the vent (Fig. 16.14). Most residential-style ridge vents are so convoluted in their airflow path as to render adequate arena air exchange impossible. An indoor riding arena is a high-moisture, dust-laden environment that has a need for much greater ventilation rates than a home's attic. Ventilation openings and rates suitable for horse facilities are provided in Chapter 6.

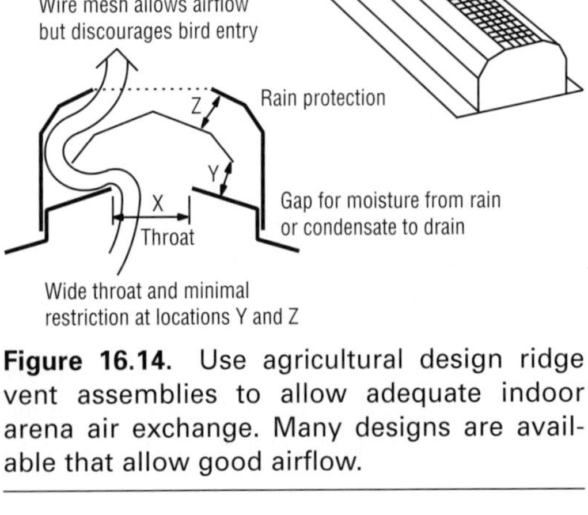
Wire mesh allows airflow
but discourages bird entry
Rain protection
Z
Y
X
Throat
Gap for moisture from rain
or condensate to drain
Wide throat and minimal
restriction at locations Y and Z

Figure 16.14. Use agricultural design ridge vent assemblies to allow adequate indoor arena air exchange. Many designs are available that allow good airflow.

Condensation

Condensation forms when arena air comes in contact with a cold surface at or below its dew-point temperature. The air temperature drops; hence, its water-holding capacity is diminished (cold air holds less moisture than warm air; see Appendix) and the water is deposited on the cold surface. Condensation commonly occurs on windows and metal roofs, which tend to be close in temperature to outside air, but will occur anywhere warm, moist air encounters a surface colder than its dew-point temperature. One line of defense against condensation is increased insulation on the offending surfaces. This is not often done in cold buildings, such as indoor arenas, except an R-5 insulation under the roof material. The primary line of defense to avoid condensation is removal of the excess moisture that has built up in the structure. Simply bring in fresh outside air, move it through the interior to pick up moisture, and then discharge it. Properly sized natural ventilation openings (see "Opening Size" section) will provide adequate air exchange to prevent moisture buildup. Occasional condensation on arena building materials can be expected on the worst cold days. This will not be a problem to wood and metal materials as long as they can dry out and remain dry most of the time. Moisture trapped next to building materials is a problem, such as wet insulation material next to a metal roof.

Chronic condensation and odor is an indication of underventilation, where adequate stale air is not being removed from the arena.

Chronic condensation and odorous air is an indication of underventilation, where adequate moisture is not being removed from the structure. Chronic condensation results in dripping roofs, saturated insulation and building materials, rust, and deterioration of building component strength. Solutions include providing supplemental heat and increasing air exchange through ventilation. Even with supplemental heat addition, which will increase the moisture-holding capacity of the arena air, ventilation will be necessary to remove the moist air and replace it with drier outdoor air. The simplest, least costly solution is to provide more natural ventilation air exchange with larger, unobstructed eave and ridge openings or to open other arena openings, such as large doors, periodically to "air" out the interior. Mechanical ventilation fan and inlet system may be used for minimum ventilation exchange of humid interior air with drier outside air.

Hot Weather Ventilation

During warm outdoor temperatures, ideally the indoor arena serves as a sun shelter and the building is opened up to admit as many cooling breezes as possible. At a minimum, provide large endwall doors that open and supplement with sidewall sliding (Fig. 16.15) or swinging panels. Large sidewall doors are often used too so that as breeze direction changes, large openings can allow air to be directed through the building. In fact, pleasing cross-breezes are usually welcome within the arena in all but cold weather. Variable weather during spring and fall conditions provides the most challenge where sidewall and endwall openings will have to be periodically adjusted over the day as temperature swings from cool to warm. In cases where the arena will get consistent year-round use in a northern climate or have primary use during hot summer in a warm climate, opening the structure for cooling breezes will be a priority. The openings discussed are in addition to the permanent ventilation openings needed for

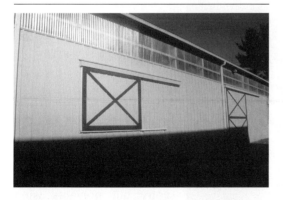

Figure 16.15. Sliding doors and panels are popular for providing large openings for admitting summer breezes to the arena.

basic air quality and moisture removal for cold weather.

During hot outdoor temperatures, the indoor arena serves as a sun roof with open sidewalls to admit as many cooling breezes as possible.

CURTAIN SIDEWALLS

Curtain sidewalls on an arena offer flexibility for providing small or large air exchange openings and admit light at relatively low cost. The curtain covers most of the sidewall area (Figs. 16.16 and 16.17). Sidewall curtain fabrics and construction techniques can be selected for attractive and durable installations. Aesthetically, opinions vary as to curtain appeal compared with that of other sidewall materials. Permanently open eave inlets are provided above the curtain so that even when it is closed, there is fresh air exchange in the arena environment.

Each curtain opening can be conveniently opened and closed with a simple winch assembly. Curtains usually open from the top down, so that when minimally opened during cool weather the air enters high at the eaves to minimize drafts at the horse and rider level. Curtains positioned high in the sidewall from eave height to within 8 feet of the floor will lessen horses' distraction with outdoor activities (Fig. 16.18). Full sidewall openings, from eave to ground, but protected by arena rail fence, should be considered for warm climates where cooling cross-breezes over horse and rider would be welcome.

Most sidewall curtain materials are translucent and will provide enhanced natural light to the arena than will solid wood or metal sidewall materials. Curtain material is obtained from agricultural building suppliers and may be single layer or multilayer "insulated" curtains, although the latter do not usually provide more than an insulating value of R-5. Sidewall curtains disadvantages include some flapping in windy conditions if string supports are not kept taut. This may be distracting to riders and new horses. Experience with curtains has shown that horses adjust within a day or two. Proper installation will mitigate most flapping and aesthetic challenges. The enhanced light and fresh air in curtain sidewall arenas have received high praise and may outweigh the disadvantages.

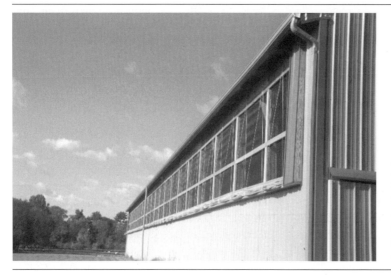

Figure 16.16. Curtain material as the upper portion of the sidewall can be used to easily provide large fresh air and light openings. They typically open from the top down.

Heated Arena

Indoor arenas can be kept at outdoor temperatures during the winter or provided with supplemental heat to maintain warmer conditions. The arena may be heated full time using space heating or a radiant heating system. Alternatively, it may be heated as needed with overhead radiant heat. Chapter 12 provides detail of heating systems typically used in stables and riding arenas, but a short overview is included in this chapter. It is costly to heat an indoor arena environment both in heating system installation and in operation and maintenance costs.

The heating systems discussed here are permanently installed systems and not portable "space" heaters borrowed from residential, office, and camping use. Those portable heaters are not recommended for use in indoor arenas because of the potential fire hazard from unattended heater operation, fumes from combustion, and/or construction ill-suited for the dusty and humid environment.

Agricultural-type heaters are designed for use in humid, dusty environments that contain flammable materials such as bedding or footing materials. Use agricultural-type heating equipment to minimize

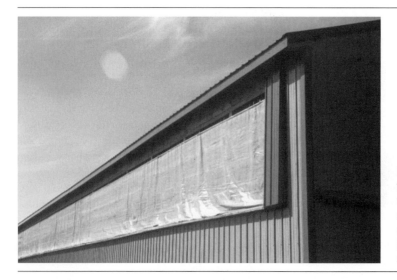

Figure 16.17. When closed, the translucent curtain sidewall material allows light entry but prevents wind entry. A continuous eave inlet opening is provided above the curtain.

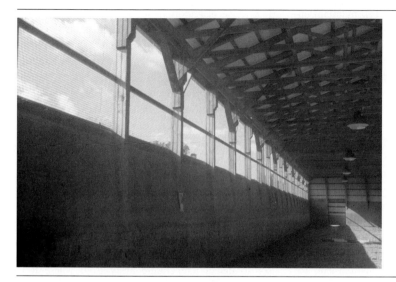

Figure 16.18. Indoor arena with curtain material on upper wall for abundant light and fresh air exchange. Bird mesh is provided to prevent bird entry at the curtain opening and as part of supporting the curtain when it is raised. Light entry and glare could be reduced through addition of shade cloth or other mesh material over the opening.

fire hazard from gas-fired units. Address safe use of space and radiant heating units by maintaining proper manufacturer-specified distances between heat elements and surrounding flammable materials, including ceiling and wall insulation materials. Arena surface footing materials are variable in flammability, ranging from organic wood products to inorganic sand.

Directed Heat in a Cold Arena

In cold climates, consider overhead radiant heat in areas where an instructor often stands, visitors view activity, or riders congregate. This directs heat where it is needed and when it is needed rather than having to maintain the entire arena at an elevated temperature (Fig. 16.19). Control of the heat may be as simple as a switch that allows the radiant heat device to turn on or off as needed, because there is no warm-up time to bring an entire building up to the desired temperature. A timer dial is useful that allows the user to select the amount of heating time and to save energy. A timer or automatic shutoff provides safety in reducing unattended operation of the heaters. Insulation of a cold (unheated) riding arena is not necessary. An R-5 roof insulation is recommended for moderate roof condensation control in cold climates.

Radiant heat can be used to heat the arena floor over long periods of time. The mass of heated floor (and footing material) will then release heat by convection and re-radiation to the surroundings. A fully

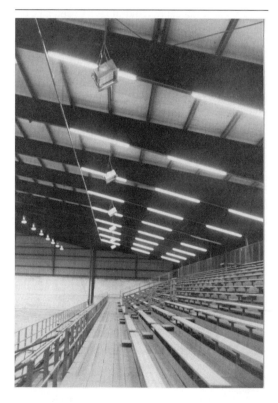

Figure 16.19. Radiant heaters are used to heat occupants of the arena at key locations, such as a spectator area. Courtesy of Detroit Radiant.

insulated building is recommended to maintain an elevated air temperature within the arena.

> *Use radiant heat to direct warmth to critical areas where occupant comfort is desirable.*

SPACE-HEATED ARENA

Supplemental heating for the whole arena airspace may be a welcome addition for arenas in cold climates. Individual unit heaters are usually the least expensive and easiest option to install. They may be gas-fired or use hot water to heat air that is discharged from the unit via a fan. Other options for space heating include hot water pipe "radiators" around the arena perimeter, but this is not a common application. Heating arena air to around 40 or 50°F is often enough to take the chill out of the environment. To determine the total supplemental heat needed, a heat balance needs to be performed, which takes into account typical outside temperature, desired indoor temperature, building insulation level, and ventilation rate for winter moisture removal (see Chapter 12 for an example supplemental heat calculation).

Unit heaters are usually positioned high in the structure in order to be unobtrusive to horse and rider traffic. The disadvantage to this is that heated air is discharged overhead and it has no natural inclination to drop down into the horse and rider zone (hot air rises). For a 60-foot by 120-foot arena, plan on providing at least two units, and preferably four units, which can be mounted to direct heated air in a racetrack fashion around the arena interior. Each unit directs heated air horizontally with small but effective fans, but it will not throw heated air all the way to the other end of a riding arena. Uniform air distribution with individual heaters is a challenge in such a large interior space where natural temperature stratification will position the warmest air near the ceiling where it offers little benefit to arena users. Ceiling (or truss) mounted paddle fans are very effective in mixing and directing this stratified warm air back down toward the floor. Heat units should be mounted for ease of maintenance where they can be accessed via ladder or lowered on a pulley system. Gas-fired units will need gas lines run to each individual heater. Typical unit heater sizes range from 70,000 to 250,000 Btuh (Btu/hr).

The noise of heat unit fans and/or air moving in distribution ducts can be a significant disadvantage of space-heating systems. Reduction of heating system noise is important for indoor arenas used for competition, demonstrations, or teaching.

Temperature control for the arena using unit heaters will likely consist of an agricultural-grade thermostat set to the desired temperature. Heaters will cycle on and off to meet the temperature set-point. A thermostat is a relatively inexpensive temperature control device, but realize that their temperature-setting dials are not highly accurate (often off by 2 to 7°F). Hang a simple, cheap thermometer near the thermostat sensor to check on controller and heater functions. Position the thermostat at about human head height to detect the temperature that a horse, a rider, and an instructor will experience. Most thermostats detect temperature via a coil mounted on the unit itself, but thermostats can have a remote sensor to detect temperature away from where it is mounted. Place the thermostat sensor (whether remote or on the thermostat unit itself) away from heater discharge air and other obvious cold and hot spots. Keep the sensor out of direct sunlight (or other radiant sources) so it does not indicate arena temperature plus radiant temperature gain. Dust accumulation on the sensor slows sensor reaction time.

For large commercial or public show arenas, the space-heating system design will become more complex and approach the type of systems used in nonagricultural commercial buildings. The challenge remains that in an agricultural-use environment, such as an indoor riding arena, heavy dust and high moisture loads will provide design and maintenance challenges. Arenas used for numerous events with substantial spectator seating may benefit from warm temperatures for patron comfort. The majority of the heat can be directed into the seating area, or radiant heat may be provided above the seating area.

Whether the heating system is simple or sophisticated, select fans, controls, and heaters designed for agricultural use. Agricultural equipment is manufactured using materials and design, such as moisture- and dust-resistant motor enclosures, that will withstand years of use in humid and dusty environments.

> Whether the heating system is simple or sophisticated, select agricultural-grade fans, controls, and heaters that are designed for use in humid and dusty environment.

More substantial sidewall and roof insulation is recommended when using supplemental heat to minimize condensation and reduce heating cost. Chapter 12 has more information on suitable insulation materials for arena environments. Ventilation will still be needed to remove winter moisture buildup. Mechanical ventilation is employed in a heated arena for more careful control of air exchange rates than can be achieved via natural ventilation (Chapter 6 includes a section on mechanical ventilation design). An automated control can be set to turn on mechanical ventilation of the heated arena when a high humidity level is reached.

Heated air will hold more moisture; so once an indoor arena environment is heated, it will need to be managed carefully for condensation control if there will be periods when supplemental heat is turned off. Overventilate the arena after heat is turned off to replace the moisture-laden air with drier outside air. If the warm, moist air is allowed to cool in the arena, the risk of condensation on cold walls and roof is greatly increased.

Ducted Air

A polytube or other fan-and-duct system (Fig. 16.20) may be used to distribute warmed or fresh air throughout a riding arena. These fan-and-duct systems are good for providing distribution of unit heater air that may be any one or a mixture of fresh air, heated air, or recirculated air. A polytube is made of clear plastic material, while a rigid duct is typically of wood, PVC pipe, or sheet metal con-

struction. The polytube or rigid duct would provide about 50 to 100 feet of air distribution from each heater with heated air discharged through holes positioned evenly along the duct length. The holes are used to direct air downward or more horizontally to provide good air distribution throughout more of the arena structure than is possible with unit heaters alone. The polytube makes a rather loud sound with fast motion as air inflates the tube, which will be disconcerting for unsuspecting horses and riders. When the indoor riding arena is in use, it is recommended that the polytube be kept inflated at all times, even if the heater is off, to avoid the potentially frightening inflation-deflation cycles. The polytube offers advantage in being inexpensive compared with a permanent duct system, so it can be replaced when it becomes dusty. Chapter 12 provides detail of duct design for warm air distribution.

LIGHT

Indoor riding arenas can be very dark environments that are not attractive to rider or horse. Provide artificial and/or natural lighting. Natural lighting includes the use of translucent wall coverings or open doors, curtains, and window panels (Fig. 16.21) on more traditional structures. Hoop structures usually have a translucent roof material (Fig. 16.10). Artificial lighting in indoor arenas is necessary for nighttime riding and for arenas with no natural lighting provision. Light levels of 20 to 30 footcandles should be sufficient for riding. White or light colored ceilings, walls, and footing material maximize reflectance and brighten the interior at little to no added expense. Dark-colored interior surfaces increase the light output needed to provide the same illumination level found in a light-colored interior.

> *Brighten the indoor arena interior with light-colored surfaces and footing material and natural light-admitting translucent panels, and then supplement with efficient high-intensity discharge (HID) electric lights.*

Artificial Light

Arena artificial lighting is usually with fluorescent or high-intensity discharge (HID) fixtures for greater light levels with much reduced electricity cost than using incandescent bulbs. Fortunately, with ceiling heights of 16 feet and higher, the bright,

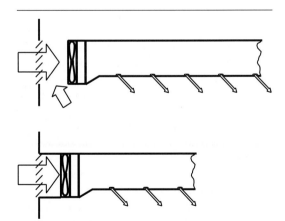

Figure 16.20. Ducts can distribute heated air throughout a fully heated arena with air coming from a preheat area (attic) or mixed with heated arena air near a heater location.

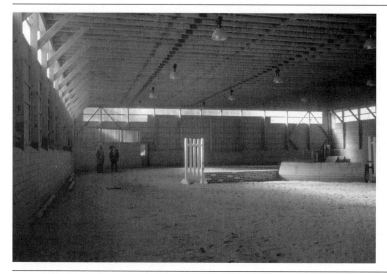

Figure 16.21. Natural lighting via translucent panels located on all four sides of the indoor arena. An elevated platform in a corner offers a relatively inexpensive construction that allows spectators a good view of arena activity. Storage is provided under the platform for training aids, and so forth.

energy-saving HID lamps may be used. HID options include metal halide lamps, which cast a bright bluish light, and high-pressure sodium lamps, which are bright with a slightly yellow glow (low-pressure sodium lamps have the very yellow glow of parking lot lights and are not recommended for indoor lighting applications). HID lamps operate at high temperatures and can add considerable heat to an arena on a hot evening. Fluorescents do not provide nearly as much heat but are not typically used above a 10- to 12-foot mounting height. More fluorescent fixtures will be needed than HID fixtures to provide similar light level. Fluorescent lamps have cold-start problems, which can be minimized with selection of cold-start bulbs and ballast; HID lamps do not have cold-start problems. See Chapter 11 for more lighting system design information and comparisons of lamp life and energy efficiency.

WALK-THROUGH LIGHTS

A set of incandescent fixtures should be installed on a "night" switch for minimal illumination. The HID lamps take around 10 minutes to come to full illumination power and are expensive to start for a short lighting period, such as for checking or just walking through the arena. Likewise, frequent on-off cycles on fluorescent fixtures will shorten bulb life.

SPECIALTY LIGHTS

For an end or section of the arena where intricate tasks are performed, such as final tacking or instruction, more light at 50 footcandles may be provided.

Security and access lighting around the arena exterior is often desirable and may be provided with HID or incandescent floodlights. Either may be equipped with motion or daylight sensors for energy savings. Emergency lights are needed in public-use arenas. Follow regulations for exit signs, and so forth.

Natural lighting

SIDEWALL TRANSLUCENT PANELS

Natural lighting can be successfully built into the structure of indoor riding arenas to cut artificial lighting electrical costs and to provide welcome brightness into a dark interior. Fortunately the arena design trend is toward providing natural light entry. Translucent panels installed high in the sidewall under the eave provide a relatively even diffuse lighting. Install at least a 36-inch height of translucent panel to provide sufficient light for riding even on cloudy days. Tailor the amount of translucent panel to your climate's bright and cloudy day patterns. A problem with arenas attached to a stable can be the limited availability of natural light from sidewalls.

Direct sunlight will pass through translucent panels, with two potentially detrimental effects in addition to the beneficial light. The first is heat buildup in the arena similar to the greenhouse effect. Although desirable in winter, this adds to heat that must be removed on hot summer days. The facility manager should determine whether heat buildup interferes with arena use if most riders are using an outdoor riding arena during summer months. Direct sunlight entry can be mitigated by eave overhangs

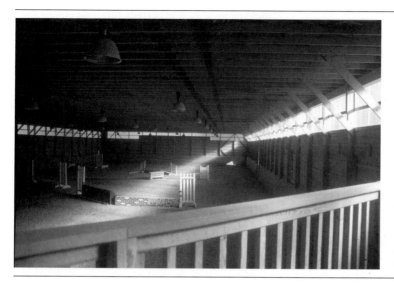

Figure 16.22. Direct light entry through translucent panels results in heat gain, which is often desirable during cold weather, and distinct light and dark floor patterns. (Photo taken from observation deck of Figure 16.21).

that shade sidewall panels from the high summer sun penetration while allowing the lower winter sun angle direct rays to penetrate (see Chapter 11). This will not alleviate winter light pattern problems.

The second problem of direct light entry into the arena via translucent panels can be distinct light and dark pattern thrown on the arena floor that can be confusing to horses (Figs. 16.9 and 16.22). Sidewall translucent panels result in a long strip of light parallel to the sidewall. Horses new to the arena may jump the pattern or shy away until they get used to it. Panels that diffuse light rather than being fully transparent

are better for reducing distinct light patterns on the floor. Eave overhangs can be designed to block some direct light entry. Overhangs provide a more finished and refined look to the building and allow roof water to be discharged away from the arena base and building foundation (see "Site Preparation" section).

Hoop structures use translucent cover material for abundant light entry. Select material that will provide a pleasantly high light level without annoying glare. More opaque cover materials can provide moderate light entry while decreasing solar gain (Fig. 16.23).

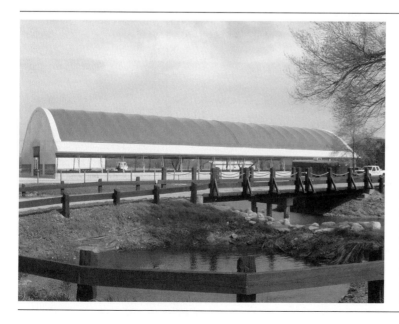

Figure 16.23. The translucent cover material of hoop structures is attractive for the abundant natural light interior. Select material that reduces glare and solar gain. Courtesy of Coverall Building Systems.

Hinged or sliding door panels will provide additional natural lighting when opened (Fig. 16.15). These are most often opened during warm weather where their use in natural ventilation is employed. Movable panels may have glazing that admits light even when closed.

Sidewall curtain material is often translucent and so provides light even when closed (Fig. 16.17). Another option for light and air entry is a mesh material rather than or in addition to a solid curtain material. Greenhouse shade cloth or similar material may be used. Shade cloth is a woven polypropylene fabric that is selected to block from 5 to 95% of the light striking it. Therefore, a portion of light is blocked for reduced glare from direct light and heat buildup. The mesh fabric reduces wind speed of air entering the arena through the large opening for benefit on windy or cool days when fresh air exchange is desirable, but reduced air velocity is more comfortable for arena occupants. Mesh no more than 80% weave for light blocking is recommended to allow adequate airflow even during the coldest weather, while providing adequate light blockage.

TRANSLUCENT ROOF PANELS

Translucent panels located in the roof cause light, water, and heat problems and are not recommended. Light patterns thrown on the floor from roof translucent panels are even more troublesome as they are spread throughout the arena interior and seem to have a more troubling influence on horses. Translucent panels do not have the same temperature expansion and contraction properties as the roofing materials around them, so that disparate material movements cause gaps to form even around the best-installed and caulked panels. Water leaks result. Finally, there is no way to block direct sunlight penetration, such as with an eave overhang, which assures heat buildup and lighting pattern influences.

COMMON ARENA DESIGN FEATURES

Viewing Area

Interior amendments that provide nonriders a way of viewing the action are most welcome. Provide an area for chairs, bleachers, viewing platform, or an enclosed lounge. Viewing areas placed on an end-wall or corner (Figs. 16.21 and 16.22) allow better field of view of ring activity than one placed flush with one long sidewall. To keep arena dust out of the viewing area, a wall with windows is needed. Lounges imply more amenities than a viewing area and can vary from spare to plush.

Rider Guards

Stirrup rails and rider wall guards are common in indoor arenas. The objective is to keep riders' stirrups and knees from contacting the columns that support the arena roof structure. Rails can be as simple as a 2×8 lumber rail nailed at stirrup height along the interior of columns. Clearly, not everyone's horse and stirrup level are at the same height, so this method has its limitations. The next step is to enclose most of the lower 4 to 6 feet of sidewall in wooden cladding, such as plywood, to provide a smooth surface. Metal-sided arenas will need this wood liner to protect horse and metal from damage.

The preferred rider guard is shown in Figures 16.24 and 16.25. This sloped guard keeps the horse hoof traffic at least 12 inches away from the wall, leaving room for rider knees and stirrups to pass along the wall without hitting the columns and wall. Horses will

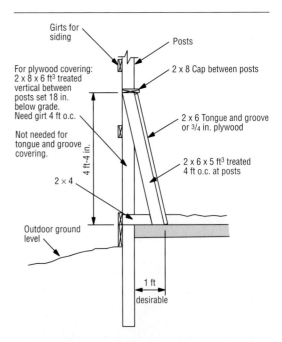

Figure 16.24. Construction detail of a lower wall guard to keep rider knees and feet from contacting the arena posts when horses track close to the wall.

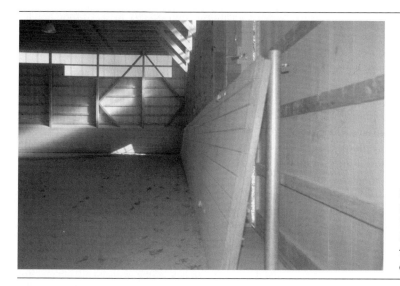

Figure 16.25. Movable arena rider guard protects riders at large sidewall door opening. Post supports both halves of the swinging guard when closed.

learn to track right next to the wall, so this wall guard needs to be maintained around the arena even at open end doors (Fig. 16.26). Swinging door guards can be provided at gates and doors. The guard wall material is most commonly made of $^{3}/_{4}$-inch exterior grade plywood but can be 2 × 6 tongue-and-groove lumber for more strength and attractiveness. The top plate on the guard should be slanted toward the arena interior to help shed dirt and dust.

A rider guard around the indoor arena perimeter is appreciated for protecting rider knees and stirrups.

Training Equipment Storage

Small storage areas in corners or an end of the arena are desirable for placement of training aids such as barrels, poles, cones, jump standards, and rails. This equipment needs short-term storage that is convenient to rider use; so providing a safe, unobtrusive place for it in the planning stage is more thoughtful than having it in the way once riding activity begins. Long-term storage of similar items is usually best in another structure. If a mezzanine viewing area is added above the storage space, then the space has two useful functions: storage and observation of arena activities.

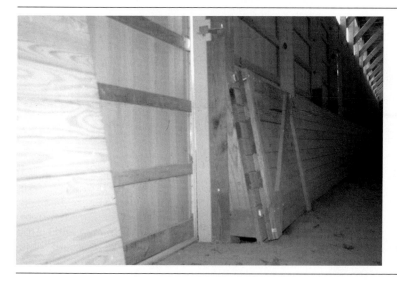

Figure 16.26. Rider guard is continuous around entire arena perimeter, so provision is made to have gated guard construction (shown here hinged back against the stationary guard) for accessing arena entry doors.

Separate Storage

Using arena area for equipment storage utilizes rather expensive construction space compared with providing an attached shed or nearby building for storage of a large quantity of equipment (Fig. 16.27). Equipment, such as tractor and harrow drag, hoses and watering equipment, and hand tools, will be needed for arena surface maintenance. Better to store them nearby than right in the arena. A storage near or within a breezeway from stable to arena may serve this function. A roof extension on one of the arena's southerly sides can serve dual purpose of covered storage and shading of direct sunlight entry through sidewall translucent panels. This attached storage may be the most cost effective option compared with a separate building.

Utilities

Access to water will be necessary for maintaining moisture in the arena footing material, for cleaning, and possibly for horse drinking water. Footing watering system options are covered in the Chapter 17. A washroom may be a necessary convenience, particularly in a public facility, unless washrooms are provided in a nearby stable or office. Electric service is required for lighting with installation of a subpanel usually required for the artificial lighting electrical load (Fig. 16.28). The subpanel needs to meet electrical code and be protected from horse access, even for loose horses in the arena. All wiring needs to be protected by conduit at all horse acces-

sible locations (Fig. 16.29) to a 12-foot height. Wiring needs to be protected from moisture and dust throughout the arena if wiring cable other than UF-B is installed. See Chapter 10 for detail on suitable wiring in damp and dusty environments, such as found in indoor riding arenas. A telephone extension may be desirable, so riding sessions are not interrupted by trips back to the stable office phone. A telephone should be nearby for use during an emergency.

Other Amenities

For arenas with virtually continuous use, convenience and comfort become important for the riders and trainers. Consider inclusion of a small area or part of a room for light food service, such as coffee and other beverages, along with small refrigerator and oven. This necessitates electric and water availability and plenty of electric outlets for appliances. Short-term tack storage is convenient for changes between training activities and lessons.

A sound system may supply background radio programs or music for competitive practice. A stereo system will need an area with reduced dust or be protected from dust with a cover that allows electronics heat dissipation. Speakers should be mounted above rider height with wiring below 12-foot height protected similar to that provided for electric cable.

Mirrors allow a rider to evaluate their own and horse position and are a welcome training aid in most disciplines, being particularly common in dressage

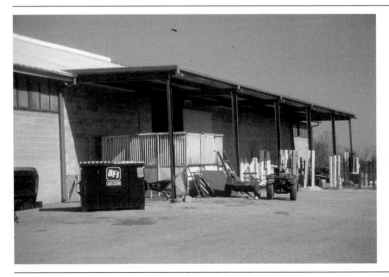

Figure 16.27. Provide dedicated storage outside of riding arena for surface grooming equipment and large supplies of training aids, such as jumps and barrels.

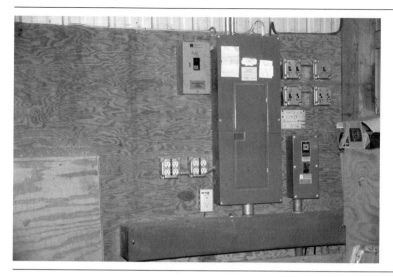

Figure 16.28. Electric service will require a subpanel to accommodate the electrical load requirements of indoor arena electric lights. The subpanel area should be inaccessible to horses at all times including for loose horses in the arena. Use covered convenience outlet and switch fixtures (not shown here).

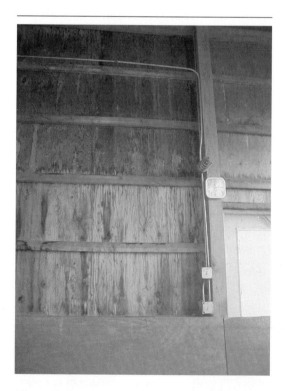

Figure 16.29. Use of moisture- and dust-resistant fixtures (not shown) and protected wiring in the indoor arena is necessary. Protection of all wiring at a height reachable by horses (up to 12 feet) is necessary, particularly in arenas where horses may be at liberty.

arenas. Mirrors need to be large to be useful (6 feet × 12 feet) and with tempered glass recommended for durability. The mirror is mounted with the long side horizontal. A mirror at least 6 feet tall should allow activity at the other end of modest-sized arena to be seen. Place the lower edge of the mirror about 5 feet above the floor to diminish breakage potential from horse and surface grooming equipment activity. Ideally, most of an endwall would have a line of mirrors along the entire width, similar to applications in a dance studio or exercise room. Reduced mirror coverage should position the mirror(s) where most riding activity can be evaluated. One large mirror in the center of the endwall can allow much of the entire arena to be in view. A mirror at the corner of the endwall will allow performance along the long side arena rail to be evaluated. Try to provide at least three mirrors across the endwall, with one at each corner and the third in the middle.

Large mirrors are costly and heavy. Support demands that each mirror have a frame of 2 × 4 or 2 × 6 lumber, depending on side length, with a backing made of ¾-in. minimum thickness exterior-grade plywood. Additional 2 × 4 frame reinforcing will be needed for large mirrors. One pre-framed option is a 4 × 8 ft mirrored sliding closet door available at home supply stores.

SITE PREPARATION

An effective stable complex includes site grading for handling surface water runoff without creating erosion and attention to subsurface drainage features.

Place the indoor arena on high ground or build up the site to keep the arena foundation above encroaching water. Avoid a site in a low-lying area or with a high water table or spring. Runoff from adjacent land that drains onto the arena site needs be diverted away using diversion ditches, interceptor drains, or dikes. Good slopes for surface drainage are up to 2%, so grade as needed. Chapter 18 contains the detail of site preparation and water drainage that is applicable to both indoor and outdoor arena sites. The only major difference in site preparation will be that an indoor arena surface is not expected to shed water and so is built flat rather than sloped. Chapter 4 provides information on locating the arena in relation to other farmstead features.

Provide drainage of rain and snowmelt from the indoor arena roof to a location away from the foundation. This can be done with gutter and downspout system or below-grade drains (Fig. 16.30). Nearby buildings need a roof gutter system or perimeter drains when the roof runoff would otherwise empty onto the indoor arena site. Even for a relatively small indoor arena at 60 feet by 120 feet, consider that a 1-inch rain event will dump a 30-inch depth of water on the 1-foot-wide area along each long sidewall of the arena. Use roof gutters and downspouts to divert this roof water to a diversion or infiltration area and away from surrounding paddocks or manure stockpile areas. Any runoff from an indoor arena roof without gutters and downspouts should be directed, via surface flow, drainage ditch, or interceptor trench, to a vegetated area such as pastureland, crop-

land, or an infiltration area to avoid a muddy mess and erosion around the arena perimeter.

Subsurface drainage is needed around building foundations to reduce frost heaving and moisture infiltration into the interior. The finished indoor arena surface will be about 12 inches above the surrounding grade to keep the building pad dry. See Chapter 7 for additional information.

> *The indoor arena protects a carefully planned multilayer riding surface that consists of a highly compacted base material and properly prepared subbase.*

RIDING SURFACE CONSTRUCTION

The indoor riding arena surface may be composed of a variety of materials, as discussed in Chapter 17. A successful riding surface is the top layer with a well-constructed series of underlying layers that support it. Construction of a good riding arena surface is preceded by attention to grading and base material selection and installation. Chapter 18 contains more detailed base layer information, but an overview is included here with special considerations for indoor arena surface construction being noted.

The indoor arena riding surface is usually constructed with three layers of material (Fig. 16.31). Between the subbase, consisting of compacted, naturally occurring subsoil at the site, and the arena footing your horse will travel on is positioned a base material layer. The base provides an important function in

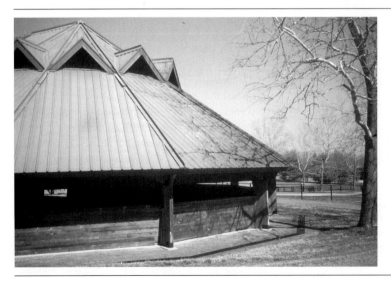

Figure 16.30. Drainage of a substantial amount of water from the arena roof is necessary. Where flat topography does not allow adequate gravity flow to a suitable location, an in-ground drainage system will be necessary.

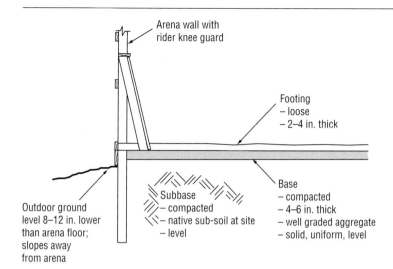

Figure 16.31. The indoor arena riding surface is a multilayer construction where the loose footing material is supported by a highly compacted level base material over a compacted subbase.

Labels in figure:
- Arena wall with rider knee guard
- Footing – loose – 2–4 in. thick
- Base – compacted – 4–6 in. thick – well graded aggregate – solid, uniform, level
- Subbase – compacted – native sub-soil at site – level
- Outdoor ground level 8–12 in. lower than arena floor; slopes away from arena

stability for the riding surface. Generally, the riding surface is a 2- to 4-inch layer of loose cushioning material, but under this a compacted 4- to 12-inch base is needed for providing traction and a solid, uniform, and level surface for the loose footing material.

Good base material characteristics include a well-graded, or widely graded, aggregate material where differently sized particles can be compacted together into a dense, uniform, and level surface. Well-graded refers to a mixture where differently sized particles are represented in relatively equal proportions from small gravel size down to silt- and clay-sized particles. This allows the fine particles to fill the voids between the large particles to form a compactable material. A suitable graded material would be composed of aggregate no larger across than about $\frac{1}{4}$ inch to avoid any potential hoof injury if some base material works its way up into the footing. Compacted clay subsoils are usually too slick when wet and prone to potholes to be suitable as the base material. Typical base materials include an engineered crushed rock material composed of limestone, bluestone, or whitestone. The subbase and base materials need to be rolled with heavy equipment, such as an 8- to 10-ton roller, for compaction solid enough to withstand horse riding activity.

A level, even subbase under the indoor arena base is desirable. Unlike outdoor arenas, where it is very important to crown the arena subbase and base with a 1 to 2% grade to facilitate surface water movement, with indoor arenas, no rain events are likely and this slope becomes unnecessary.

Essentials of Indoor Arena Base Construction
- Determine arena size.
- Select site for functional location.
- Remove topsoil.
- Build up or amend site to facilitate drainage.
- Grade and compact native subsoil for subbase.
- Construct indoor arena shell.
- Add well-graded base material, level and compact to 4- to 12-inch layer.
- Finish interior rider guard, and so forth.
- Add loose footing material as riding surface.

SUMMARY

Indoor riding arenas offer an improved environment for riding during various inclement weather events. Their construction simply provides protection of a riding surface, and in warm climates provision of only a roof over the riding area may be sufficient. In cold climates a more substantial building with sidewalls is desirable to block winter winds, and some arenas may be heated for additional user comfort. Seasonal openings, such as large doors, sliding panels, and curtains, are used on arenas to provide rider comfort during all seasons. Ventilation is provided year round via permanently open eave and ridge openings, even during the coldest weather, to maintain good air quality in the arena. Providing natural light to the arena environment results in brighter interior conditions than what is typically supplied by electric lights alone. Most arenas include electric lights for evening riding. Site preparation emphasizes maintaining a dry pad upon which the indoor arena is located. Separate indoor arena and stable buildings are recommended for better environment in both buildings and less fire risk and to diminish conflict between riding and stabling activities. Arena size will depend on intended use and budget. Truss construction is typical on arenas from 60 to 80 feet wide, while rigid frame construction is typically more economical for widths greater than 100 feet. Amenities on the arena interior include rider guards along wall support posts to protect rider knees and feet, mirrors to check horse and rider positioning during movements, separate covered storage for extra training aids, and often an observation lounge for spectators.

17
Riding Arena Surface Materials

RIDING ARENA SURFACE

Unfortunately, there are no universal recommendations for the perfect riding surface or footing material. A "perfect" riding surface should be cushioned to minimize concussion on horse legs, firm enough to provide traction, not too slick, not too dusty, not overly abrasive to horse hooves, freeze-proof during cold weather, inexpensive to obtain, and easy to maintain. Cost of footing materials is locally dependent on material availability and transportation cost. The intended use of the arena for jumping, reining, or driving, for example, also influences footing material attributes such as traction or depth of loose material. Manufactured or trademarked materials are an option that depend less on local availability and provide more guarantee of uniformity in material properties. Naturally occurring inorganic materials (sand, etc.) are offered by quarries that can provide raw materials or mixtures that meet accepted standards.

A handicap to recommending a strict formula for footing materials is that materials vary greatly around the county and country. For example, sand in one location is often very different from sand in another location. Local terms for materials can vary widely and contribute to the confusion. However, it is possible to develop some guidelines and use common sense to get a good, workable footing material. Inorganic materials (sand, stonedust, gravel, road base mix for the base) from quarries can be designated according to standard adopted nomenclature in relation to particle sizes and the distribution of sizes found in the purchased product. Particle size distribution describes a footing material in a "standard" format. The distribution is determined by shaking the footing material through a set of sieves that have increasingly smaller hole size, so that finer material ends up on the lower sieves while larger particles are held on the upper sieves.

Footing is actually a rather dynamic material. Many successful riding arena surfaces are a composite of two or more materials, often resulting from continued use. The arena surface started as one material, which broke down into smaller particles or compacted over time. Subsequently, a second material was added to the surface, manure "naturally" mixed in over the years, and the result is a good workable footing that no longer has a simple description. In addition, footing materials break down from the impact of horse hoof action. The key is to learn to manage what you have.

Other arena surfaces may start and remain as primarily one material. These arenas are topped off with fresh material as older material breaks down. Most arena surfaces will need amendment at least every couple years because arena footing material does not last forever. Plan on a complete footing replacement, or at least a major overhaul, every 5 to 10 years. Even with proper management, the best, most carefully selected footing materials rarely maintain their good attributes indefinitely.

This chapter focuses on arenas that have a moderate to high amount of horse traffic, such as at a commercial facility. A private backyard arena, used once or twice per week, would be exposed to much less wear and tear and may suffice with a simple arena design. Most importantly, it has been proven that a successful riding surface is no better than the underlying foundation of base and subbase it rests upon (Fig. 17.1). A good indoor or outdoor arena surface is just the top layer of a multilayer composite. The base material is hard-packed material similar in construction to the base supporting a road surface. See Chapter 18 for design of the base and subbase layers of arena construction. The loose footing material discussed in this chapter is installed on top of this supporting base. The footing needs to "knit" to the base material, meaning that loose footing is not allowed to freely slide along the compacted base as horses work in the arena. Knitting is naturally achieved with some footing material selection and is

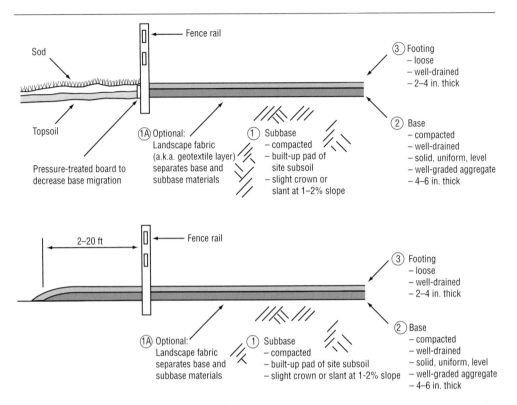

Figure 17.1. The footing material is only the top layer of riding arena construction and is dependent upon the support of a suitable base and subbase.

designed into other footing material installations (details provided in the section that follows).

Footing materials used on a farm's indoor and outdoor arenas may be different. Consider the conditions and use of each arena. For example, the indoor arena may be primarily used during cold weather months, with outdoor arena used during the other seasons. The outdoor arena may have to shed considerable quantities of water with the expectation that most footing material will stay in place, and so a well-draining, heavy material that does not float would be desirable. An indoor arena footing mixture that holds moisture longer will reduce the frequency of human-supplied watering events. The indoor arena surface material may incorporate salt for dust control via moisture retention. Alternatively, a wax, polymer, or oil coating may be added to reduce dust.

UNDERSTANDING FOOTING RAW MATERIALS

The primary principle of selecting footing materials is to obtain materials that maintain their loose nature without compaction while providing suitable stability for riding activity. Footing materials are composed of particles with properties that influence their suitability as footing materials. The major component of most footing is a mixture of naturally occurring sand, silt, and clay particles. In a sieve analysis (available from most industrial sand producers), these are listed from largest to smallest particle size. In addition to the particles of sand, silt, and clay in the footing mixture, there can be organic material (original and/or added through horse manure droppings) and perhaps additives such as coatings, synthetic fibers, or pieces of rubber. Compaction occurs when the voids between particles fill with smaller particles, thus "bridging" the matrix of particles together. Compaction is a function of the range of particle sizes and particle shapes found in the material. For the discussion that follows, "think small" while picturing common particle shape and its relation to neighboring particles.

There appear to be two main approaches to arena surface material selection. On one front are those who prefer to start with a large portion of the footing composed of the native soil and manipulate the surface with equipment, used frequently, to achieve the desired riding characteristics. The other approach designs a surface composed of delivered materials that meet criteria for the expected riding activity. Both approaches will work. The approach chosen often depends on local soil conditions and availability of locally mined raw materials. Most of the discussion that follows in this section relates to designed surfaces. When one works with the native soil as a primary component, the decision to use this material is a local one based on soil characteristics at the site. Soil is not the same throughout the country. For this discussion of arena footing materials, it is instructive to outline characteristics of suitable materials, which then allows evaluation of the suitability of local soil.

The range of particle sizes is the first key component for selecting footing materials. When footing is primarily composed of materials with one particle size, it cannot compact. In the extreme, this can be such a loose footing that it is unstable without much "purchase" for changes in direction or speed while riding. In contrast, when a widely graded material is used, then many particle sizes are present (up to the maximum size you specify). With this wide distribution of particle sizes, the smallest particles fill the gaps between the larger particles, so that eventually the materials are effectively contained in a smaller volume, or compacted.

Aggregate particle shape is the second key component in footing material selection. Sharply angular materials (like manufactured sand or stone dust) are more prone to compaction than "sub-angular" particles. Sharply angular materials can fit tightly together and have smaller void spaces between the particles than the less angular particles. Sub-angular particles have already had the sharpest corners broken off, so they do not fit as tightly together and provide larger void spaces between particles. To help visualize this, picture a brick placed next to adjacent bricks. Visualize new bricks that are sharply angular placed tightly and evenly so that the spaces between adjoining surfaces are even and very narrow. Now visualize bricks worn over time into a sub-angular shape with broken corners. Placing these sub-angular bricks tightly against each other will leave more space between bricks. A riding surface that is composed of sub-angular particles will be relatively

stable because the wide range of particles can nest together without rolling (round particles will roll) but will not compact because the rounded edges have voids between them that provide cushion. Manufactured particles fit together like pieces of a puzzle and have no air space, and therefore no cushion.

Particles need some angularity to offer resistance to movement between particles. Round particles would appear to offer the biggest void space between adjacent particles, thus being less compactable. But a footing primarily composed of round particles is not suitable because there is too little stability between particles. Picture a giant-scale footing composed of ball bearings or marbles. Beach and river sand have rounded particles through the wear of water action that has removed most angular corners. These rounded particles only have stability near the shoreline where they are saturated with water. Sub-angular particles offer resistance to movement between particles without the rolling action found with rounded particles. The sub-angular particle shapes are typical of naturally occurring mined materials. Naturally occurring sands have had the sharpest corners of their originally sharply angular particles broken off. These mined materials are more durable and provide better traction and stability because of their shape and are less prone to becoming dusty than manufactured materials. Crushed stone or gravel is manufactured and will be sharply angular until it erodes over time through use as the arena footing. This erosion of the sharpest corners of particles eventually makes them sub-angular, but the former corners leave fines that have potential to loft as dust. Not everyone lives within affordable delivery distance of mined sand, so understand and learn to manage what is available in your area.

Another aspect of particle shape relates to the fine particles within the footing matrix, which can be composed of silt or clay particles, depending on the gradation of sand that you choose. Within the finest particles of arena footing, the flat particle shape of clay is more prone to becoming slippery when wet because these particles easily slide over each other compared with the more angular silt and sand particles. A footing mixture with a large portion of clay or silt particles will be dusty when dry because these superfine particles loft easily and can be slippery when wet. In addition, the small clay particles easily "cement" the larger particles together by filling the void spaces between.

When compactable material is desired, such as for an arena base, for a stall floor base, or under a building foundation, use a widely graded manufactured material that has angular particle sizes that range from very fine to the largest size you specify (usually no larger than ¼ inch; any larger can bruise a horse's hoof). Crushed stone is the product most useful as a compactable base material.

When a noncompactable but stable footing surface is desired, choose an evenly graded material so that the majority of particles are within a limited size range. Choose a material with sub-angular particle shape. Type of riding activity will partially determine the stability needed in the riding surface. Evenly graded material will have a range of particle sizes, mostly in the middle range of suitable arena particle sizes, but it does not have the extremes that contain the fines (leading to dust and compaction) and large particles.

A feature that is becoming more important in footing material selection is the abrasiveness of the material on horse hooves. With a relatively nonabrasive material, such as wood products or shredded leather, horses may remain unshod if their primary riding area is in this type of footing. Conversely, sand, stonedust, and other sharply angular, aggregate materials can be abrasive to the hoof wall.

COMMON FOOTING MATERIALS

Sand

Sand is the common ingredient in many arena surfaces and ranges from fine sand at 0.05-millimeter diameter to coarse sand at 2.00-millimeter diameter. Sand alone may be used, but it is often combined with other particle sizes or other materials. Be careful to apply the proper depth of sand. With its deep, loose traction, sand deeper than 6 inches is stressful to horse tendons. Start with about 2 inches and add a ½ inch at a time as necessary. (Start with only 1½ inches for arenas used primarily for driving horses.) Newly laid sand contains air pockets that absorb shock and rebounds. However, despite its solid, inorganic nature, sand will erode and compact into an unsuitable surface over time.

Sand dries out fairly rapidly because it drains well, so frequent watering is essential. Some managers add a water-holding material, such as a wood product or commercial additive, to the sand footing material to hold water between watering events, thus reducing dust.

Certain specifications of sand are required for good footing material. Riding arena surfaces should contain cleaned and screened, medium-coarse, hard, and sharp sand. Fine sand will break down more readily into particles small enough to be lofted as dust. "Cleaned" means the material has been washed of silt and clay, making the sand less compactable and less dusty. "Screened" means large, undesirable particles have been removed and a more uniform-sized material remains that will be less prone to compaction. "Hard" is quartz sand, which will last up to 10 years. Obtained from a quarry, "sub-angular" sand has sharp particles compared with the rounded particles found in river sand. The sub-angular particles of naturally occurring mined materials are old deposits of sand that have weathered from natural forces of water (typically) into particles that are still angular for traction as an arena surface. Manufactured sand is very fine, crushed rock and is also angular, but not as hard as real sand. Angular sand provides better traction than rounded sand particles, which behave similar to millions of ball bearings underfoot.

Sand is often one of the cheapest materials to use for arena footing material; yet the hard, angular washed sand that is most suitable as a riding surface is among the most expensive. "Waste" or "dead" sand contains considerable quantities of the silt and clay particles that are the by-products of "clean" sand and is unacceptable for good arena footing. Cleaned, washed sand alone is too loose for some riding disciplines that require sharp turns and stops, such as barrel racing and cutting. Wetted sand provides much more traction than dry sand, but frequent and abundant watering is needed and this is not realistic in some locations.

Allowing 5 to 10% fines (passing 200 screen) in the chosen sand product provides particles that help bind the larger sand particles. More fines than this, and the sand mixture becomes very dusty and slippery when wet. Providing 5% fines will allow some binding activity while decreasing dust potential; as the sand wears, the fine particle percentage will increase. For arena surfaces designed to use native topsoil, 10% to 30% of the mixture may be "dirt" with the balance sand. Unfortunately, the fines in either of these mixtures will loft as dust if not managed for dust suppression (see "Dust Management" section of this chapter). Fibers, natural or synthetic, may be used to bind loose sand with less risk of adding dustiness but cost greater than the addition of fines or local soil. A combination sand-soil arena is popular with western riding events where high traction is needed for speed events so the footing can be kept moist and more compacted or harrowed into a loose mixture for sliding stops and cutting work.

Other materials, such as wood and rubber, may be mixed with sand to overcome some difficulty encountered when using sand alone. Wood products added to sand footings will add moisture-holding capacity and improve traction while adding some cushioning. Rubber adds cushion to a sand footing and can prolong the useful life of the sand through decreased abrasion of sand particles on sand particles. Although rubber can add some cushion to worn sand footing, for old and eroded sand the better long-term fix is to discarded the failed surface material and replace with a new mixture. Rubber is a relatively expensive addition to a footing that has outlived its useful life and is best replaced.

Stonedust

Stonedust provides good traction, drains well, and can be an attractive surface if kept watered and harrowed. It will be almost as hard as concrete if allowed to dry and compact, requiring attentive moisture management for indoor use. Stonedust is very dusty if not kept constantly moist throughout the entire depth of footing. For footing material, the stonedust (also known as blue stone, rockdust, limestone screenings, decomposed granite, or white stone) should be within a narrow range of grade sizes so that it does not compact easily. Stonedust is a finer version of the road base material used in arena base preparation. If the stonedust in your area is well graded and is suitable as a compacted base material, it will be difficult to keep loose as a footing material. In contrast, when stonedust is not compactable, it can make a suitable arena footing material.

Stonedust mixed with rubber will provide a less compactable footing than stonedust alone while keeping the high traction stonedust offers for quick changes in direction and speeds, such as jump take-off and landing activity.

Wood Products

Wood products may be used as the primary footing material or mixed with other footing materials.

Wood chips or coarse sawdust will provide some cushioning and moisture-holding capacity to an all-inorganic footing (sand, stonedust). Wood products are quite variable, not only from location to location around the country but even from load to load at the same wood mill. Any wood product will eventually decompose because it is organic, and smaller and softer wood products will break down into smaller particles that will eventually lead to compacted footing. Expect to add more wood products every couple years as the older wood decomposes. Eventually, some footing may have to be removed to maintain an appropriate depth.

Manufactured wood products may be used as the predominant footing component. All-wood footing offers cushioning in a material with fibers that interlace for traction. Wood footing materials contain pieces larger and longer than wood chips or sawdust that are more durable and require little maintenance when installed correctly. Wood footing has ½- to 1-inch slender pieces, or wood "fiber" mixed with some finer wood for knitting the wood footing to the base material. All-wood footing is often installed on a 1-inch layer of wetted and washed angular sand to further tie the wood pieces into the highly compacted base surface. Hardwood pieces will last longer than softwood products. Do *not* use walnut and black cherry hardwood products because they are highly toxic to horses. For this reason and for quality control in eliminating contaminants in the shipment (large wood chunks, nails, staples from ground pallets, etc.) it is recommended to buy wood footing from a manufacturer that specializes in supplying horse arena footing. An advantage of all-wood footing is the reduced abrasiveness on horse hooves compared with sand- and stonedust-based footing materials. The material must be kept moist to maintain adhesiveness of the wood pieces with each other. Fully dried all-wood footing can become slippery as the wood becomes more brittle and does not as effectively interlace for traction. In contrast, all-wood footing with large pieces (for example, chunk bark or wood greater than 1-inch square, not slender) becomes slippery when overly wet.

Rubber

Rubber from recycled shoes or tires can be ground or shredded into small particles. Rubber source

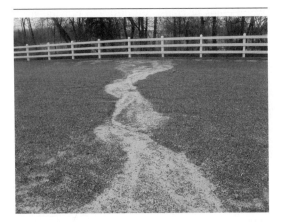

Figure 17.2. Rubber pieces can float to the top of a footing mixture after large rainfall events. The rubber will have to be mixed back into this stonedust mixture with surface conditioning equipment.

may vary, so use products from a horse footing material supplier. Make sure to get a guarantee that the shredded product will not contain metal (from steel-belted tires) or other foreign materials, or check the load upon delivery. Ground rubber is usually mixed with sand or other surface material to minimize compaction and add some cushion into the surface. A rubber product will not degrade like wood but will break down into smaller pieces through grinding against sand and horse hooves. Its ability to darken an outdoor arena surface color reduces glare and helps thaw the surface faster during winter by absorbing more solar radiation. Pure rubber tends to be too bouncy and the black color provides significant heat on outdoor arena users. Indoor arena users may notice the rubber odor, but horses are not prone to eat it. Rubber pieces float and with heavy rainfall can separate and be out of the footing material mixture (Fig. 17.2). Simply reincorporate with surface conditioning equipment. Rubber is added to a sand or stonedust footing at the rate of 1 to 2 pounds of rubber per square foot. Crumb-shaped rubber pieces are suitable to reduce compaction in a sand-dirt or stonedust mixture. Flat rubber pieces (or fibers) will help knit together an all-sand clean footing that needs more stability. The rubber fibers essentially knit together the entire depth of footing profile to create a material that does not shift as readily as pure sand.

CHALLENGING FOOTING MATERIALS

Topsoil

Topsoil is hard to define because of differences in local soil types, but the properties that make it useful in growing crops or sod make it unsuitable for arena footing. Topsoil is not recommended because it is a widely graded material and therefore tends to compact. Topsoil is a mixture of clay, loam (silt), sand, and organic material that provides too many fine particles, leading to dust problems when dried. Organic material breaks down further over time, adding to the dust problem. Topsoil with a large clay portion will be slippery when wet and hard when dried. Not all topsoils are well draining and so require more time than the surface materials discussed earlier to become suitable for riding after a drenching rain. Dirt arenas continue to be successfully used when the native soil contains large quantities of sand particles (more than 50%) or is mixed with sand (see "Sand" section).

Stall Waste

Stall waste (manure and bedding mixture) can be used as an arena footing for the very short term and is admittedly a cheap material. It will be dusty because it is almost entirely organic material that breaks down rapidly into small particles that lead to compaction. Filth of lofted dust and potential for attracting flies can be a concern. Odor is unpleasant if the stall waste contains large amounts of manure. Ammonia gas given off by the decomposing urine and feces is not healthy for the horse respiratory system. On outdoor arenas, stall waste is slippery when wet. Even on indoor arenas, when kept wet enough to dampen the dust, the stall waste surface tends to be slippery. It will need to be replaced at least annually.

LOCALLY AVAILABLE MATERIALS

Arena footings composed of shredded leather, industrial by-products, and mine waste have all been used and may be a cheap local source of footing materials. Match the good footing criteria presented earlier to the properties of the local material to help determine how desirable the material will be.

A FOOTING RECIPE TO TRY

This sand and wood product combination has been used successfully at the Pennsylvania State University and in many private arenas.

Recipe for 1000 square feet of arena surface:

Sand at 100-lb/ft^3 density
12 tons for 3 inches deep
8 tons for 2 inches deep

Sawdust at 15-lb/ft^3 density
1.25 tons (or 6 yards) for 2 inches deep
½ to ¾ ton (or 3 yards) for 1 inch deep
(a "yard" is a cubic yard or 27 ft^3)

CHARACTERIZING FOOTING MATERIALS

Table 17.1 presents characteristics of several common footing materials. The characteristics represent those selected specifically for good arena footing (e.g., dust potential). You can see why wood products would be added to a footing to increase moisture-holding capacity and why rubber pieces or sand would be added to reduce compaction. Figure 17.3 offers a look at the footing particle size distributions that were found in six indoor riding arenas located at commercial boarding facilities in central Pennsylvania. (Particle size distribution determines the various ranges of particle diameters in a composite material such as arena footing.) Note that the two "sand" arenas were very different in their particle size distribution. This emphasizes why you should be specific as to the desired type of sand (or

any other material) in an arena footing. Some materials are sold with a particle size distribution analysis. It is important to keep the fines, or particles below 0.1-millimeter diameter, to a minimum in the mixture. Dust is caused by clay and silt particles, which are 0.001 to 0.005 millimeter in diameter, and should be kept below 5% of the mixture. Fine and very fine sands, which are 0.05 to 0.25 millimeter in diameter, also contribute to dust when allowed to dry. The more the fines, the more the dust potential.

DUST MANAGEMENT

Riding arenas, and particularly indoor arenas, are plagued with dust problems. Dust causes eye and nose irritations and contributes to respiratory damage in both horse and rider. It is estimated that an idle horse inhales 16 gallons of air per minute and during strenuous exercise can inhale up to 600 gallons per minute. Minimizing the amount of dust in this air should be a primary goal in footing material choice and subsequent management to suppress dust. In addition to horse and handler respiratory irritation, dust coats any structure and equipment near the arena. Dust rises from the surface when a large percentage of fines break loose and float into the air. Naturally, lightweight particles are more

Table 17.1. Characteristics of Riding Arena Footing Materials

Material	Primary Use	Cushion or Compaction Resistance	Traction Improved	Dust	Drainage	Water Retention	Slippery When Wet	Freezing Potential	Durability	Abrasive	Maintenance	Cost
Sand	Footing	H	M	L	H	L	N	L	H	H	L	M
Wood products[a]	Footing / Additive to increase moisture retention	H	M	V	M	H	V	V	M	L	M	L–M
Stonedust	Footing / Compacted for base	M	H	H	H	L	N	L	H	H	M	L–M
Rubber pieces[a]	Additive to reduce compaction	H	M	L	H	L	N?	L	M	L	L	H
Soil	Additive for stability	L	V	V	V	V	Y	H	L	M	H	L
Stall waste	Footing	M	L	H	L	H	Y	V	L	L	H	L

Note: L, low; M, medium; H, high; V, variable; Y, yes; N, no.

[a]Potential contaminants are diminished when materials are purchased from a specialty horse footing material supplier.

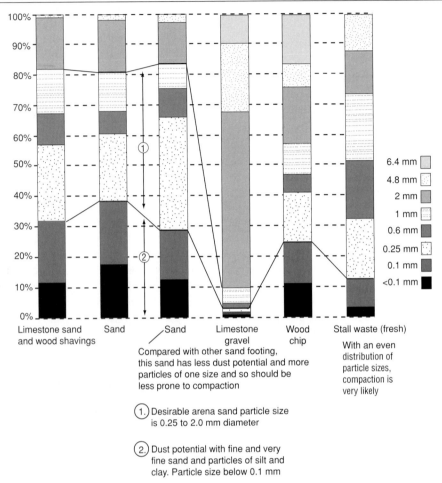

Figure 17.3. Particle size distributions of six indoor riding arena footing materials. Minimizing the amount of fine material will decrease dust potential.

prone to suspension than heavier particles. Decrease lightweight particles in three ways:

1. Eliminate fine particles, such as silt, clay, or fine sand, in the footing mixture by careful footing material selection. Even coarse materials such as sand and wood products will break down over time into many fine particles, so maintenance is critical to reduce dust. In some footing mixtures, 10 to 30% of these materials are deliberately added for traction and water-holding capacity; but realize the implications for more diligent management for dust suppression. With a high percentage of fines, the arena footing material should be partially or wholly replaced. Remove manure deposited on the arena surface before it gets mixed in. Manure will break down into fine particles contributing to the dust problem.

2. Moisten particles to increase their weight with simple, cheap, and environmentally friendly water. With no rain occurring in indoor arenas, the facility manager must be in charge of moisture control. Moisture retention and evaporation is site and season dependent, so weekly checks on moisture level are important. Materials that can hold more water will increase the time between watering events (more about watering in the next section of this chapter).

3. Provide an additive to bind particles together. Many riding surface additives are available. Moisture retainers can be used or the surface amended to capture and hold more moisture on a dry site. Wood chips, and other organic mate-

rials, retain moisture well and can be a first line of defense. Synthetic or natural (e.g., coconut) fibers can be used to intertwine with footing particles to bind the materials together. Crystals resembling cat litter can absorb relatively large quantities of water and then release that moisture into the surrounding footing material as it dries out. Water additives can slow evaporation, increase moisture penetration, or encourage microbes to grow on footing materials for their moisture and binding activity. Peat moss holds considerable water and, when managed to be kept constantly damp, it is effective at binding a footing mixture. Once peat moss dries, it no longer has binding ability and becomes loose and potentially slippery. Fully dried peat moss is hydrophobic and takes considerable effort to re-wet.

Oil-based products (such as palm, coconut, mineral, and soybean oil) can weigh down or glue together fine particles similar to the effects of water application. The first application of oil is used to coat all the footing particles to increase their weight. Subsequent annual or biennial application of oil is of much reduced quantity to coat newly formed particles that have abraded off the original footing particles. The plant-derived oils can become rancid over time. Application of used motor oil is an environmental hazard. Costing more but lasting longer, wax or pharmaceutical-grade petroleum coating is a good option. The latter has characteristics similar to Vaseline. The petroleum coating lasts about 10 years between applications, is UV resistant, and will not become rancid.

Salt may be used to draw moisture out of the air and into the footing material. Calcium chloride ($CaCl_2$) and magnesium chloride ($MgCl_2$) are less expensive and more effective compared with common table salt sodium chloride (NaCl). The effectiveness relates to calcium chloride and magnesium chloride having three available ions for binding water molecules, while sodium chloride has only two ions. Salt application has lost favor for use as a moisture retention additive because it dries out hooves and, being a salt, is corrosive to metal such as indoor arena siding and structural supports when lofted with the dust. (These salts are still effectively and commonly used to reduce the freezing temperature of the footing material during cold weather in northern climates.) Salt application rate is 20 to 50 pounds per 1000 square feet of arena surface area.

With watering or rainfall, the salt leaches out of the footing and needs to be replenished.

WATER USE AND TECHNIQUES

Watering the footing material reduces dust levels and can put some traction back into loose, sandy or wood-based footing. Frequent deep watering will be part of normal arena maintenance, so planning ahead to make it a less arduous task will have long-term benefit. The objective is to keep the material moist all the way through.

Water to keep the footing evenly moist to a 3-inch depth. Once the arena is at a moisture that is suitable for your riding purpose, use a garden-supply store meter to determine that moisture content and strive to achieve that moisture on subsequent waterings. Water an arena as you would a garden. It does not need to be flooded, nor does just wetting the top fraction of an inch do any good. Give it a good watering with plenty of water in frequent, short periods. The dry spells are for water absorption into the footing material(s). In fact, leave about four hours or overnight before using the arena again to allow moisture to soak in. Once the correct moisture is achieved, subsequent waterings will only be needed to remoisten the topmost surface that will be drying faster than the footing underneath. The water schedule will naturally depend on season (air temperature), wind, and sun exposure of outdoor arenas and the indoor arena air temperature and moisture level. Watering when the arena surface begins to show signs of dustiness will preserve moisture in the underlying layer. Check moisture level weekly and more often when drying conditions prevail, such as during times of combined low humidity, high temperature, or greater wind speed over the arena surface. On outdoor arenas, direct sunlight dries the top footing layer on a daily basis.

Watering systems include those requiring continuous or frequent human involvement for proper application of the water and those that are automated and, once installed or setup, require little human attention during the watering event. Watering that requires a high level of human involvement include hand-held spray nozzle, garden sprinkler, and tractor-mounted sprayer (Fig. 17.4). More automated systems included ceiling- or post-mounted spray nozzles and self-traveling irrigation.

Handheld hose watering takes considerable time and can be uneven in moisture addition. The benefit

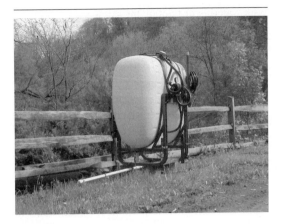

Figure 17.4. A tractor- or pickup-mounted water spray tank: a way to partially automate wetting arena surface materials.

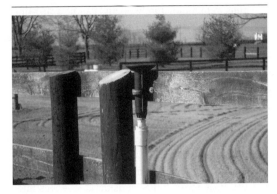

Figure 17.6. Horticultural-type sprinklers can be used in indoor and outdoor arenas to automate the surface watering process.

is that the person watering can accommodate wet and dry patches of arena surface with more or less water. Garden sprinklers can be set out for timed operation and moved to cover the entire arena surface over time. This allows other chores to be performed by the operator but is likely to be less uniform in coverage than the handheld technique. Puddles are common when a sprinkler stays in one area too long. Tractor or pickup mounted watering can be done in concert with surface conditioning (Fig.17.5). A frost-proof hydrant should be located near the arena to supply hose- or sprinkler-applied water. A hydrant is a con-

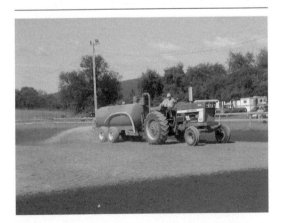

Figure 17.5. Large amounts of water may be necessary to keep outdoor arena surface dust under control. To more fully suppress dust, more than just the topmost surface layer needs to be wetted.

venient tap for filling a water tank that is pulled by truck or tractor through the arena.

Automated arena watering is provided by a permanently installed sprinkler system located along the perimeter of an outdoor arena or throughout the roof framing of indoor arenas, or by mechanized field watering equipment in both indoor and outdoor arenas. The width of the arena and the available water source are important factors in determining what type of system will be most effective.

Horticultural- or agricultural-grade sprinkler systems (gear-driven rotors or impact heads) are suitable for providing fairly even watering to the riding arena surface. Ceiling-mounted sprayers (indoor arena) produce a mist of water and have a good, uniform coverage. Frost-proof installations are needed under freezing conditions. Landscape sprinklers can be installed around an outdoor arena perimeter to reach the entire surface with water (Fig. 17.6). Indoor or outdoor sprinklers are spaced on the basis of anticipated coverage pattern of the particular spray nozzle. Side-mounted sprinklers require substantial flow rates to spray water distances greater than 50 feet. Greater spray distances provide uneven water application with strips of unwetted surface between adjacent wetted circles or half-circles. For indoor arenas, the side-mounted sprinklers' uneven water distribution results in too much water applied in some areas, which is a problem because the indoor arena base is not constructed to shed water. The sprinklers may be activated as needed or controlled by a timer.

Arena surface materials may be wetted by mechanized field watering equipment. A flexible hose traveling system is an effective option for sites with larger arenas or with low volume water sources. One disadvantage is that the traveling hose has to be set up each time it is used. Once set up, it operates unattended with an automatic shutoff after the sprinkler cart on the traveling hose arrives back at the hose reel. Advantages include more even water distribution than with perimeter-mounted sprinklers and potential to double its usefulness by watering both indoor and outdoor arenas. Installation and maintenance costs of automatic systems are the highest of the footing watering options, but labor is significantly reduced.

Winter watering is a challenge in freezing climates. Too much water and the footing is frozen hard; too little water and dust prevails. This is a particular challenge for indoor arenas where riders expect that the surface will be usable year round. Managers may opt to reduce water additions to the indoor arena as freezing weather approaches. The advantage of having a footing material that does not compact is even more important when freezing is possible. Excess water can pass through a well-drained material such as sand and not bind particles together into a solid mass. Many indoor arena managers use salt to lower the footing's freezing point during the winter and discontinue its use during warmer weather.

SURFACE MAINTENANCE

Horse traffic patterns during arena use will cause the footing material to become uneven. The high-traffic path along the arena rail will take the most abuse. Depending on the riding discipline, high-traffic areas are also located along the arena diagonals, near barrels or poles, and the centerline. The footing within the high-traffic area will be thrown out of the path by hoof action, while any remaining footing will be more compacted where it is most needed. It is not uncommon for the footing material to be almost entirely gone from the high-traffic area with the horses working off the base material. This is very undesirable; footing is supposed to provide a cushion above the highly compacted base material. Horse hooves contacting the base will cause permanent ruts in the base that are expensive to repair. Footing near jumps also compacts. Surprisingly, the position where riding instructors stand is among the most compacted footing in an arena.

Uneven footing and compacted areas at the rail and elsewhere are resolved with a dragging device

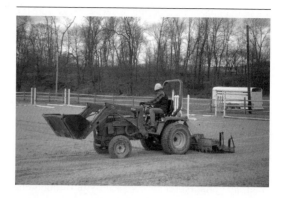

Figure 17.7. Equipment will be needed for frequent conditioning of the riding surface to redistribute footing for an even coverage of the base material and, in some cases, to loosen compacted surface materials.

to redistribute or break up the footing material (Fig. 17.7). Dragging should be done even before traffic patterns begin to be detected. Plan to drag the arena at least once per week even for arenas that are lightly used for riding three times a week or more. Arenas under heavily scheduled use will need the surface dragged once or more daily. Once a deep path of disturbed footing is established, it is difficult to alleviate. Ruts along the rail are common, but frequent redistribution of the footing will keep the rut from becoming chronic. Accumulation of footing at the fenceline of an outdoor arena can slow surface water drainage. To make the dragging less time consuming, use appropriate equipment that is easy to hook up and adjust to conditions.

Several options for dragging arena footing back into position are available. A tractor-pulled chain-link fence section (with added weight) or light harrow is adequate for loose footing such as wood products. Dragging devices that cannot be lifted will drag footing material out of the arena gate as it exits unless it is stowed prior to exit. Finer but heavier footing materials, such as sand and stonedust, will need a harrow with short tines. The tines are dull "spikes" that are flat on the bottom. Adjustable tines are highly recommended so they may be set to redistribute and loosen the entire depth of footing while not disturbing the base material. Adjustment of harrow tines is a real advantage in surface conditioning to match desired conditions, to match depth of footing as it wears and compacts, and for use in more than one arena footing material. Make sure the tines are set or purchased short enough so that they do not penetrate the underlying base material. The base is an expensive part of the arena construction and costly to repair if it is accidentally dredged up into the footing material. Heavier harrows benefit from a three-point tractor hitch arrangement to raise and lower the device for entry and exit from the arena.

SUMMARY

With no common recipe for successful riding arena surface material, understanding the physical principles that one is trying to achieve with the footing can lead to better selection of materials. Once installed, learn to manage the footing materials, because each material and mixture of materials will have advantages and shortcomings. Footing will change over time; therefore, be adaptable and manage the footing material accordingly. Understand the principles of surface maintenance and indication of when footing material needs to be amended or replaced. Footings with sand as a major component are usually successful. Choose hard, angular, and washed sand for stability with loose footing composition. The addition of about 5% fines will help bind sand together but with increased need for management of dust. Good footing requires regular and consistent management in dust control and surface finishing.

18
Outdoor Riding Arena Design and Construction

An outdoor arena of 100 feet by 200 feet is considered useful for a variety of riding uses. Arenas that are smaller than 60 feet by 120 feet have limited use for vigorous activity. Of course some disciplines have common arena sizes (Table 18.1), such as a standard dressage arena of 20 meters by 60 meters (66 feet by 190 feet). The arena will take up land area larger than the arena riding surface dimensions because the construction will include additional pad and water drainage features beyond the riding arena perimeter.

SITE COMPONENTS AND LOCATION

Outdoor riding arena components consist of the riding surface and the underlying base layers of material that support the riding surface, and although optional, there is usually a fence or rail to designate the riding arena perimeter. Additional components often include a sprinkler system for dust control and lighting for after-dark riding. Spectator seating may be provided.

With an outdoor arena, site selection, especially in relation to water management, is essential. Select as level a site as possible to reduce excavation costs. Even a level site will need to be built to facilitate drainage of precipitation on the riding surface. All arenas will need to be sloped to effectively shed water.

The outdoor arena "site" will include features external and upslope to the actual riding surface that facilitate drainage. Grade the site or install perimeter drainage so that surface water and groundwater do not reach the arena site. It is far more important to divert incoming surface water from the arena site than to install elaborate drainage features under the arena surface.

Site location considerations include being close enough to the stable for convenience of users. Arena activity can be stimulating to turned-out horses, and pastured horses can provide distraction for horses working in an arena. Choose a location away from paddocks and pastures, when possible. Arenas that will be used for competition should be separated from traffic or activity to lessen the noise and distraction for competitors. Provide an all-weather driveway access to the arena site for horses and surface maintenance equipment.

THE SIMPLEST ARENA

The most simple outdoor arena construction would consist of a well-graded and -drained site using only compacted subsoil as a base. Strip topsoil from arena area, adjust grade of subsoil as needed to facilitate drainage, compact subsoil, add leveled sand as footing, and ride. Initially start with between 1½ and 2 inches of sand (depending on riding discipline) and see how this compacts and works. Add another ½ inch at a time until a suitable footing is achieved. It is much easier to add another ½ inch of any material than it is to remove material once it is deemed to be too deep. This type of two-layer arena construction, with only a compacted subbase and loose footing material, will suffice for casual riding. The simple two-layer arena will not have a suitable riding surface for all weather conditions. The addition of a base layer under the footing will provide more stability for the riding surface and is recommended for all but the most infrequently used outdoor arenas.

In order to provide a year-round riding surface, careful site preparation is involved. Site selection and preparation will be among the most important decisions in relation to arena durability and maintenance cost.

ARENA USE

The number of horses and the type of use will determine the complexity and expense level of your arena

Table 18.1. Arena Dimensions Suggested for Competition Activities[a]

Arena Type	Width (ft)	Length (ft)
Suggested Sizes		
Barrel racing	150	200
Calf roping or steer wresting	100	300
Team roping	150	300
Pleasure riding	60–100	120–200
Regulation Sizes		
USEF[b] small	110	220
USEF[b] standard	120	240
USDF[c] small (20 m × 40 m)	66	132
USDF[c] standard (20 m × 60 m)	66	190

[a]Continue site grading 2 to 20 feet in all directions beyond riding surface area as an arena pad to dissipate forces of arena use and to accommodate water drainage off site.

[b]United States Equestrian Federation; formerly National Horse Show Association (NHSA).

[c]United States Dressage Federation.

construction. If it will not be used every day, a simple construction (described earlier) may suffice. But a busy boarding or showing stable will need the more elaborate multilayered base surfaces and perhaps more careful drainage system for year-round, daily use. Highly used arenas should consider the most durable construction that may initially be more expensive but offers lower cost and reduced maintenance in the long run. Even simple, infrequently used arenas will benefit from considering the construction principles presented here in order to avoid costly reconstruction and maintenance headaches. Grading and drainage remain as important issues despite the simplicity of the construction or limited riding use. *Underfoot*, a very useful booklet by the U.S. Dressage Federation (USDF; see Additional Resources) can be helpful to contractors not familiar with arena construction techniques. Contractors familiar with road construction practices will be comfortable with outdoor riding arena construction because similar techniques apply.

SLOPE FOR PRECIPITATION MOVEMENT

Provide the riding arena 1% to 2% slope in all directions with the crown, or the highest point, down the arena centerline. This center crown design provides the shortest path for water travel off the arena as long as runoff water can be handled where it collects. A shorter water flow path means less chance for surface material movement in contrast to higher volume

water flows over longer paths with other arena slope designs. The 2% grading is usually preferable and will seem flat to horse and rider but provides enough slope to allow water to run off the site. Some horses will be able to detect this change in grade, and for highly disciplined riding, such as dressage, a 1 to 1½% slope is preferred. In lower precipitation areas, a 1% slope can be tolerated. In some cases, the site topography is not conducive to high center crown drainage, so the arena can be uniformly sloped 1 to 2% in any one direction. Providing the slope in the direction of the shortest dimension will likely be the least costly in terms of grading and will minimize the surface material movement mentioned earlier. The use of survey equipment is required to obtain this 1 to 2% slope, which is nearly indistinguishable by eye. (Indoor arenas are not crowned for precipitation drainage and may be flat.) Water does not lie. If water ponds somewhere within the riding arena (Fig. 18.1), then that is a low spot and an elevation or slope change is needed to fix the situation.

LAYERS

In many ways, building an outdoor riding arena surface is similar to building a road. Both depend on quality workmanship in excavation, base compaction, and material layering. The main difference is that the arena's topmost surface is a loose footing material rather than asphalt. Careful site preparation and compaction of the subbase and base materials

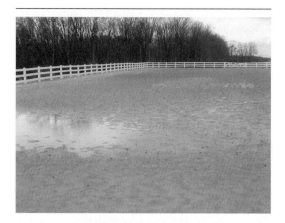

Figure 18.1. With inadequate crown (or slope) to the outdoor riding arena surface, water will pond in a low spot. Without adequate base preparation, low-lying areas form in locations of heavy arena use.

using proper techniques are necessary for durable roads or arenas. It is recommended that the outdoor arena be constructed to move rainwater and snowmelt horizontally off the riding surface and away from the site rather than a design that allows vertical water movement down through the base layers into drains. The discussion that follows assumes construction for horizontal water movement.

Essentials of Outdoor Arena Construction
- Determine arena size.
- Select site for functional location.
- Remove topsoil.
- Build up or amend site to facilitate drainage.

- Grade and compact native subsoil for subbase.
- Add well-graded base material; slope and compact to 4- to 12-inch layer.
- Install perimeter fence or rail (optional).
- Add loose footing material as riding surface.

Arena construction cost varies considerably, but a very rough estimate is that about $10,000 in materials alone will be needed for a full-sized dressage arena. This cost is simply for a 6-inch stonedust base material and 2 inches of sand footing dumped at the site. This rough cost does not account for long freight hauling if the proposed arena site is in an area without naturally occurring materials that are suitable for arena base and footing materials. This expenditure is for material alone and does not include additional cost for grading the site and construction of the arena using the delivered materials.

Building an outdoor riding arena surface is similar to building a road because both depend on quality workmanship in excavation, compaction, and material layering.

Subbase Pad

Build a subbase (pad) that is sloped in support of the layers above it that are expected to drain water. All topsoil is removed from the arena, drainage swales, and other areas influenced by the arena construction. The swales are often created as subsoil borrow areas for building up the subbase pad under the riding surface. The pad needs to be 2 to 20 feet longer in all directions, or well beyond the perimeter fencing, than the planned final arena size (Fig. 18.2).

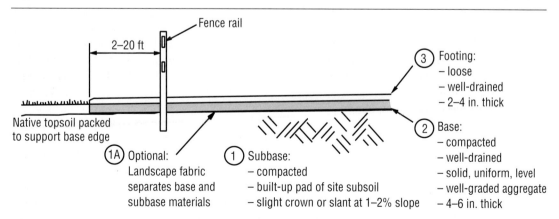

Figure 18.2. Outdoor riding arena construction is sloped for surface water drainage and includes a well-compacted subbase and base construction to support the riding surface material.

This recommendation is relatively easy to achieve because the subbase grade is generally extended beyond the riding surface as part of the drainage swales.

The subbase is sloped 1 to 2% to move surface water off the arena site. This subbase needs to be compacted as densely as possible with at least an 8-ton roller; larger is even better. A bulldozer or front-end loader will not provide sufficient compaction. It is generally more cost effective to bring in the roller for proper compaction than to spend the effort it takes to compact small lifts of subsoil with many passes of unsuitable packing equipment. The subbase should be a minimum 92% compaction. Compaction increases the density of the subbase, which makes it impervious to the effects of rain, freezing, and horse activity. Potholes, or weak points, in the arena foundation will be less likely to form.

Base

The base supports the weight and concussion of the horse traffic and is essentially the foundation for the arena. It also provides protection to the subbase.

MATERIALS

Base material can be of limestone, bluestone, or whitestone composition. Depending on region, other names for base material may prevail, but requesting "road base" mix is a good starting point. An "engineered" crushed rock material is recommended. The material is an aggregate of many particle sizes that is not slippery and will not swell once compacted or wet. Base material must be a well-graded material that can pack well and needs to be able to drain water horizontally away from the topmost arena footing. The goal is to shed water although even a properly compacted base will allow about 5 to 15% of applied water to percolate through. With a poor-draining subbase, the base material has to function as a medium over which water will flow horizontally.

Use base material with aggregate no larger than ¼ inch so that stones large enough to injure horse hooves do not work their way up into the footing material. Choose a base mixture that contains at least 10% material that will pass a #200 screen to ensure effective cementation between the larger particles. Preferred is a material with 15 to 16% material that passes the #200 screen for suitable binding of the base materials. Mixtures with a high proportion of sand or uniform particle size will not compact.

Where possible, choose a base material of contrasting color relative to the chosen arena surface footing material color. This will help in visual evaluations for maintenance of arena trouble spots. One can see whether base material has worked its way into the footing. Footing material options are discussed in Chapter 17.

CONSTRUCTION

Extend the base, as was the subbase, 2 to 20 feet beyond the arena fenceline. This is done to prevent the edges of the arena from crumbling off as horses work along the rail, similar to a paved shoulder of a road. The 2-foot dimension is the minimum acceptable dimension that allows horse hoof impact along the arena rail to be dissipated through the surrounding base material. A 10- to 20-foot dimension, if supplied with footing material, can accommodate horses warming up around the outside track. Compact the base material as close to 100% compaction as possible; 95% compaction is typical. The base should be smooth and look almost like asphalt when properly prepared. In fact, some arenas use coarse asphalt as their arena base. Install arena fence holes and posts prior to the footing layer installation.

The base is typically a 4- to 6-inch compacted depth of well-graded material. The softer the subbase, the more the base depth needed. The more use and abuse of the arena surface, the deeper the base needed. A jumping arena or one used with many horses at a time may need a 6- to 12-inch compacted base. The base is sloped the same as the subbase. Maintenance of the base layer will be needed in even a properly constructed arena. Trouble spots may develop in high-traffic or impact areas if the base is damaged during routine surface maintenance or if the base is not allowed to dry and harden after a deep watering or heavy rainfall.

One of the last steps in arena site construction is an even layer of topsoil added back on the drainage swales for grass establishment. The topsoil is installed to butt against and support the full depth of the base material edge. This interface is rolled and compacted into an integral junction as part of the final landscaping. This design of the base edge is more cost effective in using native material than constructing a timber retainer. Where site conditions will not allow 2-foot extension of the arena pad,

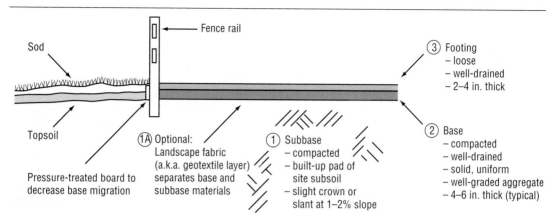

Figure 18.3. A board or timber at arena perimeter can be used to hold base and footing material when extending the arena pad at least 2 feet beyond the riding surface is not feasible.

wood timbers may be used to support the edge of the base material at the arena perimeter fenceline (Fig. 18.3). Maintenance of the edge of the base will be necessary as water shed from the arena surface will work its way between the timber and base material causing base material washout. Adding the timber retainer is an improvement over no support of the base edge if the base does not extend beyond the fence perimeter.

PorOuS BASE OPTION

For Olympic-caliber arenas that need to have the low 1% slope and are used during and immediately after significant rain events, a more porous base (with only 7 to 8% of material passing a #200 screen) may be supplied that allows about 25 to 30% of surface-applied water to percolate through (compared with the 5 to 15% water movement though the more common arena construction designed to shed rainwater). For this more porous arena construction, most rainwater can be shed via the shallow 1% arena crowned slope, but up to a third of the water will flow through the base to a gravel layer for horizontal water movement off the arena site. The subbase is sloped at 2% to better move water off the site through the gravel layer. This 2% slope is changed through built-up material to transition to the 1% base and surface material slope. This is clearly an expensive arena construction.

Geotextile Layer

A layer sometimes incorporated into outdoor arena construction is a geotextile or landscape fabric

between the base and subbase materials (see Fig. 18.2). The fabric is sturdy enough to keep the two materials in place and prevent mixing of the components. Because of rainwater drainage, which tends to carry small particles downward, and freeze-thaw cycles, which can hoist materials upward, material movement is more of a problem in outdoor arenas than indoor arenas. With the addition of the geotextile layer, the well-graded aggregate of the base does not eventually work its way downward into the subbase, and any rocks in the subbase are not as likely to work their way toward the arena surface. It also tends to be easier to compact the base when a geotextile is used on top of the subbase. The fabric also provides tensile reinforcement within the arena base construction that is traditionally strong in compression and weak in tension. The result is an arena base where surface loads are spread over a larger area, thus reducing localized base failures. These characteristics will lessen pothole formation. Rolls of geotextile material are laid over the subbase with a 12- to 18-inch overlap at edges of adjoining fabric pieces. A 4- to 5-ounce polyester nonwoven filter fabric is recommended for arena construction. Geotextile pores will clog with fine soil particles, so they are not recommended for use where water is expected to flow through them. For arena construction, water is diverted at the sloped surface and is not expected to flow downward through the base layers. The addition of a geotextile layer adds roughly 10% to arena construction cost.

WATER MANAGEMENT

Water runoff from adjacent land needs to be diverted from the arena area by diversion swales, drains, or by placing the arena on high ground. Precipitation on the surface needs to be drained down through the footing layer and directed away horizontally by the base because it cannot effectively percolate through the highly compacted base and subbase construction. Obviously, a high water table that breeches the arena surface is undesirable. Site selection should avoid saturated soil areas by not building in a low-lying area or flood plain, despite how attractive they might be as level sites.

Drains in or under the arena are not recommended and would be redundant if the practices mentioned earlier are followed. It is much more important to slope water away and divert incoming water than to rely on drains under the arena. Drains in the arena surface will clog. Drains under the arena surface are unnecessary if the arena is built up higher than surrounding land, the surface is sloped to drain off rainwater, and any excess water has been diverted and drained away from the arena edges.

Ensure that water will flow around your arena, not through it, and that precipitation water can flow off:

- Divert surface water flowing from adjacent land away from the arena.
- Construct to be above soils saturated with groundwater.
- Encourage precipitation to flow off the arena by sloping the surface.

Surface Water

Diversion ditches catch and/or divert surface water coming toward the arena from higher areas to save the arena from flooding. Sod-covered swales are shallow, wide ditches that are located to the side of the riding surface pad (Fig. 18.4). They often start at 6 to 12 inches deep and about 8 to 20 feet wide, depending on the water they are expected to handle. They slope 1 to 2% toward an area where water can be discharged or collected. If possible, the sides should be sloped at approximately 1:3 (vertical:horizontal) to the deepest bottom part of the swale and should be planted to sod. The swale bottom should be wide enough to allow mowing for ease of maintenance. Steeper slopes may be covered with a large-diameter drain rock. If a drain rock needs to be installed, then the ditch should be fenced to prevent horse injury on the uneven rock

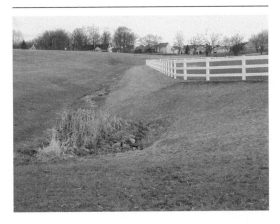

Figure 18.4. Divert surface water from the outdoor arena site with a swale or other suitable diversion.

surface. Likewise, fencing to keep horse hooves from tearing and pocking the ground of the sod swale will prolong its usefulness. The swale will likely be wetter than surrounding territory and so is more prone to sod damage from horse traffic. The drainage diversions around the arena perimeter provide a 20- to 25-foot buffer between activities in the arena and surrounding paddocks.

Drainage catchment is also needed to contain the precipitation water being shed from the riding arena. Drainage ditches for outdoor arenas can be constructed so that they are essentially an infiltration area, or vegetative filter. It may be a long, grassed, and gently sloping channel (swale) or a broad, flat area with little or no slope surrounded by a berm or dike. The sloping channel is more likely at a horse facility. Infiltration areas do not need to be elaborate, but management is required for maintenance of the vegetative cover. The swales discussed earlier often serve a dual purpose in collecting arena surface water in addition to catching and diverting surface water coming into the site from surrounding territory.

Groundwater

Underground water will weaken the foundation (base and subbase) of the arena. A French drain is a buried rock bed with a (optional) perforated water pipe positioned at its lowest level. It assists groundwater travel by collecting excess water in one location and using gravity flow to transport that water to an outlet located where excess water can be conveniently handled. It is positioned outside the perimeter of the arena pad. Provide up to 2% grade to the French drain system from the highest collection point to the outlet. French drain systems require some major excavation to build and yet provide simple removal of excess groundwater near an arena. One potential problem with buried drain rock is clogging with fine soil particles. Wrapping the drain rock inside a geotextile envelope is common practice. Although a geotextile will allow water passage while screening out most fine particles, it will eventually clog and prevent water movement into the French drain. French drains may be located below a swale so that surface and groundwater impoundment are treated at once.

Poor Drainage Site

Saturated soil will not support horse-riding activity and offers extreme challenge in proper arena construction. Avoid poorly drained sites and property. There are sites and soil conditions that will not be able to support building or riding arena activity without major water management alterations. Poorly drained, saturated soils do not have strength to support weight. Think of the difference between walking through relatively dry soil and walking through the same soil when saturated, which we call "mud." Mud cannot support weight, and it moves horizontally in displacement and leaves in its wake footprints, potholes, and ruts.

Saturated sites may be unavoidable for some horse farms. For arena sites with very poorly drained soil or a high water table, either the arena pad needs to be raised well above the saturated soil conditions or interceptor trenches need to be added at the arena perimeter to drop the groundwater table. With interceptor trenches the water handling is below ground, while with a raised arena pad water runoff from the arena is handled via open, narrow ditches. One advantage to the built-up arena pad is the ability to see and monitor water drainage in the ditches and output area. Either solution can be engineered to work well in maintaining reasonably dry subbase and base arena layers.

LOWER GROUNDWATER

Installation of interceptor trenches lowers the site groundwater table so that the arena "pad" can be high and dry above the saturated zone (Fig. 18.5). Install interceptor trenches, about 6 feet in depth filled with coarse gravel with a perforated pipe near the bottom, at the arena perimeter. When there is a

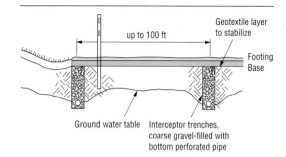

Figure 18.5. Interceptor trenches may be used to lower the groundwater table on a saturated site.

clear downhill drainage perspective, no matter how shallow, to the chosen arena site the interceptor trenches may be installed on just the long arena sides. On sites that are considered flat, interceptor drains on both long and short sides of the arena site may be needed to move encroaching groundwater away from the site. Slope the interceptor trench at 1% grade to an area where the collected water may be discharged; this may be downhill, into a stream (this is "clean" groundwater, not surface water with particulates and nutrients), or into a pit similar to septic system design. For sites that have uphill topography that allow surface and groundwater to pool at the junction of sloped terrain and the arena's relatively flat terrain, the interceptor drain is necessary to divert both surface and groundwater. Interceptor trenches can be positioned up to 100 feet apart so that lateral water movement from the arena center is no more than 50 feet. For extrawide arenas, a third interceptor trench is installed along the arena midline before arena base layer construction begins. These trenches are for catching and diverting groundwater, so there is no expectation that significant amounts of water will flow down through the arena base material and into an under-arena trench.

In addition to the interceptor trenches that effectively lower the groundwater table, use a geotextile material above the compacted subbase to provide a more stable support for the base material than the native soil can provide. Geotextiles provide lateral tension support between layers. Obviously, with the deep interceptor drains around the arena perimeter and geotextile layer, this design results in an expensive arena construction that is only cost effective in fairly extreme circumstances where the arena needs to be useful under most weather conditions. The initial caveat to *not* build in a low-lying area (with saturated soils) should appear even more justified.

RAISED PAD

The second option for poorly drained sites is to build up the site so that the bottom of the arena base is 6 to 12 inches above original grade. This elevation is the same recommendation for a building's site drainage. This lifts the subbase and base above the saturated zone to provide soil that will have sufficient bearing strength for riding arena use. The arena is constructed with a slope to drain rainwater from the arena pad. On absolutely flat ground with a high water table, once the topsoil is removed, large volumes of fill material needs to be brought to the site to lift the arena subbase up to the original grade and then another 6 to 12 inches higher as a dry platform to support the base. Moving a large amount of fill to elevate large outdoor arenas will not be reasonable or cost effective in some locales.

GRAVEL LAYER

Some success has been achieved on sites with less chronic drainage problems with a rock-drain layer between the subbase and base (Figure 18.6). This rock-drain layer is to divert groundwater from infrequent encroachment of the arena surface from below. The layer consists of gravel rock where most will pass through a 3/8 -inch screen. This type of gravel may be sold as a mixture of #5 and #7 stone, sometimes referred to as "57s." A 6-inch gravel layer is placed on top of the compacted subsoil; a geotextile layer may be needed to maintain separation of the subbase and gravel layers. This porous construction provides horizontal drainage of water. One note of

caution is that on a site with a consistently high water table, this aggregate gravel layer will become routinely saturated and create a capillary "fringe" that draws water up into the base material, which is undesirable. This aggregate layer of gravel rock is only effective to divert rare groundwater and encroaching surface water away from the outdoor arena site. A gravel layer may also be part of arena construction that allows water percolation through the base material, although this is uncommon.

PERIMETER ARENA FENCE

Most outdoor riding arenas have a fence to define the arena boundary, but it is not mandatory, particularly on private arenas. Dressage arenas typically use a rail on the ground. There is great variety to the design of the fence or rail used. The objective of the arena fence is to serve as a guide for horse and rider. It provides the horse a sense of enclosure for staying in the riding area. The boundary may be a simple suggestion of the arena perimeter with a relatively low, one-rail design on some show rings, or it may be as substantial as paddock fencing used around turnout areas. Indeed, some arenas are used as turnout, although this practice is not recommended because of the relatively high cost of arena surface construction and the wear and tear and manure deposition from turnout horses.

Generally, the riding arena fence should be constructed of substantial posts, visible enough to withstand the horse bumping into it, and aesthetically pleasing. Most arena fences are of post-and-rail construction using wood, rigid vinyl, or metal pipe. Put rails on fence interior for a smoother surface without posts to knock rider knees and feet. Show arena fences often minimize the number of rails

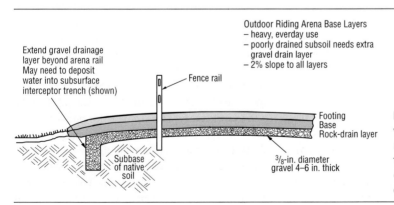

Figure 18.6. Outdoor arena with poorly drained subsoil may benefit from an additional gravel layer for drainage in the multilayer construction.

blocking spectator view. Depending on arena use, it may be desirable to have the perimeter fence high enough to discourage the horse from jumping it. Providing a slight outward lean (10%) to the fence will keep horses along the rail while offering some room for rider knees. This lean is more common on round pen construction than in outdoor riding arenas. Wire-strand fence is uncommon because of its limited visibility and danger of horse or rider entanglement. Horse mesh fence with a visible top rail offers a safe fence with little risk of horse entanglement. Mesh design offers good visibility for spectators of all heights, whether seated or standing, and excludes loose pets and children. The same principles of safe materials and sturdy construction apply to arena fence as to paddock fence, as outlined in Chapter 15. Install sturdy posts, which usually means driven, pressure-treated wooden posts, because they are the foundation of the fence. Use visible rails. Corners of the arena fence may be rounded to guide the horse or square for training purposes.

Arena gates are often constructed of material similar to the perimeter fence to make them less distracting. Two gates should be installed within the perimeter fence, located on opposite fence lines where possible. This allows option for different horse entry and exit patterns, particularly useful for a show arena between classes. Arena surface maintenance equipment may use a dedicated gate to avoid conflict between horse and vehicle access (Fig. 18.7). Supply a human-only gate or fence gap

near judging stands or other area of human activity for convenient arena access without opening a large horse and vehicle gate (see Chapter 15).

Dressage arenas often use railroad ties or other large-dimension lumber rather than fence to designate arena perimeter. Three-foot-long, 1-inch diameter retaining bars are driven through, three to a tie, to secure the ties. Dressage arenas are rectangular and without rounded corners.

UTILITIES

Electricity and water will be needed at the outdoor arena site. Electricity is relatively inexpensive to supply to the site and has uses such as for lighting and a sound system. Water will be needed for wetting the arena surface material for dust suppression.

Electricity

Lighting is provided to outdoor arena sites to extend the amount of useful time for which the arena may be used. In most cases, the lighting is not designed to be uniformly bright throughout the surface but only to provide enough light to see the surface and obstacles (Fig. 18.8). For a simple design, place arena lights on at least four poles located along the long sides at the quarter-points (¼ of the way from each end toward the middle). Locate two lamps per pole directed to light an area to the right and left of the pole toward the center of the arena. Lamps at least 12 feet above the ground will be above rider height and reduce direct glare; taller heights of 16 to 18 feet are more desirable for better light distribution. More

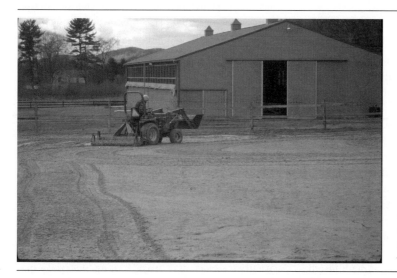

Figure 18.7. Arena fence gates need to be wide enough to allow easy passage for surface conditioning equipment.

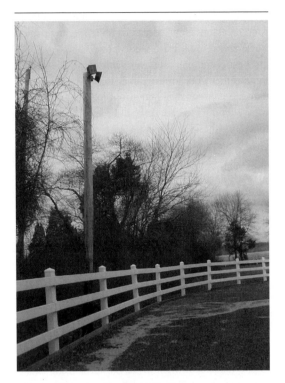

Figure 18.8. Mount HID lights on tall poles for providing at least a minimum amount of illumination without direct glare for night riding.

extensive lighting can be designed where bright, uniform lighting is desirable. High-intensity discharge (HID) lamps with reflectors are the most useful for this outdoor lighting application. See Chapter 11 for lamp and fixture options.

Water

A frost-proof hydrant should be located near the arena to supply hose- or sprinkler-applied water. A hydrant is a convenient tap for filling a water tank that is pulled by truck or tractor through the arena. Automated arena watering can be provided by a permanently installed sprinkler system located along the perimeter or mechanized field watering equipment. The width of the arena and the available water source are important factors in determining what type of system will be most effective.

Horticultural- or agricultural-grade sprinkler systems (gear-driven rotors or impact heads) are suitable for providing fairly even watering of the outdoor riding arena surface. They are typically set up to spray water in a half-circle pattern with installa-

tion along both long sides of the arena. The sprinklers are spaced on the basis of anticipated coverage pattern of the particular spray nozzle. These systems, though offering the convenience of automatic operation, require substantial flow rates to spray water distances of greater than 50 feet and so will not be suitable for arenas wider than 100 feet. Even at the 50-foot spray distance, water application becomes more uneven with strips of unwetted surface along the arena midline or between adjacent half-circles. The sprinklers may be activated as needed or controlled by a timer.

Arena surface materials may be wetted by mechanized field-watering equipment. A flexible hose traveling system is an effective option for sites with larger arenas or with low-volume water sources. One disadvantage is that the traveling hose has to be set up each time it is used. Advantages include more even water distribution than with perimeter-mounted sprinklers and potential to double its usefulness by watering both indoor and outdoor arenas.

SPECTATOR AREA

Seating and weather protection for spectators will be appreciated. Seating can be as simple as benches and outdoor furniture. A simple, roofed structure with open sidewalls can suffice for sun and precipitation protection. An elevated viewing area, even two to three steps above ground, improves visibility of the entire arena. Site topography should also be considered when siting the ring, because a spectator viewing structure can be built into slopes adjacent to the arena. Depending on weather conditions during outdoor arena activities, the viewing area can have radiant heat, circulation fans, and evaporative cooling for improved comfort.

ARENA MAINTENANCE

Surface Grooming

Maintenance grooming of the outdoor arena riding surface serves two functions. The first is to keep the footing material in good condition for riding and the second, but equal in importance, is to protect the integrity of the arena base construction. The arena footing material is "dragged" to redistribute footing material that has migrated or compacted because of hoof action. Additionally, weather events may wash footing materials into uneven patterns. The goal is to provide a uniformly deep layer of cushioning surface footing material over the entire arena base. When footing has thinned, it will risk base integrity by allowing horse hoof action to impact directly on the base, eventually creating ruts in the base material. Ruts or other low spots in the base are highly undesirable for maintaining even footing material conditions. Remember that the base is a highly compacted material designed as a supporting surface for the footing. Horses working off the base material do not have the desirable cushioning provided by the footing material. This is most obviously a problem with footing thrown off high-traffic areas such as around the arena rail.

Surface grooming involves frequent movements of displaced footing material with mechanized and handheld tools. Generally, a specific surface-grooming tool is either pulled behind or attached to a tractor. A three-point hitch attachment between tool and tractor may be used for convenience in positioning and lifting the tool. The tool is specific to the type of footing material, with more penetrating grooming needed for heavier materials, such as sand and screenings, while lighter tools are effective in redistributing lighter footing materials, such as wood products or crumb rubber. Different tools require widely different operator skill levels. Experience will play a role in effective surface preparation. It is important to use as noninvasive a tool as possible to maintain the footing material and integrity of the base. The tool should not dredge the base material up into the footing material. Adjust the tine height to prevent the tool from contacting the base material. Some tools allow height adjustment for various footing material requirements.

Handheld tools are used in addition to even the most sophisticated mechanization to replace footing material that has washed off the arena because of heavy rain events or for detailed work around perimeter fence posts and entry gate areas. More information on footing properties and maintenance is available in Chapter 17.

Keeping Surface Material in the Arena

Footing is thrown off the heavily trafficked area along the fence rail via hoof action. Water flow on the arena surface will transport lighter footing material. The first line of defense is to drag the material back frequently; but despite this, surface material

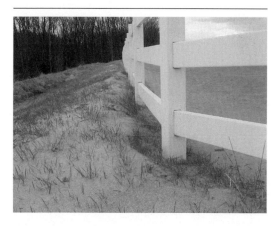

Figure 18.9. Outdoor arena surface will need frequent conditioning to keep the loose footing material evenly redistributed from the effects of horse traffic and water runoff that throw or flow, respectively, the material just outside the arena perimeter.

can build up just outside the arena fence (Fig. 18.9). Generally, with arenas that are constructed with a pad of compacted base extending beyond the arena perimeter fence, the footing material thrown or washed outside the arena will be significantly easier to get back into the arena compared with an arena design where the footing and base materials end at the working arena edge. The material can be simply raked or pushed back into the arena along the compacted base material than having to be lifted and thrown back into the arena.

A retaining board at footing level along the outside of the arena fence will help keep the surface material on the arena pad. Use a 2 by 6 pressure-treated board or landscape timber (or equivalent) installed at grade resting on the compacted base material. The retaining board does increase arena construction cost and disrupts surface water drainage. Water needs to be able to drain off the arena while not washing a lot of material with it. Some hand work with shovel and rake will still be required to replace footing thrown outside the arena perimeter even with a retaining board in place.

Drain holes can be placed under the board or timber to facilitate water drainage off the arena surface (Fig 18.10). Notch 2 by 6 boards about every 4 to 8 feet with small weep holes of ½ -inch depth and the width of a chain saw blade to provide drainage. Bevel the lower corner of both the end faces of 4 × 6

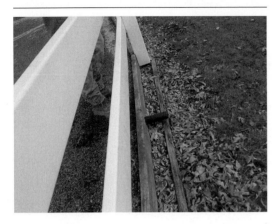

Figure 18.10. Boards may be used to help contain footing from leaving the arena surface. Gaps for water movement under the board will be needed. Shown here is a pipe moving water through the footing board. Lower board is supporting the base material above grade in a poorly drained location.

landscape timbers so that a triangular opening is provided when two timbers butt ends against each other. The board or timber resting on the base is not a well-sealed junction, and water does percolate under the board or timber at many locations along its length. Naturally, some footing will wash and work its way through the drain gap and over the board or timber. Good management and maintenance dictates that this be periodically relocated back into the arena.

Entry Gate

One trouble spot for outdoor arena maintenance is the entry gate area. Often a low spot develops from intensive horse use and vehicle traffic for arena surface conditioning (Fig. 18.11). Provide extra care in grading for surface water diversion and arena precipitation movement in this area. Use of geotextile fabric layer around the gate area will help distribute load and stabilize the material layers (see "Geotextile Layer" section). Locating the entry

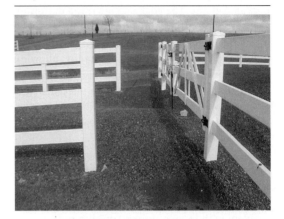

Figure 18.11. Pay special attention to grading for water drainage around heavily used areas such as the arena gate.

ramp to the arena at a high point on the riding surface will also eliminate the possibility of water flowing off the arena onto this highly traveled area.

SUMMARY

An outdoor riding arena is incorporated into virtually all horse farms. Arena construction starts with a solid-packed subsoil material topped by an even harder packed base material of well-graded aggregate. These underlying layers support the riding surface material and are critical to the arena's long-term success. Arena design is very similar to road building in function of the material layers and the attention to water drainage to maintain the integrity of the construction. Of prime importance for outdoor arena design is to divert all surface and groundwater from the arena site and to slope the arena surface slightly to shed precipitation. Individual arena uses and existing site conditions will dictate specific arena design and construction criteria. Arena surface grooming is required to maintain proper riding conditions and to ensure longevity of arena construction.

Appendix
Psychrometrics

PSYCHROMETRIC CHART AND AIR CHARACTERISTICS

A psychrometric chart presents physical and thermal properties of air in a graphical form. Air contains moisture and energy that relate to its physical properties and the psychrometric chart ties these properties together. Understanding psychrometrics can be very helpful in troubleshooting and finding solutions to environment problems within stables and riding arenas. Understanding psychrometric charts will help you visualize environmental control concepts, such as why heated air can hold more moisture or, conversely, how allowing moist air to cool will result in condensation. This appendix explains how characteristics of moist air are organized in a psychrometric chart. Three examples are used to illustrate typical chart use and interpretation. Properties of moist air are explained in the "Air Property Definitions" sidebar for your reference during the following discussions.

A psychrometric chart packs a lot of information into an odd-shaped, rather complicated, graph. If we consider the components piece by piece, the usefulness of the chart will be clearer; refer to Figure A.1, which is a simplified version of the more realistic psychrometric chart shown in Figure A.2. Boundaries of the psychrometric chart are a dry-bulb temperature scale on the horizontal axis, a humidity ratio (moisture content) scale on the vertical axis on the right-hand side, and an upper curved boundary to the left that represents saturated air or 100% moisture-holding capacity. The chart shows other important moist air properties as diagrammed in Figure A.3 on the less obvious axes: wet-bulb temperature; enthalpy; dew-point or saturation temperature; relative humidity; and specific volume. See the "Air Property Definitions sidebar" for an explanation of these terms. Moist air can be described by finding the intersection of any two of these properties. This is called a "state point." From the state point, all the other properties can be obtained. The key is to determine which set of lines on the chart represent the air property of interest. Some practice with examples will help. Use Figures A.1 and A.3 with the psychrometric chart in Figure A.2 to verify whether you can find each air property.

Psychrometric charts are available in various pressure and temperature ranges. Figure A.2 is for standard atmospheric pressure (1 atmosphere at sea level or 14.7 pounds per square inch) and temperatures from 30 to 120°F, which are adequate for most horse housing applications. Psychrometric properties are also available as data tables and equations.

An understanding of the shape and use of the psychrometric chart will help you diagnose air temperature and humidity problems. Note that cooler air (located along the lower left region of the chart) will not hold as much moisture (as seen on the y-axis' humidity ratio) as warm air (located along right side of chart). A "rule of thumb" within what we consider normal environmental conditions is that a 10°F rise in air temperature can decrease relative humidity 20%. Use of a psychrometric chart shows that this is roughly true. For example, to decrease relative humidity in a winter stable during a critical time period, we could heat the air.

USE OF PSYCHROMETRIC CHART

Example 1. Practice Finding Air Properties

A psychrometer (see "Instrument" sidebar) gives a dry-bulb temperature of 78°F and a wet-bulb temperature of 65°F. Determine other air properties from this information. Two useful air properties for environmental analysis in stables and indoor arenas would be relative humidity and dew-point temperature. Relative humidity is an indicator of how much moisture is in the air compared with desirable moisture conditions, and dew-point temperature

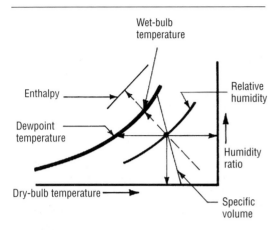

Figure A.1. Properties of moist air on a psychrometric chart in simplified form. Wet-bulb temperature and enthalpy use the same chart line but values are read off separate scales.

indicates when condensation problems would occur should the (dry-bulb) temperature drop.

Find the intersection of the two known properties, dry-bulb and wet-bulb temperatures, on the psychrometric chart, Figure A.2. This example is shown in Figure A.3, so you may check your work. The dry-bulb temperature is located along the bottom horizontal axis. Find the line for 78°F, which runs vertically through the chart. Wet-bulb temperature is located along diagonal dotted lines leading to scale readings at the upper curved boundary marked "saturation temperature." The intersection of the vertical 78°F dry-bulb line and the diagonal 65°F wet-bulb line has now established a state point for the measured air. Now read relative humidity as 50% (curving line running from left to right up through the chart) and dew-point temperature as 58°F (follow horizontal line, moving left, toward the upper curved boundary of saturation temperatures).

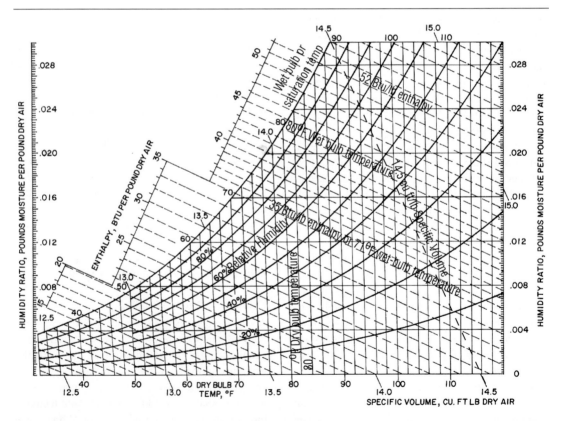

Figure A.2. Psychrometric chart showing properties of air, including heat and moisture relationships.

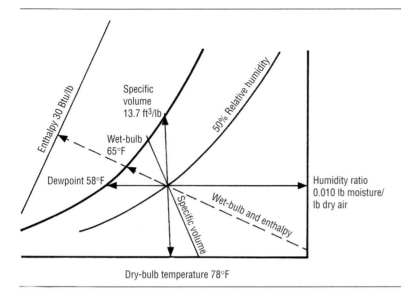

Figure A.3. Diagram of Example 1 for practice in finding psychrometric properties of air. Verify these values on psychrometric chart (Fig. A.2).

What might we conclude from this information? The relative humidity of 50% is acceptable for most horse housing and other livestock applications. If we allowed the air temperature (dry-bulb) to decrease to 58°F (dew-point) or below, the air would be 100% saturated with moisture and condensation would occur. The humidity ratio, as seen on the vertical *y*-axis scale, is a reliable indicator of air moisture level because it reflects the pounds of moisture contained in a pound of dry air and does not fluctuate with dry-bulb temperature readings as does relative humidity. The humidity ratio for air in this example is about 0.0104 lb moisture/lb dry air (move right horizontally from state point to humidity ratio scale). The humidity ratio is a good indicator of the amount of moisture in the air whereas the relative humidity is temperature dependent, as demonstrated in the next example.

Example 2. Winter Ventilation to Control Moisture Buildup

Often, air is heated as it is introduced into a stable work area or other indoor environment. This raises the air temperature but decreases the relative humidity. Consider a situation where a hygrometer (see "Instrument" sidebar) was used to determine that outdoor air was at 40°F (dry-bulb) temperature and 80% relative humidity. This air was heated to 65°F (dry-bulb) before being distributed throughout the building. Figure A.4 depicts this example's process.

Find the state point for the incoming cool air on the lower left portion of the psychrometric chart (point A in Fig. A.4). Note that other properties of the 40°F air include a wet-bulb temperature of 38°F, a dew-point temperature of about 34°F, and humidity ratio of 0.0042 lb moisture/lb dry air. Heating air involves an increase in the dry-bulb temperature, with no addition or reduction in the air's water content. The heating process moves horizontally to the right along a line of constant humidity ratio; between points A and B in Figure A.4. Heating the air to 65°F (dry-bulb) has resulted in decreasing the relative humidity to about 32%. The heated fresh air is dry enough to be useful in absorbing moisture from the environment. (Verify that the heated air at point B continues to have a dew-point of 34°F and humidity ratio of 0.0042 lb moisture/lb dry air.) The heated air, with its lower relative humidity, can be mixed with moist, warmer air already in the stable. As fresh air moves through an animal-occupied environment, it will pick up additional moisture and heat before it reaches the ventilation system exhaust (Fig A.5). Suppose in this stable we measured the exhausted air conditions at 75°F (dry-bulb) and 70% relative humidity, represented by point C in Figure A.4. Note that in this exhausted air, the humidity ratio has tripled to 0.013 lb moisture/lb dry air. This

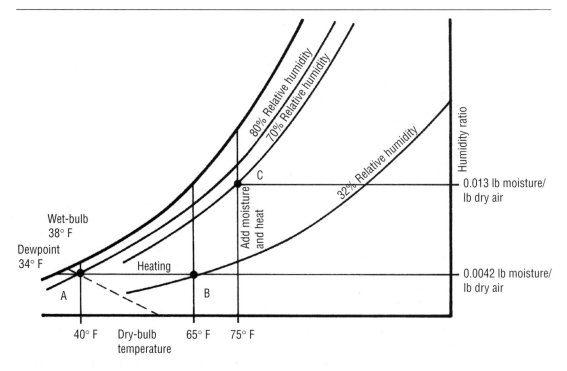

Figure A.4. Diagram of Example 2 demonstrating supplemental heat addition to a stable. Outdoor air at 40°F, 80% relative humidity (point A) is heated to 65°F (point B) for use in ventilation. Exhaust air (point C) at 75°F and 70% relative humidity contains three times the moisture of the fresh air (points A and B).

means that much more water is ventilated out of the stable in the warm, moist exhaust air than is brought in by the cold, high–relative humidity incoming air. Removing moisture from the stable or riding arena environment is one of the major functions of a winter ventilation system in order to maintain good air quality. Note that if heating system was now turned off and ventilation stopped to trap the warmed air in the building, then the air would cool and eventually reach dew-point temperature, resulting in condensation on surfaces because the air can no longer hold as much moisture.

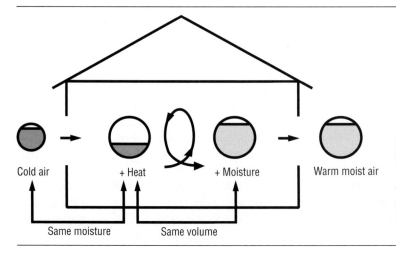

Figure A.5. Heated air holds more moisture and may be used as a "sponge" to pick up moisture from the stable and then exit the building while more dry fresh air enters.

Example 3. Evaporative Cooling for Hot Weather

Evaporative cooling uses heat contained in the air to evaporate water. Air is forced through a wetted material using fans or water is misted into warm air so that heat in the air evaporates the water. Air temperature (dry-bulb) drops while water content (humidity) rises to near the saturation point. Evaporation is often used in hot weather to cool ventilation air entering barns. The evaporatively cooled air is brought into the stable and mixed with warmer, lower humidity air in the stable for an overall cooling effect. Refer to Figure A.6 to follow this example process on the psychrometric chart. Evaporative cooling moves upward along the line of constant enthalpy or constant wet-bulb temperature; for example, from point D at 95°F and 30% relative humidity to point E cooled to 71°F for a 24°F reduction in air temperature. Evaporative cooling is most effective in locations with hot and relatively dry air. Notice that hot dry air (points D to E) has more capacity for evaporative cooling than does hot humid air (point F at same hot air temperature but double the relative humidity, at 60%, to G, with only a 12°F temperature decrease). Fortunately, despite the persistent American urban myth of hot humid summer days with 90°F and 90% humidity, the summer air is at a much reduced humidity during the hottest afternoon hours and evaporative cooling can be effective.

Air Property Definitions

The air surrounding us is a mixture of dry air and moisture and it contains a certain amount of heat. We are used to hearing about air temperature, relative humidity, and the dew-point temperature in discussions of weather conditions. All these properties and more are contained in a psychrometric chart. Chart shape and complexity take some getting used to. Refer to Figures A.1 and A.2. You will find that the upper curved boundary of the chart has one temperature scale, yet can represent three types of temperature: wet-bulb, dry-bulb, and dew-point. This upper curved boundary also represents 100% relative humidity or saturated air.

Dry-bulb temperature is the commonly measured temperature from a thermometer. It is called "dry-bulb" because the sensing tip of the thermometer is dry (see "wet-bulb temperature" for comparison). Dry-bulb temperature is located on the horizontal x-axis of the psychrometric chart, and lines of constant temperature are represented by vertical chart lines. Because this temperature is so commonly used, assume that temperatures are dry-bulb temperatures unless otherwise designated.

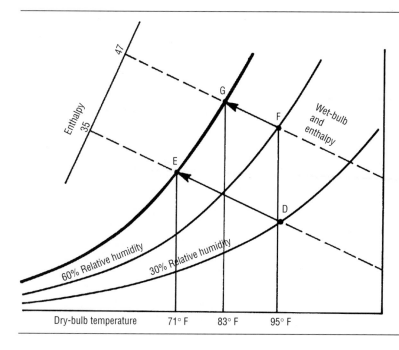

Figure A.6. Diagram of Example 3 showing evaporative cooling process. Hot dry air is evaporatively cooled from points D to E. Another example showing hot humid air cooled from points F to G. Notice greater evaporative cooling capacity with dry air.

Relative humidity *is a measure of the amount of water that air can hold at a certain temperature. It is "relative" to the amount of water that air, at that same temperature, can hold at 100% humidity, or saturation. Air temperature(dry-bulb) is important because warmer air can hold more moisture than cold air. Air at 60% relative humidity contains 60% of the water it could possibly hold (at that temperature). It could pick up 40% more water to reach saturation. Lines of constant relative humidity are represented by the curved lines running from the bottom left and sweeping up through to the top right of the chart. The line for 100% relative humidity, or saturation, is the upper left boundary of the chart.*

The Humidity ratio *of moist air is the weight of the water contained in the air per unit of dry air. This is often expressed as pounds of moisture per pound of dry air. Because the humidity ratio of moist air is not dependent on temperature, as is relative humidity, it is easier to use in calculations. Humidity ratio is found on the vertical y-axis, with lines of constant humidity ratio running horizontally across the chart.*

Dew-point temperature *indicates the temperature at which water will begin to condense out of moist air. Given air at a certain dry-bulb temperature and relative humidity, if the temperature is allowed to decrease, the air can no longer hold as much moisture. When air is cooled, the relative humidity increases until saturation is reached and condensation occurs. Condensation occurs on surfaces that are at or below the dew-point temperature. Dew-point temperature is determined by moving from a state point horizontally to the left along lines of constant humidity ratio until the upper, curved, saturation temperature boundary is reached.*

Enthalpy *is the heat energy content of moist air. It is expressed in Btu per pound of dry air and represents the heat energy due to temperature and moisture in the air. Enthalpy is useful in air heating and cooling applications. The enthalpy scale is located above the saturation, upper boundary of the chart. Lines of constant enthalpy run diagonally downward from left to right across the chart. Lines of constant enthalpy and constant wet-bulb are the same on this chart, but values are read from separate scales. More accurate psychrometric charts use slightly different lines for wet-bulb temperature and enthalpy.*

Wet-bulb temperature *is determined when air is circulated past a wetted sensor tip. It represents the temperature at which water evaporates and brings the air to saturation. Inherent in this definition is an assumption that no heat is lost or gained by the air. This is different from dew-point temperature, where a decrease in temperature, or heat loss, decreases the moisture-holding capacity of the air, causing water to condense. Determination of wet-bulb temperature on this psychrometric chart follows lines of constant enthalpy, but values are read off the upper, curved, saturation temperature boundary.*

Specific volume *indicates the space occupied by air. It is the inverse of density and is expressed as a volume per unit weight (density is weight per unit volume). Warm air is less dense than cool air, which causes warmed air to rise. This phenomenon is known as thermal buoyancy. By similar reasoning, warmer air has greater specific volume and is hence lighter than cool air. On the psychrometric chart, lines of constant specific volume are almost vertical lines, with scale values written below the dry-bulb temperature scale and above the upper boundary's saturation temperature scale. On this chart, values range from 12.5 to 15.0 cubic feet/pound of dry air. Greater specific volume is associated with warmer temperatures (dry-bulb).*

Instrument

A couple of handheld instruments are described that are useful in monitoring air properties in horse facilities.

Psychrometer is an instrument used to determine dry-bulb and wet-bulb temperatures. The traditional way to measure relative humidity is a two-step process: both wet-bulb and dry-bulb temperatures are obtained and then converted to relative humidity using a psychrometric chart. The dry-bulb temperature is measured with a standard thermometer. The wet-bulb temperature is determined from a standard thermometer modified with a wetted fabric wick covering the sensor bulb. Sufficient airflow is provided over the wick material so that as distilled water (to prevent salt buildup) evaporates from the wet wick, the temperature falls and the thermometer reading reflects the wet-bulb temperature. Air movement can be provided through an aspirated box (with a fan) or by whirling the dry-bulb/wet-bulb thermometer through the air. Psychrometers are considered highly accurate but have been replaced for most casual observations of temperature and humidity by hygrometers.

Hygrometer is an electronic instrument that measures relative humidity directly, rather than using a psychrometer and psychrometric chart. The hygrometer sensor has a matrix material in which electrical properties change as water molecules diffuse in and out in response to air moisture content. Other hygrometer sensor materials indicate electrical changes as water molecules adhere to their surface. Sensor material changes are interpreted and displayed by the hygrometer. Careful calibration is essential. The sensor materials may not tolerate conditions near saturation, so reliability of many relative humidity sensors is questionable when the relative humidity rises above 95%. Most hygrometers also provide a measure of dry-bulb temperature. A relatively inexpensive, pocket-sized hygrometer provides digital dry-bulb temperature and relative humidity readings. These devices can take several minutes to display a correct reading and provide relative humidity measurements with an accuracy of 3 to 5%. Generally, hygrometer prices have decreased and reliability improved over the past several years.

Additional Resources

General Horse Facilities References
Horse Facilities Handbook, MWPS-60. 2005.
Eileen Wheeler, Bill Koenig, Jay Harmon, Pat
    Murphy, and David Freeman
Midwest Plan Service
122 Davidson Hall
Iowa State University
Ames, IA 50011
800-562-3618 or 515-294-4337
www.mwpshq.org

*Horsekeeping on a Small Acreage: Designing and
    Managing Your Equine Facilities* 2005.
Cherry Hill
Storey Books, Pownal, VT

Stables and Other Equestrian Buildings. 1997.
Keith Warth
J.A. Allen, London

Chapter 2: Horse Stable Layout and Planning
*Complete Plans for Building Horse Barns Big and
    Small.* 1997.
Nancy Ambrosiano and Mary Harcourt
Breakthrough, Ossining, NY

*Stablekeeping: A Visual Guide to Safe and Healthy
    Horsekeeping.* 2000.
Cherry Hill
Storey Books, Pownal, VT

Chapter 3: Construction Style and Materials
*Horse Housing: How to Plan, Build and Remodel
    Barns and Sheds.* 2002.
Richard Klimesh and Cherry Hill
Trafalgar Square, North Pomfret, VT

Hoop Structure Ventilation
*Ventilating Greenhouse Barns, Guidelines for
    Livestock Production,* G-102.

Eileen Wheeler
Agricultural Engineering Building
The Pennsylvania State University
University Park, PA 16802
814-865-7685
server.age.psu.edu/extension/factsheets/g/

Farm Building Construction
Structures and Environment Handbook, MWPS-1.
MidWest Plan Service
122 Davidson Hall
Iowa State University
Ames, IA 50011
800-562-3618 or 515-294-4337
www.mwpshq.org

Chapter 4: Horse Farm Site Planning
Pasture Management
Pasture and Hay for Horses. Agronomy Facts 32.
    1992.
Marvin Hall and Pat Comerford
College of Agricultural Sciences
Publications Distribution Center
112 Agricultural Administration Building
The Pennsylvania State University
University Park, PA 16802
814-865-6713
pubs.cas.psu.edu

"Pastures for Horses," HIH 730.
R.A. Russell, J.E. White and R.J. Antoniewicz
Chapter in *Horse Industry Handbook*
American Youth Horse Council, Inc.
577 N. Boyero Ave.
Pueblo West, CO 81007
800-TRY-AYHC
www.ayhc.com

Horse Owner's Field Guide to Toxic Plants. 1996.
Sandra M. Burger and Anthony P. Knight
Breakthrough, Ossining, NY

Chapter 5: Stall Design
Att Bygga Häststall-en idéhandbok [*To Build a Horse Stable—An Idea Handbook*]. 2001.
Michael Ventorp and Per Michanek
Institutionen for Jördbrukets Biosystem och Teknologi
Sveriges Lantbruksuniversitet
Alnarp, Sweden

Chapter 6: Ventilation
Chimney Vents
Horse Barn Ventilation, 96-031. 1997.
Harry Huffman
Ministry of Agriculture and Food
Ontario, Canada
www.gov.on.ca/omafra/english/engineer/facts/96-031.htm

Ventilation Guidelines for Livestock Housing
Heating, Cooling and Tempering Air, MWPS-34. 1990.
Mechanical Ventilating Systems, MWPS-32. 1990.
Natural Ventilating Systems, MWPS-33. 1989.
Midwest Plan Service
122 Davidson Hall
Iowa State University
Ames, IA 50011
800-562-3618 or 515-294-4337
www.mwpshq.org

Respiratory Health
"Housing the Horse" (D. S. B. Sainsbury) and "Stable Environment in Relation to the Control of Respiratory Diseases" (A. F. Clarke)
Chapters in *Horse Management*, 1987
John Hickman, editor
Academic Press, London

Chapter 7: Flooring Materials and Drainage
Mattress Floor Construction
Manufacturers such as: www.stablecomfort.com and www.comfortstall.com

Chapter 8: Manure Management
Manure Storages
Livestock Waste Facilities Handbook, MWPS-18. 1985.
Midwest Plan Service
122 Davidson Hall
Iowa State University
Ames, IA 50011

800-562-3618 or 515-294-4337
www.mwpshq.org

Commercial-Scale Composting
On-Farm Composting Handbook. NRAES-54. 1992.
Robert Rynk, editor
Natural Resources, Agriculture, and Engineering Service Cooperative Extension
P.O. Box 4557
Ithaca, NY 14853-4557
607-255-7654
www.nraes.org

Fly Control
Pest Management Recommendations for Horses
P. Kaufman, D. Rutz and C. Pitts
College of Agricultural Sciences
Publications Distribution Center
112 Agricultural Administration Building
The Pennsylvania State University
University Park, PA 16802
814-865-6713
pubs.cas.psu.edu

Manure Nutrient Values
Horse Manure Characteristics Literature and Database Review. 2003.
L. Lawrence, J. Bicudo, and E. Wheeler
Proceedings of the International Symposium for Animal, Agricultural, and Food Processing Wastes IX (pp. 277–284)
American Society of Agricultural and Biological Engineers
2950 Niles Road
St. Joseph, MI 49085
269-429-0300
www.asae.org

Manure Production and Characteristics, Standard ASAE D384.2.
American Society of Agricultural and Biological Engineers
2950 Niles Road
St. Joseph, MI 49085
269-429-0300
www.asae.org

Chapter 9: Fire Safety
Guarding Against Hay Fires, ANR-964. 1985.
C. B. Ogburn

Alabama Cooperative Extension System
122 Duncan Hall Annex
Auburn University, AL 36849
334-844-5690
www.aces.edu/publications

Fire Control in Livestock Buildings, NRAES-39.
  1989.
W. C. Arble and D. J. Murphy
Natural Resources, Agriculture, and Engineering
  Service Cooperative Extension
P.O. Box 4557
Ithaca, NY 14853-4557
607-255-7654
www.nraes.org

Extinguishing Fires in Silos and Hay Mows,
  NRAES-18. 2000.
D. J. Murphy and W. C. Arble
Natural Resources, Agriculture, and Engineering
  Service Cooperative Extension
P.O. Box 4557
Ithaca, NY 14853
607-255-7654
www.nraes.org

Fire safety information, including extensive
  extinguisher specifications, is available at the
  Hanford Fire Department
  www.hanford.gov/fire/index.htm

National Fire Protection Association
1 Batterymarch Park
Quincy, MA 02269-7471
617-770-3000
www.nfpa.org

Chapter 10: Utilities
Agricultural Wiring Handbook
National Food and Energy Council
P.O. Box 309
Wilmington, OH 45177-0309
937-383-0001
www.nfec.org

Farm Buildings Wiring Handbook, MWPS-28. 1992.
Midwest Plan Service
122 Davidson Hall
Iowa State University
Ames, IA 50011
800-562-3618 or 515-294-4337
www.mwpshq.org

National Electrical Code (NFPA 70)
National Fire Protection Association
1 Batterymarch Park
Quincy, MA 02269-7471
617-770-3000
www.nfpa.org

Chapter 11: Lighting
Lighting Design for Livestock Buildings. 1997.
J.P. Chastian, L.D. Jacobson, and J Martins
Proceedings of the Fifth International Livestock
  Environment Symposium V
American Society of Agricultural and Biological
  Engineers
2950 Niles Road
St. Joseph, MI 49085
269-429-0300
www.asabe.org

*Supplemental Lighting for Improved Milk
  Production.* 1998.
J. P. Chastain and R. S. Hiatt
Electric Power Research Institute, Inc. (EPRI)
3412 Hillview Ave.
Palo Alto, CA 94304
www.epri.com

Chapters 14 and 15: Fence Planning and Fence Materials
Fencing Materials
*Fencing Options for Horse Farm Management in
  Virginia.* 1999.
Larry A. Lawrence
Virginia Cooperative Extension
www.ext.vt.edu/news/periodicals/livestock/
  aps-99_04/aps-0050.html

High-Tensile Wire Fencing, NRAES-11. 1981.
Natural Resources, Agriculture, and Engineering
  Service Cooperative Extension
P.O. Box 4557
Ithaca, NY 14853-4557
607-255-7654
www.nraes.org

EquiSearch
Information about horse fencing (and other topics)
  with links to material manufacturers and
  contractors, and theAmerican Fence Association
800-822-4342

www.equisearch.com/farm/special/2001/09/07/
    fences
www.americanfenceassociation.com

Pasture Management
Pasture and Hay for Horses, Agronomy Fact 32
    (see Chapter 4)

All-Weather Paddock Construction Detail
Using All-Weather Geotextile Lanes and Pads,
    AED-45. 1999.
K. Janni, T. Funk, and B. Holmes
Midwest Plan Service
122 Davidson Hall
Iowa State University
Ames, IA 50011
800-562-3618 or 515-294-4337
www.mwpshq.org

**Chapters 17 and 18: Riding Arena Surface
Materials and Design**
*The Equine Arena Handbook: Developing a User
    Friendly Facility.* 1999.
Robert Malmgren
Alpine, Loveland, CO

*Under Foot: The USDF Guide to Dressage Arena
    Construction, Maintenance and Repair.* 1992.
United States Dressage Federation

220 Lexington Green Circle
Suite 510
Lexington, KY 40503
859-971-2277
www.usdf.org

All-Weather Surfaces for Horses. 1999.
Ray Lodge and Susan Shanks
J.A. Allen, London

Installation Instructions for All-Wood Arena
    Footing Materials and Base Construction
Fiber Systems
www.engineeredwoodfiber.com/horses/installation.
    html

Appendix
**Evaluating Livestock Housing Environments
(3 part series). 1995.**
Principles of Measuring Air Quality, G-80
Instruments for Measuring Air Quality, G-81
Evaluating Mechanical Ventilation Systems, G-82
Eileen Wheeler and Robert Bottcher.
Agricultural Engineering Building
The Pennsylvania State University
University Park, PA 16802
814-865-7685
server.age.psu.edu/extension/factsheets/g/

Index